Molecular Epidemiology

The Practical Approach Series

Related **Practical Approach** Series Titles

* indicates a forthcoming title

Please see the **Practical Approach** series website at
http://www.oup.com/pas
for full contents lists of all Practical Approach titles.

Essential Molecular Biology V2 2e*
Radioisotopes 2e*
Epitope Mapping
Protein Purification Applications 2
Protein Purification Techniques 1
Bioinformatics: sequence, structure
  and databanks
Functional Genomics
Essential Molecular Biology V1 2/e
Combinatorial Chemistry
Immunoassay
Monoclonal Antibodies
RNA Viruses
Differential Display
Fmoc Solid Phase Peptide Synthesis
DNA Viruses
Virus Culture
Immunodiagnostics
DNA Microarray Technology
High Resolution Chromatography
Chromosome Structural Analysis
Gel Electrophoresis of Proteins 3/e
In Situ Hybridization 2/e
HPLC of Macromolecules 2/e
Chromatin
Mutation detection

Molecular Genetic Analysis of
  Populations 2/e
PCR3: PCR In Situ Hybridization
Genome Mapping
MHC 2
MHC 1
Affinity Separations
Immunochemistry 2
Immunochemistry 1
Signalling by inositides
Protein Structure Prediction
DNA Cloning 4: Mammalian
Systems
DNA Cloning 3: Complex Genomes
Gene Probes 2
Gene Probes 1
Ion Channels
Pulsed Field Gel Electrophoresis
HIV Volume II
HIV Volume I
Non-isotopic Methods in Molecular
  Biology
Medical Parasitology
DNA Cloning 2: Expression Systems
DNA Cloning 1: Core Techniques
PCR 1

No. 251

Molecular Epidemiology
A Practical Approach

Edited by

Mary Carrington
NCI-FCRDC
Bldg. 560, Rm 21-76, Miller Drive,
Frederick, MD 21702
USA

and

A. R. Hoelzel
Department of Biological Sciences,
University of Durham, South Road,
Durham DH1 3LE
U.K.

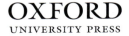

OXFORD
UNIVERSITY PRESS

OXFORD
UNIVERSITY PRESS

Great Clarendon Street, Oxford OX2 6DP

Oxford University Press is a department of the University of Oxford.
It furthers the University's objective of excellence in research, scholarship,
and education by publishing worldwide in

Oxford New York

Athens Auckland Bangkok Bogotá Buenos Aires Cape Town
Chennai Dar es Salaam Delhi Florence Hong Kong Istanbul Karachi
Kolkata Kuala Lumpur Madrid Melbourne Mexico City Mumbai
Nairobi Paris São Paulo Singapore Taipei Tokyo Toronto Warsaw

with associated companies in Berlin Ibadan

Oxford is a registered trade mark of Oxford University Press in the UK and
in certain other countries

Published in the United States by Oxford University Press Inc., New York

British Library Cataloguing in Publication Data
Data available

Library of Congress Cataloguing in Publication Data

ISBN 0 19 963811 X (Hbk.)
ISBN 0 19 963810 1 (Pbk.)

10 9 8 7 6 5 4 3 2 1

Typeset in Swift by Footnote Graphics, Warminster, Wilts
Printed in Great Britain on acid-free paper
by The Bath Press, Bath, Avon

Preface

Molecular epidemiology is a rapidly growing field encompassing a range of disciplines, which include molecular biology, population biology, genetics, and statistics. In an era when many fields of study have 'gone molecular', epidemiology is one where the benefits are especially clear, in particular now that we can begin to take advantage of the tremendous resource provided by the human genome project. It is our hope that the studies collected in this volume will facilitate the further development of this emerging field, and help contribute to the important tasks of disease assessment and control. Identification of a relevant sample pool, collection of clinical specimens, and compilation of detailed clinical data are the first steps in an epidemiological study. This book focuses on some of the essential methods that follow the organisation of samples and clinical data. These include the genetic characterisation of infectious agents, identification of host genetic characteristics that may be involved in susceptibility or resistance to the agent, and the analysis of data in a way that facilitates meaningful interpretations. Chapters 1–3 highlight concepts and methods at the forefront of studies of infectious diseases, and include a synopsis of general epidemiologic design and analysis, as well as current techniques for molecular typing of microbial pathogens. Chapters 4–6 focus on recent advances in studying host genetics, including methods for the detection of mutations and polymorphisms, identification of linkage among alleles of genes on a given chromosome, and the use of DNA pooling to increase efficiency in association studies of genetically complex traits. Chapters 7 and 8 deal with the relationship between pathologies and immune system genetics, and on the use of DNA sequence information to garner insights into the evolution of infectious pathogens, and the evolution and function of the immune system. We thank the authors for the quality of their contributions and for their patience during the editorial process.

We dedicate this volume to the memory of Dr. Norman R. Hoelzel.

Mary Carrington
Rus Hoelzel

Contents

List of protocols *page* *xiii*

Abbreviations *xv*

Introduction to molecular epidemiology *xvii*

Charles S. Rabkin and Nathaniel Rothman

    References *xix*

1 Epidemiological methods for studies of genetic factors that influence infectious diseases *1*

Eric A. Engels and Thomas R. O'Brien

  1 General considerations *1*

  2 Types of epidemiological studies *2*

  3 Cohort study *4*

      Cohort studies: cumulative incidence *5*

      Cohort studies: incidence *7*

      Example of cohort study *8*

      Attributable risk *9*

  4 Case-control studies *10*

      Example of case-control study *12*

  5 Cross-sectional studies *14*

  6 Interpretation of epidemiological associations *15*

  7 Confounding *17*

  8 Bradford Hill's criteria for causality *18*

  9 Statistical considerations *20*

  10 Further statistical considerations *21*

  11 Interaction *23*

  12 Identifying candidate genes for epidemiological studies *24*

  13 The future of genetic epidemiology *25*

     References *26*

2 Molecular differentiation of bacterial strains *29*

Eric W. Brown

  1 Introduction *29*

2 PCR-based fingerprinting of the bacterial chromosome   *33*

Preparation of genomic DNA from Gram negative and Gram positive
eubacterial species   *34*

Reaction conditions   *37*

The 'ribotype' method   *38*

Repetitive PCR fingerprinting   *40*

RAPD-PCR   *41*

Gel electrophoresis of amplicons   *43*

Analysis and interpretation of PCR fingerprint data   *44*

3 RFLP analysis of the bacterial chromosome   *44*

General considerations   *46*

Preparation of genomic DNA for RFLP analysis   *46*

Enzymes   *47*

Polyacrylamide gel electrophoresis (PAGE)   *48*

Analysis and interpretation of genomic restriction data   *50*

4 PFGE analysis of the bacterial chromosome   *50*

General considerations   *52*

Genomic DNA quality   *53*

Restriction enzymes employed in PFGE   *54*

Electrophoretic conditions   *55*

Analysis and interpretations   *56*

5 DNA sequence analysis of the bacterial ompA gene   *57*

Amplification of the bacterial *omp*A locus   *58*

Cloning and DNA sequencing of *omp*A PCR products   *59*

Interpretation of *omp*A nucleotide sequence variation   *62*

6 Conclusion   *63*

Acknowledgements   *64*

References   *64*

3 Detection and quantification of heterogeneous viral targets: HIV as a model   *67*

Shirley Kwok

1 Introduction   *67*

2 Impact of sequence heterogeneity on PCR   *68*

3 Primer and probe design for HIV   *69*

Sequence selection   *69*

Reaction conditions and cycling parameters   *70*

4 Assay sensitivity and specificity   *70*

5 Preventing false positives from PCR carryover   *71*

6 Amplification target: DNA vs. RNA   *72*

7 Qualitative vs. quantitative assays   *73*

8 Importance of internal controls and quantitation standards   *73*

Construction of the IC/QS   *74*

Quantitation of the QS   *74*

9 Evaluation of assay performance   *75*

10 Qualitative HIV DNA assay   *75*

Sample collection for HIV DNA amplification   *75*

DNA extraction from cells   *77*

Preparation of DNA from dried blood spots   78
DNA amplification   79
Colorimetric microwell plate detection   81
Interpretation of results   83

11 Quantitative HIV RNA assay   83
Sample collection for plasma HIV RNA amplification   83
Extraction of viral RNA with GuSCN   84
RNA amplification   87
Quantification of amplified products   88
Interpretation of results   90
Controls   91

12 Quantitative DNA asay   91
Quantification of total genomic DNA   91
Quantification of HIV DNA   93

13 Real time detection formats   93
TaqMan® technology   93
Dye intercalation   94

Acknowledgements   95

References   95

4 Mutation detection by single-stranded conformation polymorphism and denaturing high performance liquid chromatography   97

Michael Dean, Bernard Gerrard, and Rando Allikmets

1 Introduction   97
2 Single-stranded conformation polymorphism (SSCP) and heteroduplex analysis (HA)   98
Optimization of the PCR reaction   98
SSCP sample preparation   100
Optimization of SSCP/HA detection   101
Multiplexing   101
Interpretation of results   102
Applications   103
Other methods   103
3 Denaturing high performance liquid chromatography (DHPLC)   103
Application of DHPLC to mutation detection   108
Sensitivity of detection   108
Conclusions   108
Interpretation of results   110
Genotyping   110

References   110

5 DNA pooling methods for association mapping of complex disease loci   113

Lisa F. Barcellos, Soren Germer, and William Klitz

1 Introduction   113
2 Quantification of DNA samples for pooled amplification   115
3 Genetic analysis of microsatellite markers using pooled DNA samples   117

4 Analysis of pooled microsatellite data   *121*
    Correction methods for stutter and differential amplification   *122*
    Example of a case-control study using pooled DNA amplification   *126*
    DNA pooling using nuclear family-based samples   *127*
    Analysis of microsatellite allele image patterns from DNA pools   *127*
5 SNP allele frequency determination using kinetic PCR   *129*
6 Experimental design considerations   *134*
    Selection of markers for full genome association screen   *137*
    Study guidelines   *138*
    Technical considerations   *139*
7 DNA pooling in the era of the human genome sequence   *140*
Acknowledgements   *141*
References   *141*

6 Single-sperm typing: a rapid alternative to family-based linkage analysis   *145*
Michael Cullen and Mary Carrington

1 Introduction   *145*
2 Isolation of single sperm   *147*
3 Whole genome amplification of haploid DNA   *152*
4 PCR amplification using PEP reaction products as a source of DNA   *154*
    Amplification of polymorphic short tandem repeats (STRs)   *155*
    Amplification of single nucleotide polymorphisms (SNPs)   *162*
5 Discriminating alleles by gel electrophoresis   *167*
6 Interpretation of sperm typing data   *172*
    Single-sperm haplotype scoring   *173*
    General approaches for analysing recombination data   *174*
References   *177*

7 PCR-based methods of HLA typing   *181*
Henry A. Erlich and Elizabeth A. Trachtenberg

1 Introduction   *181*
2 The HLA loci   *182*
3 HLA allelic sequence diversity   *183*
4 Nomenclature   *184*
5 HLA typing: a brief history   *185*
    Serological and cellular methods   *185*
    DNA-based techniques   *185*
6 HLA typing requirements   *204*
7 The problem of new alleles and of ambiguity   *204*
Acknowledgements   *205*
References   *205*

8 Evolutionary analysis of molecular sequence data   *209*
Austin L. Hughes, Jack da Silva, and Federica Verra

1 Introduction   *209*

2 Comparing sequences   *210*
    Rationale for statistical models   *210*
    Comparing amino acid sequences   *212*
    Comparing DNA sequences   *212*
    Synonymous and non-synonymous substitution   *213*
    Mean nucleotide diversity   *216*

3 Reconstructing phylogenies   *216*
    Overview of the problem   *216*
    Methods of phylogenetic reconstruction   *219*
    Testing phylogenies   *221*

4 Applications   *222*
    Phylogenetic analysis   *222*
    Testing for positive selection   *224*
    Nucleotide diversity and population structure   *228*

    References   *231*

List of suppliers *233*

Index *239*

Protocol list

PCR-based fingerprinting of the bacterial chromosome

Rapid preparation of cell lysates from Gram negative bacteria   *34*

Rapid freeze–fracture preparation of cell lysates from Gram positive bacteria   *35*

Preparation of high quality chromosomal DNA for restriction endonuclease analyses and other applications where high quality DNA is needed   *36*

A general PCR set-up strategy for amplification-based DNA fingerprinting   *38*

RFLP analysis of the bacterial chromosome

Digestion of DNA for RFLP analysis   *47*

Polyacrylamide gel electrophoresis of restriction digests   *49*

PFGE analysis of the bacterial chromosome

Preparation of DNA in agarose plugs   *53*

Digestion of bacterial DNA for PFGE analysis   *54*

Pulsed field gel electrophoresis (PFGE) analysis   *55*

DNA sequence analysis of the bacterial *ompA* gene

A method for the preparation and storage of competent bacterial cells   *60*

A strategy for the molecular cloning of PCR products   *61*

Qualitative HIV DNA assay

Preparation of cell pellets from whole blood for HIV DNA PCR   *75*

Preparation of Ficoll-Hypaque separated cells for DNA PCR   *76*

Extraction of DNA from PBMCs   *77*

Dried blood spot extraction   *78*   .

DNA amplification   *80*

Preparation of coated microwell plates   *81*

Colorimetric microwell plate detection for the qualitative DNA assay   *82*

Quantitative HIV RNA assay

Processing plasma for HIV RNA PCR   *84*

Extraction of RNA from plasma: standard method   *85*

Extraction of RNA from plasma: ultrasensitive method   *86*

Amplification of HIV RNA for quantitative assay   *87*

Colorimetric detection of amplified products for the quantitative assays   *88*

Results calculation for the quantitative RNA assay   *89*

Quantitative DNA assay

Total DNA determination   *92*

Quantification of HIV DNA   *93*

Single-stranded conformation polymorphism (SSCP) and heteroduplex analysis (HA)
PCR set up and optimization   *99*
Preparing an SSCP/HA gel   *100*

Denaturing high performance liquid chromatography (DHPLC)
DHPLC analysis   *109*

Quantification of DNA samples for pooled amplification
DNA quantitation using fluorescence detection   *116*

Genetic analysis of microsatellite markers using pooled DNA samples
PCR amplification of microsatellite markers   *118*
Elimination of A-overhang from PCR products   *119*
Preparation of denaturing polyacrylamide gel for electrophoresis   *119*
Sample preparation and gel electrophoresis using automatic sequencer   *120*

SNP allele frequency determination using kinetic PCR
SNP allele frequency determination on pooled DNA samples   *132*

Isolation of single sperm
Wash and stain sperm   *149*
Isolate individual sperm by fluorescence activated cell sorting   *150*

Whole genome amplification of haploid DNA
Primer extension pre-amplification (PEP)   *153*

PCR amplification using PEP reaction products as a source of DNA
First round of PCR amplification (STRs only)   *159*
Second round (nested) PCR amplification (STRs only)   *161*
Radiolabelling oligonucleotide primers with [γ-^{32}P]dATP   *162*
Single round PCR amplification from PEP product (SNPs only)   *164*
Optional second round (nested) PCR amplification (SNPs only)   *165*

Discriminating alleles by gel electrophoresis
Preparing polyacrylamide gels   *168*
Sample preparation and polyacrylamide gel electrophoresis   *170*
Sample preparation and non-denaturing gel electrophoresis   *171*
Silver staining of DNA in polyacrylamide gels   *171*
Ethidium bromide staining of DNA in polyacrylamide gels   *172*

HLA typing: a brief history
High-throughput PCR amplification for HLA typing   *191*
Immobilized probe strip hybridization   *194*
Dot blot membrane preparation   *198*
Data interpretation   *200*

Abbreviations

ACRS   amplification created restriction sites
ADPL   allele discrimination by primer length
AFLP   amplification fragment length polymorphism
AIDS   acquired immunodeficiency syndrome
ARMS   amplification refractory mutation system
ASA   allele-specific amplification
ASO   allele-specific oligonucleotide hybridization
C   crosslinking (% acrylamide to bis-acrylamide)
CAE   capillary array electrophoresis
CEPH   Centre d'Etudes du Polymorphisme Humaine
CHEF   contour-clamped homogeneous electric field
DGGE   denaturing gradient gel electrophoresis
DHPLC   denaturing high performance liquid chromatography
ERIC   enterobacterial repetitive intergenic consensus
EST   expressed sequence tag
FACS   fluorescence activated cell sorting
HA   heteroduplex analysis
HIV   human immunodeficiency virus
IC   internal control
IDDM   insulin-dependent diabetes mellitus
IGS   intergenic spacer
ME   minimum evolution
MHC   major histocompatibility complex
ML   maximum likelihood
MP   maximum parsimony
NJ   neighbour-joining
OTU   operational taxonomic unit
PAGE   polyacrylamide gel electrophoresis
PBMC   peripheral blood mononuclear cell
PBS   phosphate-buffered saline
PCR   polymerase chain reaction
PEP   primer extension pre-amplification

PFGE	pulsed field gel electrophoresis
PIC	polymorphic information content
QS	quantitation standard
RAPD	randomly amplified polymorphic DNA
REP	repetitive extragenic palindrome
REP-PCR	repetitive PCR fingerprint analysis
RFLP	restriction fragment length polymorphism
SE	standard error
SNP	single nucleotide polymorphism
SSCP	single-stranded conformation polymorphism
SSO	sequence-specific oligonucleotide
SSP	sequence-specific priming
STR	short tandem repeats
STS	sequence-tagged site
UNG	uracil-*N*-glycosylase

Introduction to molecular epidemiology

Charles S. Rabkin and Nathaniel Rothman
Division of Cancer Epidemiology and Genetics, National Cancer Institute, Bethesda, MD 20892, USA

Epidemiology is the study of the distribution and effects of disease determinants in human populations. Molecular biology is the study of the physical and chemical reactions of living cells, and when applied to diseases is the study of biochemical derangements which underlie the diseased state. The emerging discipline of 'molecular epidemiology' is the result of confluent developments in these seemingly disparate approaches to understanding human disease.

The 'molecular' aspect of molecular epidemiology refers to the application of molecular biological approaches to epidemiological problems. The variety and power of molecular methods are rapidly expanding our capability to dissect aetiologic mechanisms of disease. These approaches represent an ever-increasing proportion of epidemiological studies, generate some of the most interesting observations, and warrant continued emphasis for future epidemiological research.

Likewise, the 'epidemiological' aspect of molecular epidemiology refers to utilizing the tools and perspective of epidemiology to comprehend observations in molecular biology. An increasingly sophisticated variety of powerful molecular techniques are being applied to generate a virtual explosion of data on exposures and outcomes whose significance must be determined. For example, population studies of relationships between numerous genetic polymorphisms and disease risk will produce many novel associations, some spurious and others meaningful. Discerning and interpreting this massive amount of information is necessitating new approaches in bioinformatics, functional genomics, and statistical analysis. Epidemiological methods are valuable to translate laboratory observations to understanding disease process in free-living individuals, identify which of these phenomena are aetiologically important, and relate their interplay in coherent pathways of causation.

A functional definition of molecular epidemiology was stated by Schulte as 'the use of biological markers or biological measurements in epidemiological research' (1). In this context, a biomarker is considered to be any substance, structure, or process that can be measured in the human body or in its products, that may influence or predict the occurrence or outcome of disease (2). Under this formulation, all biomarkers are regarded as within the purview of molecular epidemiology, including those based on the measurements of proteins and exogenous and endogenous chemicals as well as those based on the measurement of nucleic acids. While the concept of a distinct discipline may be new, epidemiological research has long used biomarkers, in studies of infectious disease (e.g. antibodies) and cardiovascular disease (e.g. serum lipids), to name but two examples.

Biomarkers have been classified according to various schemata, but a simple, functional taxonomy divides them into measures of exposure, early biological effect, susceptibility, and disease (3). This categorization also helps to crystallize the rationale for using biomarkers to enhance the epidemiological study of disease, which includes:

(a) Improve assessment of exposures.
(b) Identify underlying mechanisms of disease and disease transmission.
(c) Identify subgroups of the population that are more susceptible to the effects of pathogens or pathogenic substances.
(d) Identify subgroups of cases with more homogeneous disease to better clarify the role of various aetiologic agents.

Although newly developed biomarkers may offer novel opportunities for application in epidemiological studies, a crucial component of molecular epidemiology involves their characterization and the validation of their usefulness in large population studies. This procedure includes defining and testing the conditions necessary to optimally collect, process, and store the relevant biological sample and determination of laboratory accuracy and precision (4). Biomarker misclassification can lead to either overestimation or underestimation of associated risk. Most often, biomarker misclassification that does not differ between cases and controls tends to bias disease risk estimates towards the null. The attenuated risk estimate will also result in diminished statistical power. Thus, careful consideration of assay quality is essential for all classes of assays.

An example can be seen in the fundamental importance of test reliability in studies of the association of human papillomavirus (HPV) infection with cervical neoplasia. As outlined by Schiffman (5), early studies utilizing HPV-testing methods with moderate measurement error failed to reveal the true magnitude of this association. These workers had performed two similar case-control studies of cervical intraepithelial neoplasia (CIN), which methodologically differed primarily by the much greater reliability of HPV testing in the second study. The findings were startlingly different, for odds ratios associating HPV infection with CIN (3.7 vs. 20.1), ten or more lifetime sexual partners (1.9 vs. 11.6), and as a cofounder of the association of CIN with lifetime number of sexual partners (1.0 vs. 2.8) (5). The attributable proportions of CIN explainable by HPV infection were 36% vs. 77–90%, transforming the interpretation of HPV's role from a risk factor to the central, causal agent. Current understanding of cervical cancer aetiology was greatly clarified by these improvements in molecular epidemiological methods.

Measurement error may be particularly problematic in studies of gene–

environment interaction. Garcia-Closas and colleagues have demonstrated how exposure misclassification can lead to substantial bias in the estimation of an interaction effect and increased sample size requirements (6). In their hypothetical example, even a 5% sensitivity error in genotyping and a 20% sensitivity error in environmental measurement increases the minimum number of cases (and a similar number of controls) required to detect a twofold multiplicative interaction from 720 to 2044. Further, the observed interaction parameter is attenuated to 1.46 from the actual value of 2. Thus, the validity of molecular epidemiological studies is highly dependent upon the accurate assessment of both genetic and environmental exposures.

This volume provides a broad overview of the diverse approaches encompassed by this emerging discipline. Chapters 1–3 highlight concepts and methods at the forefront of studies of infectious diseases, and include a synopsis of general epidemiological design and analysis, as well as current techniques for molecular typing of microbial pathogens. Chapters 4–6 are focused on recent advances in studying host genetics, including methods for the detection of mutations and polymorphisms, identification of linkage among alleles of genes on a given chromosome, and the use of DNA pooling to increase efficiency in association studies of genetically complex traits. Chapters 7 and 8 deal with the relationship between pathologies and immune system genetics, and on the use of DNA sequence information to garner insights into the evolution of infectious pathogens, and into the evolution and function of the immune system.

The wealth of information generated by the Human Genome Project and the corresponding efforts in microbial genomics are providing researchers with extraordinary new opportunities to further understand the aetiology of disease. Molecular epidemiology is rapidly evolving through the application of more relevant markers of exposure and better identification of subgroups at increased risk of early disease processes and progression. The application of the next generation of biological markers in high quality molecular epidemiology studies that are designed, conducted, analysed, and interpreted appropriately holds great promise. These developments should lead to enhanced understanding of the underlying pathogenesis of disease and suggest improved primary, secondary, and tertiary prevention strategies.

References

1. Schulte, P. A. (1993). In *Molecular epidemiology: principles and practices* (ed. P. A. Schulte and F. P. Perera), pp. 3–44. San Diego: Academic Press.
2. Proceedings of the Workshop on Application of Biomarkers to Cancer Epidemiology. (1997). Lyon, France, 20–23 February 1996, pp. 1–318. IARC Sci Publ.
3. The role of biomarkers in reproductive and developmental toxicology. (1987). January 12–12, 1987, Washington DC. *Environ. Health Perspect.*, 74, 1–199.
4. Rothman, N., Stewart, W. F. and Schulte, P. A. (1995). *Cancer Epidemiol. Biomarkers Prev.*, 4, 301.
5. Schiffman, M. H. and Schatzkin, A. (1994). *Cancer Res.*, 54, 1994s.
6. Garcia-Closas, M., Rothman, N. and Lubin, J. (1999). *Cancer Epidemiol. Biomarkers Prev.*, 8, 1043.

Chapter 1

Epidemiological methods for studies of genetic factors that influence infectious diseases

Eric A. Engels and Thomas R. O'Brien

Viral Epidemiology Branch, Division of Cancer Epidemiology and Genetics, National Cancer Institute, 6120 Executive Blvd, Rockville, MD 20852, USA

1 General considerations

Epidemiological studies are concerned with the relationship within populations between exposures and outcomes. A strong relationship between an exposure and outcome provides evidence that the exposure, at least in part, is a cause of the outcome. Numerous types of exposures are of potential interest to epidemiologists. These types include, but are not limited to, environmental exposures (e.g. toxic chemicals or radiation), exposures defined by socioeconomic status or occupation (which can be markers for more specific exposures that are difficult to measure), and endogenous exposures (e.g. blood pressure or hormone levels). An additional type of exposure is provided by infectious agents, i.e. micro-organisms such as viruses, bacteria, or parasites. Infectious diseases, by definition, require exposure to an infecting organism for the development of disease. Nonetheless, although contact with the micro-organism is *necessary* for infectious diseases, it is often not *sufficient*. Not everyone who is exposed to an infectious organism becomes infected, and not everyone who becomes infected develops disease.

For infectious diseases, one may thus consider cofactors that act with the micro-organism in determining outcome. *Genetic makeup* of the host represents a unique type of exposure and is emerging as an important cofactor in infectious disease epidemiology. Numerous studies have demonstrated that individuals may have different risks for infectious disease because they have different alleles at certain genetic loci. In this regard, genetic epidemiological studies can address two relevant questions related to infectious disease aetiology. First, among individuals exposed to an infectious agent, what effect does genetic makeup have on the risk of becoming *infected*? And secondly, among infected individuals, what effect does genetic makeup have on the risk of developing clinically apparent *disease*?

The observational nature of epidemiological studies makes them more complex than experimental studies, such as randomized clinical trials. In a well-planned clinical trial, the random assignment of subjects into exposed (i.e. treatment) and unexposed (i.e. placebo or comparison) groups usually renders the two groups comparable for important determinants of outcome other than the exposure of interest. However, in observational studies, extraneous determinants of outcome are usually present but rarely allocated equally. If these extraneous factors are left uncontrolled, they may lead to *confounding* and erroneous results (confounding is discussed in more detail in Section 7). Furthermore, in a randomized trial, blinding of investigators and subjects to treatment assignment insures that comparable information is collected from each group. In observational epidemiological studies that utilize retrospectively reported information, reports may be influenced by the subjects' or investigators' knowledge of the outcome.

In light of these considerations and others discussed below, modern epidemiology has developed rigorous methods for study design and data analysis in an effort to insure the validity of epidemiological results. These methods are covered in detail in a number of excellent texts (1–3). The purpose of this chapter is to provide the non-epidemiologist with an overview of epidemiological design and analysis that will be useful in collaborative efforts. In our experience, the most successful epidemiological studies of genetic factors that influence infectious diseases require the co-ordinated efforts of a team of investigators with expertise in genetics, infectious diseases, and epidemiology.

2 Types of epidemiological studies

The subject of epidemiological studies is the relationship between exposure and outcome for all individuals within a large *population*. However, for practical reasons it is usually impossible to study all individuals within a population of interest. Epidemiological studies are therefore most often based on a *sample* obtained from the study population. Conclusions regarding exposure and outcome in the population are based on generalizing from observations made on the study sample. The validity of these conclusions largely rests on how well the sample represents the overall population.

The techniques of *classical epidemiology* provide methods to determine the impact of genetic makeup on infectious diseases. In classical epidemiological studies, individuals are sampled from the population without respect to familial relationships, and these are also known as *genetic association studies*. The two main types of classical epidemiological studies are the *cohort study* and the *case-control* study (a third type of study, *cross-sectional* study, will be discussed briefly below).

Cohort and case-control study design samples from the study population in complementary ways. In a cohort study, individuals who have not yet developed the outcome of interest are sampled from the population and followed forward in time to determine whether they develop the outcome. If genetic makeup is of interest, the cohort may be constructed based on whether or not individuals within the sample have a particular genotype. Alternatively and more commonly, genotype may be determined retrospectively among members of a cohort already being followed.

In comparison, for a case-control study, individuals are sampled from the population on the basis of their outcome status, i.e. whether they have the outcome of interest ('cases') or not ('controls'). The exposure status (e.g. genotype) of cases and controls is then retrospectively determined. Both cohort and case-control studies allow determination of the risk of disease among exposed subjects relative to unexposed subjects. In other words, both types of study allow assessment of the association between exposure and outcome.

For epidemiological investigations, the cohort and case-control study designs each have advantages, which are summarized in *Table 1* and discussed in more detail below. The prospective nature of the cohort study allows determination of the absolute rate at which events occur, as well as the period between infection and development of disease (the *incubation* period). For example, through cohort studies of human immunodeficiency virus (HIV)-infected patients it has been determined that those who are heterozygous for the chemokine receptor allele *CCR5-Δ32* develop acquired immunodeficiency syndrome (AIDS) about two years later than those who are homozygous for the wild-type allele (4). Cohort studies that are conducted prospectively also eliminate the possibility that the quality of reported exposure information will vary between subjects who develop a disease and those who do not (*recall* bias), although recall bias is not a concern for measurement of genotypes. Cohort studies permit examination of a large number of outcomes, whereas each case-control study is limited to a single outcome.

Case-control studies are generally more efficient than cohort studies when the disease is rare. On the other hand, cohort studies are more efficient when the exposure is rare. Case-control studies eliminate the necessity of costly follow-up of a large number of subjects. Case-control studies allow simultaneous ex-

Table 1 Comparison of cohort and case-control studies

Epidemiological issue	Cohort study	Case-control study
Determination of absolute risk for outcome	Possible	Not possible
Determination of incubation period	Possible	Not possible
Recall bias in assessing exposure	Not usually a problem	May be a problem
Selection bias	Not usually a problem, but may be a problem if some subjects lack specimens	May be a problem
Multiple exposures or outcomes	Assess effects of various exposures on multiple outcomes	Assess effects of multiple exposures on single outcome
Efficiency	Most efficient if exposure is rare	Most efficient if outcome is rare
Cost	Relatively expensive	Relatively inexpensive

amination of multiple exposures for their effects on risk for a single outcome of interest. *Selection bias*, which occurs when the relationship between exposure and outcome is mismeasured because of distortions in the way individuals are selected into the study sample, is usually a more important problem for case-control studies than cohort studies.

When genetic makeup is an exposure of interest, several unique considerations arise. First, genotyping of subjects is contingent on availability of adequate biological specimens. An opportunity for *selection bias* then arises for cohort studies, if specimens are available for only a subset of subjects and if the availability of specimens is related to both the genotype of interest and the outcome. Secondly, once specimens are available, laboratory methods allow genotyping at many loci simultaneously. Because genotype at any of these loci would be an exposure of interest, the cohort study, like the case-control study, does provide the ability to examine the effects of multiple exposures in an efficient manner.

3 Cohort study

The cohort study allows the epidemiologist to measure the association of interest in an appealingly direct way. The investigator includes individuals in the study sample based on whether they have the exposure of interest. In a *prospective* cohort study, these included individuals are then followed forward in time to record whether they develop the outcome of interest. For example, one may examine the effect of a particular genotype on the risk of schistosomiasis-induced bladder cancer by beginning with a sample of individuals with schistosomiasis and classifying them into different arms of the cohort study based on their genotype. One would then follow this cohort forward in time to determine the relative or absolute difference in bladder cancer risk in the groups defined by the different genotypes.

Individuals followed in an existing cohort study can serve as a source of subjects for a new cohort study. For instance, by evaluating genotypes for intravenous drug users already under follow-up, one could use this group as the study sample for a new cohort study examining the effect of genetic makeup on risk of acquiring HIV infection.

A disadvantage of some cohort studies is the need to follow included individuals forward in time while waiting to determine whether the outcome occurs. This follow-up may be time-consuming and expensive. Furthermore, loss of individuals from the study will decrease the ability of the investigator to measure an association, and it might also lead to biased results if loss to follow-up differs by exposure status.

A *retrospective* cohort study design can minimize some of the cost and time problems involved in follow-up in cohort studies. In a retrospective cohort study, individuals are still included based on their exposure status. However, all of the outcome events have already occurred when the investigator initiates the study, so the investigator does not have to conduct prospective follow-up or wait for events to occur. A retrospective cohort study for the effects of genetic makeup on the outcome of interest would depend on the availability of reliable information on the history of cohort members and of biological specimens for all subjects, so that all cohort individuals could be classified by genotype exposure.

The cohort study design is advantageous when the exposure of interest (e.g. a particular genotype) is rare. This advantage arises because the cohort study design allows one to select increased numbers of individuals with this rare genotype for inclusion in the study sample. Including more individuals with the rare genotype increases the precision with which the association between genotype and outcome can be measured. Additionally, cohort studies allow one to examine the effect of variation at a genetic locus on multiple outcomes of interest. For example, one could use the same cohort study sample of HIV-infected individuals to estimate the effect of a single genotype on risk of AIDS, lymphoma, or Kaposi's sarcoma.

3.1 Cohort studies: cumulative incidence

For each group in a cohort study, risk for the outcome of interest can be measured in several ways. One useful way to quantify risk is to identify a particular time point and measure the proportion of subjects in each arm of the cohort study who develop the outcome before this time point. This measure is known as the *cumulative incidence*. For example, during an outbreak of an acute infectious disease, an epidemiologist might examine the proportion of subjects who become infected or ill during the period of the outbreak. To calculate cumulative incidence in epidemiological studies, it is often desirable to construct a table that cross-classifies the sampled individuals on the basis of exposure and outcome status. *Table 2* shows the general form of such a table.

In *Table 2*, a = number of exposed individuals with the outcome, b = number of unexposed individuals with the outcome, c = number of exposed individuals without the outcome, and d = number of unexposed individuals without the outcome. *Table 2* also presents hypothetical data from a cohort study examining

Table 2 Cohort study

General form of data	Exposed	Unexposed
Outcome	a	b
No outcome	c	d
Cumulative incidence of outcome	a / (a + c)	b / (b + d)

Specific example (hypothetical data)

Among persons with hepatitis C infection:	Genotype A/A or A/B	Genotype B/B
Cirrhosis	190	120
No cirrhosis	810	880
Cumulative incidence of cirrhosis	190/1000 = 0.19	120/1000 = 0.12
Risk difference	0.19 − 0.12 = 0.07	
Risk ratio	0.19/0.12 = 1.6	

the effect of a genetic exposure (having one or two copies of an allele A) on cumulative incidence of cirrhosis, among persons infected with hepatitis C virus. Several *measures of association* can be calculated based on such an enumeration of sampled individuals by exposure and outcome: the *risk difference*, the *risk ratio*, or the *odds ratio*.

The risk difference (often abbreviated RD) provides information on the absolute difference in cumulative incidence between those with the exposure and those without the exposure.

$$\text{risk difference} =$$

$$(\text{proportion of exposed with outcome}) - (\text{proportion of unexposed with outcome}) =$$

$$[a / (a + c)] - [b / (b + d)].$$

In the hypothetical example in *Table 2*, the risk difference is 0.07, indicating that hepatitis C virus-infected individuals with an A allele have a 7% higher risk (in absolute terms) of developing cirrhosis than do those lacking the A allele.

The risk ratio measures the cumulative incidence among the exposed group *relative* to cumulative incidence among the unexposed group. The risk ratio (RR) is also known as the *relative risk*.

$$\text{risk ratio} =$$

$$(\text{proportion of exposed with outcome}) / (\text{proportion of unexposed with outcome}) =$$

$$[a / (a + c)] / [b / (b + d)].$$

In the worked example in *Table 2*, the risk ratio is 1.6, indicating that risk in those with A alleles is greater by a factor of 1.6 than risk in those lacking an A allele.

Finally, for cohort studies (and also for case-control studies) one can calculate the odds ratio (OR). Like the relative risk, the odds ratio is a measure of relative difference in risk associated with exposure.

$$\text{odds ratio} = (\text{odds of outcome in exposed}) / (\text{odds of outcome in unexposed}) =$$

$$(a/c) / (b/d) = (ad) / (bc).$$

The odds ratio is less intuitively understood than the risk ratio, but when an outcome is rare, the odds ratio provides a good approximation of the risk ratio. Under this circumstance, one may interpret an odds ratio of 3 or 0.5, for example, as indicating a 'tripling' or 'halving' of risk. The odds ratio has one advantage over the risk ratio. As discussed in more detail below, logistic regression models are often used in epidemiological studies to control for the effect of possibly confounding variables on the exposure–outcome relationship of interest. The odds ratio, not the risk ratio, is the parameter that is estimated by the logistic regression model.

In general, a risk difference greater than 0 or a risk ratio or odds ratio greater than 1 suggests that the exposure is associated with an increased risk for the outcome, and one would say that the exposure is *positively associated* with the outcome. Conversely, when the risk difference is less than 0 or the risk ratio or odds ratio is less than 1, the study is said to demonstrate a *negative association*. It is important to note that a positive or negative association, no matter how strong, does not by itself prove that the exposure causes or protects against the outcome. As discussed below, one must consider whether the observed association may be due to chance or a bias in the data.

3.2 Cohort studies: incidence

A second way that risk can be compared in cohort studies considers the *time to occurrence* or *rate of occurrence* of the outcome. This approach arises naturally when individuals are followed for different periods of time before they develop the outcome or are *censored* (censoring occurs when the study ends or when subjects leave the study without developing the outcome). In a cohort study one may thus calculate the *incidence* of an outcome (also called an *incidence rate*). Incidence is measured as the number of outcome events per person-time interval, where person-time is calculated by summing up the duration of follow-up for each person in the group, before they develop the outcome or are censored. For example, if one observed 6 cases of malaria during 56 person-years of follow-up, the incidence would be 0.11 cases per person-year (i.e. 6/56 = 0.11). For cohort studies these considerations lead naturally to the type of table shown in *Table 3*.

The incidence rate ratio, defined as $(a/T_1) / (b/T_2)$, provides a useful measure of the relative difference in incidence, incorporating the known differences between the groups in the length of time individuals were at risk.

Table 3 Cohort study (calculation of incidence rate)

	Exposed	Unexposed
Number of persons with outcome	a	b
Total number of person-years	T_1	T_2
Incidence rate	a/T_1	b/T_2

When considering the time to outcomes in cohort studies, *Kaplan-Meier* curves are a useful means of displaying data. An example of a Kaplan-Meier curve is presented in *Figure 1*. These curves allow one to determine whether the exposure has an immediate effect on outcome risk, a late effect, or an effect that is constant over time, by examining how much the curves separate over time. Elementary statistics texts describe the derivation of these curves and tests for evaluating whether the curves differ from each other (see ref. 5, pages 188–209).

Finally, when considering the time to the outcome, it is also useful to examine the *hazard* for the outcome. Although the technical details are complex, the hazard may be considered a measure of the *instantaneous* risk for the outcome among those individuals in the study group who have not yet developed the outcome. Graphically, for a cohort group whose experience is summarized in a Kaplan-Meier curve, the hazard at any time point is related to how steeply the Kaplan-Meier curve is dropping at that time point. Of particular interest in this regard are *relative hazards* (also referred to as *hazard ratios*), which measure the

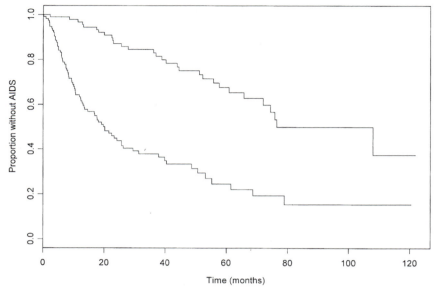

Figure 1 An example of Kaplan-Meier curves is shown for two hypothetical groups of HIV-infected subjects in a cohort study. The curves illustrate the proportion of subjects in each group who have not yet developed the outcome, acquired immunodeficiency syndrome (AIDS), at each time during follow-up. These two groups might be defined, for example, by different alleles at a locus of interest. The group whose curve is lower has a higher AIDS incidence, since at each time the proportion of subjects without AIDS is lower for this group than for the other group.

relative difference between two groups in the instantaneous risk for the outcome. Hazard ratios find wide application in survival analyses and can be derived using Cox proportional hazards regression (6, 7). Details of a full survival analysis are complex and should best be approached with collaboration from an epidemiologist or biostatistician.

3.3 Example of cohort study

There has recently been substantial interest in the effect of polymorphisms in chemokine and chemokine receptor proteins on the course of HIV infection. HIV uses chemokine receptors as co-receptors to enter macrophages and CD4+ lymphocytes, cells in which the virus replicates. Individuals with variant chemokine receptors may be protected from becoming HIV-infected, or may progress slowly to HIV-disease end-points once infected.

Smith and co-workers used a retrospective cohort study design to examine the association between risk of HIV-disease progression and variants of two chemokine receptors, CCR2 and CCR5 (8). Their study examined the *CCR2-64I* allele, a single nucleotide substitution in the wild-type CCR2 gene that changes a valine to an isoleucine in the transmembrane domain of the receptor. Also, the study examined *CCR5-Δ32*, which is an allele that contains a 32 bp deletion in the *CCR5* gene resulting in a non-functional CCR5 receptor on the cell surface. Individuals homozygous for *CCR5-Δ32* allele are highly protected from HIV-infection.

Smith and colleagues pooled together individuals from several separate cohort studies. 891 study subjects had been followed since HIV seroconversion. These subjects were typed at the *CCR2* and *CCR5* loci. They were evaluated for the occurrence of AIDS or death. The investigators used a Cox proportional hazards regression analysis, which provided estimates of the magnitude of association between each genotype and risk (measured as relative hazard) and the statistical significance of each association (p-value; for a discussion of statistical significance, see Section 9).

The *CCR2-64I* allele was associated with decreased risk for disease progression. Based on a Cox proportional regression analysis, individuals heterozygous or homozygous for the *CCR2-64I* allele appeared to be less likely to develop AIDS (relative hazard 0.80, p-value 0.04) or death (relative hazard 0.76, p-value 0.08), compared to individuals homozygous for the wild-type *CCR2* allele.

There were no HIV-infected individuals homozygous for the *CCR5-Δ32* allele. Compared with individuals homozygous for the wild-type *CCR5* allele, hetero-zygotes had a reduced risk for progressing to AIDS (relative hazard 0.68, p-value 0.002) or death (relative hazard 0.67, p-value 0.02).

The *CCR2* and *CCR5* loci are tightly linked on chromosome 3. In the Smith study, *CCR2-64I* and *CCR5-Δ32* were found to be in linkage disequilibrium, in that no individual was identified with both *CCR2-64I* and *CCR5-Δ32* on the same chromosome (for a discussion of linkage disequilibrium see Section 7). *Table 4* illustrates the independent effects of the two loci on outcomes and shows that individuals with either a *CCR2-64I* allele or a *CCR5-Δ32* allele have a decreased risk of AIDS or death, compared with individuals with neither allele.

Table 4 Example of cohort study (data from ref. 8)

CCR2 alleles[a]	CCR5 alleles[a]	AIDS		Death	
		Relative hazard	p-value	Relative hazard	p-value
+/+	+/+	1.00	–	1.00	–
64I/+ or 64I/64I	+/+	0.64	0.001	0.58	0.005
+/+	Δ32/+	0.61	0.0003	0.57	0.002
64I/+	Δ32/+	0.72	0.07	0.79	0.06

[a] +, wild-type allele.

For the individuals heterozygous for both *CCR2-64I* and *CCR5-Δ32* (who had these variant alleles each present on *separate* chromosomes; last row of table), the presence of both variants did not appear to offer added protection against AIDS or death beyond that offered by either *CCR2-64I* or *CCR5-Δ32* separately. However, the small number of these double heterozygotes (seventeen) limited the strength of this conclusion.

3.4 Attributable risk

An additional useful means of quantifying the association between exposure and outcome in a cohort study is provided by the *attributable risk*, which is the excess risk present among those exposed compared with those unexposed. In absolute terms, the attributable risk is the same as the risk difference between exposed and unexposed. In relative terms, the attributable risk can be expressed as a percentage of the risk in those exposed:

$$\text{percentage attributable risk (\%)} =$$
$$100 \times (\text{risk in exposed} - \text{risk in unexposed}) / (\text{risk in exposed}).$$

Here risk can be measured either by cumulative incidence or by incidence.

For example, consider the effect of a genotype A_1 on the risk for cirrhosis among hepatitis C-infected individuals, relative to the usual genotype A_2 present in most individuals. If cirrhosis incidence is 0.5 per 100 person-years among individuals with genotype A_1 and 0.3 per 100 person-years among those with genotype A_2, then the percentage attributable risk for genotype A_1 is $100 \times (0.5 - 0.3) / (0.5) = 40\%$. This result implies that 40% of the risk of cirrhosis among individuals with genotype A_1 arises because they possess genotype A_1 (assuming that the relationship between genotype and cirrhosis risk is causal). Large values of the percentage attributable risk imply a strong effect of the genotype on risk for the outcome.

4 Case-control studies

The case-control study design complements the cohort design and, in some settings, offers several important advantages over the cohort study (see Section 2 and *Table 1*). One setting in which the case-control study is advantageous is when the outcome is rare, because this design allows one to select study subjects on the basis of whether the outcome has occurred. In contrast, to study a rare outcome in a cohort study, one would need to recruit large numbers of individuals into the study at its outset. Also, the case-control study eliminates the need to wait for the outcome, because one identifies cases and controls for study after the outcome of interest has already occurred. As noted above, the follow-up entailed in cohort studies may require long waiting and substantial expense to ensure that subjects in the cohort are not lost to follow-up.

A second setting in which the case-control design is advantageous is when one is interested in evaluating the effects of multiple exposures on a single outcome of interest (*Table 1*). For example, by identifying cases and controls for inclusion in the study, the investigator in a case-control study obtains a sample of individuals for whom it is possible to evaluate genotypes at several separate loci. Odds ratios can be calculated for alleles at each locus and for more complete genotypes across several loci considered together. It may be more difficult to evaluate multiple exposures in a cohort study. For example, the subjects may have been selected on the basis of a particular exposure or specimens may not be available for testing. On the other hand, a cohort study readily allows one to examine multiple outcomes, which the case-control design does not allow.

As shown in *Table 5*, the relevant process of cross-classifying subjects by exposure and outcome is similar to *Table 2* presented above for cohort studies.

Table 5 Case-control study

General form of data	Exposed	Unexposed	Odds for exposure
Outcome	a	b	a/b
No outcome	c	d	c/d

Specific example[a]

	Exposed (D543N G/A or A/A)	Unexposed (D543N G/G)	Odds for exposure
Tuberculosis	68	337	68/337 = 0.20
No tuberculosis	42	375	42/375 = 0.11
Odds ratio			0.20/0.11 = 1.80

[a] Data from ref. 9. Exposures represent various alleles at the D543N polymorphism in the *NRAMP1* gene. For further discussion of this study, see also Section 4.1 and Table 6.

For case-control studies, only the odds ratio (ad / bc in *Table 5*) provides a valid measure of association between exposure and outcome. *Table 5* presents data from a case-control study that examined the association between polymorphisms in the *NRAMP1* gene and tuberculosis risk (9); this study is discussed in greater detail below (Section 4.1). In *Table 5*, the odds ratio in the worked example is 1.8, indicating that tuberculosis risk in those with D543N G/A or A/A is 1.8 times higher than risk in those with D543N G/G.

It is important to note that absolute risk (as measured by cumulative incidence) cannot be determined in a case-control study. Because individuals are actually sampled based on their outcomes, the proportion with the event (cumulative incidence) in the sample is arbitrary and does not reflect the proportion with the event in the population. As a result, the risk difference and risk ratio are meaningless in case-control studies, since they are derived directly from the cumulative incidence. Importantly, when the outcome is rare, the sample odds ratio in a case-control study does provide a good approximation of the population risk ratio.

Determining which individuals in the study population can be eligible controls and devising a mechanism to select them in a representative manner are critical elements in the design of a case-control study (10). In order to avoid bias, the controls must be chosen in a manner that makes them representative of the population from which the cases are sampled. For example, when studying the effect of a gene on risk for infection with a micro-organism of interest, it is important to select controls from a population whose exposure to infection is comparable to that of the cases. In a study of genetic factors that affect risk for acquiring HIV infection, one might use HIV-infected intravenous drug users as cases; one would then select controls from a population of drug users who had remained HIV-uninfected despite drug use of comparable frequency to cases. In a similar way, when studying genetic effects on risk of Kaposi's sarcoma among individuals co-infected with HIV and human herpesvirus 8 (a virus implicated in the pathogenesis of Kaposi's sarcoma), one might choose cases from individuals who had developed Kaposi's sarcoma and use as controls individuals who did not have the tumour despite infection with the two viruses.

Differences between the populations from which cases and controls are selected can lead to *selection bias*. For instance, consider the consequences of selecting cases and controls without regard to race in a study examining genetic effects on risk for AIDS among drug users in the United States. If access to high-quality health care in the United States differs for drug users of different races, one can imagine that cases might be predominantly African American, but controls might be predominantly white. This possibility could seriously alter the measured effect of genes of interest on AIDS risk if the allele frequencies vary in different races (see discussion of confounding in Section 7). One may therefore wish to *match* on race, selecting individuals as controls who have the same race as cases. Special analytical methods for measuring association are needed when cases and controls have been matched in selection (see ref. 1, pages 147–61). Alternatively, if one anticipates that there will be at least some whites and African Americans among both cases and controls, one might utilize an unmatched study design and use regression methods, which can help adjust for the effects of racial differences (ref. 1, pages 359–399).

4.1 Example of case-control study

An example of a case-control study of genetic effects on infectious disease outcome is provided by a paper by Bellamy and colleagues, who examined the relationship between alleles of the *NRAMP1* (natural resistance associated macrophage protein 1) gene and susceptibility to tuberculosis among individuals living in the Gambia (9). In the Gambia and other areas of sub-Saharan Africa, infection with *Mycobacterium tuberculosis* is almost universal, although the overt disease, tuberculosis, occurs in only about 10% of infected individuals. One may thus consider that infection with *M. tuberculosis* is a necessary but not sufficient cause of tuberculosis, and that genetic determinants of disease might exist. Although the precise function of the protein encoded by *NRAMP1* is unknown, variants of the mouse homologue of this gene are associated with increased susceptibility to infection with mycobacteria and other intracellular pathogens, suggesting that alleles of the *NRAMP1* gene in humans could be associated with variation in tuberculosis risk.

Bellamy and colleagues (9) focused on specific polymorphisms in regions within or near the human *NRAMP1* gene: $5'(CA)_n$, a microsatellite polymorphism in the 5' region of the gene; INT4, a single nucleotide change in intron 4; D543N, a single base substitution that changes aspartic acid to asparagine; and 3'UTR, a deletion in the 3' untranslated region of the gene. The investigators examined the frequency of these variants among Gambians with active pulmonary tuberculosis (cases) and blood donors matched by ethnic group to the cases (controls). Assuming that blood donors are infected with *M. tuberculosis* (but lack disease) and are similar to cases in other respects, then the odds ratio between each of the alleles of *NRAMP1* and tuberculosis status provides a measure of the association between these alleles and risk of developing overt disease given infection.

Table 6 Example of case-control study (data from ref. 9)

Polymorphism[a]	Tuberculosis cases	Controls	Odds ratio[b]	Chi-square statistic[b]	p-value
5'(CA)$_n$					
199/199	263	303	1.0	6.96	0.008
199/other	125	99	1.45 (1.05 − 2.01)		
Other/other	13	8	1.87 (0.71 − 5.02)		
INT4					
G/G	320	360	1.0	7.69	0.006
G/C	78	48	1.83 (1.22 − 2.75)		
C/C	3	3	1.13 (0.18 − 7.01)		
D543N					
G/G	337	375	1.0	8.18	0.004
G/A	68	41	1.85 (1.20 − 2.85)		
A/A	0	1	0.00 (0 − 19.35)		
3'UTR					
TGTG +/+	244	301	1.0	8.32	0.004
TGTG +/del	150	100	1.85 (1.35 − 2.54)		
TGTG del/del	11	16	0.85 (0.36 − 1.97)		

[a] +, wild-type allele.

[b] Odds ratios are adjusted for ethnic group. Chi-square statistics (based on the Mantel-Haenszel statistic) and the corresponding p-values reflect this adjustment.

Each of the four polymorphisms was statistically significantly associated with tuberculosis risk, as shown in *Table 6*.

For example, the data on the 5'(CA)$_n$ microsatellite polymorphism show that the 199 allele is associated with decreased tuberculosis risk, because lacking two 199 alleles is associated with higher risk for tuberculosis. Specifically, data presented in *Table 6* indicate an odds ratio of 1.45 for having only one 199 allele and 1.87 for having zero 199 alleles. (A *microsatellite* is a short sequence of DNA that can be present in the genome in a variable number of repetitions, thereby providing a polymorphic locus for genotyping.)

Of note, linkage disequilibrium was present among these polymorphisms, so their effects on tuberculosis risk were not independent (see discussion of linkage disequilibrium in Section 7). The 201 base pair allele of the 5'(CA)$_n$ polymorphism was strongly associated with the INT4 C allele, and the D543N A allele was always associated with the 3'UTR del allele. When the INT4 and 3'UTR polymorphisms were examined together, their effects were found to be additive, in that individuals who had both INT4 C and 3'UTR del alleles had the highest risk for tuberculosis (odds ratio 4.07, compared with individuals who had neither allele).

Even this well-conducted case-control study does not prove that variation in the *NRAMP1* gene actually causes differential risk for tuberculosis. Additional epidemiological studies confirming the findings of Bellamy *et al.* (9) and laboratory studies to elucidate the function of the *NRAMP1* gene remain necessary.

5 Cross-sectional studies

A third type of epidemiological study is the *cross-sectional* study. In a cross-sectional study, the investigator obtains a representative sample of study subjects from the population, without regard to either exposure status (as is done for a cohort study) or outcome status (as is done for a case-control study). Sampling is thus simpler than for cohort and case-control studies, and the study sample obtained forms a 'cross-sectional' snapshot of the population at a given time. For example, one might include in the study sample all patients who are enrolled in a clinic at a defined time point, considering them representative of patients who attend the clinic at all other times. Exposure and outcome are then assessed for each individual in the study sample, and a table cross-classifying individuals by exposure and outcome is constructed (*Table 7*).

For cross-sectional studies, one may calculate the risk difference ($[a/(a + c)] - [b/(b + d)]$), risk ratio ($[a/(a + c)] / [b/(b + d)]$), and odds ratio ($ad / bc$).

In *Table 7*, data are presented from a study by Nadel *et al.* (11), who used a cross-sectional study design to examine the relationship between disease severity in meningococcal infections and variations in the promoter region of the tumour necrosis factor-α gene. The investigators included in their study all children admitted to a hospital with meningococcal disease over a two-year period. They found that possession of the TNF2 allele was associated with an increased likelihood of severe disease: 67% of those with a TNF2 allele had severe disease, compared with 42% of those without this allele (relative risk 1.6 associated with the TNF2 allele).

Although convenient and inexpensive to perform, cross-sectional studies suffer from several disadvantages. First, if the outcome is rare, few individuals in the sample will have the outcome and the study will have little ability to evaluate the relationship between exposure and outcome. Secondly, in a cross-sectional study the investigator has relatively little control over which persons with the outcome are included in the study sample. This lack of control becomes a problem if the outcome leads in some instances to rapid death from disease. In such a

Table 7 Cross-sectional study

General form of data	Exposed	Unexposed
Outcome	a	b
No outcome	c	d

Specific example[a]

Among persons with meningococcemia:	One or two copies of TNF2 allele	No copies of TNF2 allele
Severe disease	22	27
Non-severe disease	11	38
Risk ratio for severe disease	$(22/33) / (27/65) = 1.6$	

[a] Data from ref. 11.

case, the cross-sectional study might not include persons who quickly die from disease and might include too many persons who have an indolent form of disease. This form of *selection bias* may affect estimates of the relationship between exposure and outcome, so that the measure of association observed in the sample (whether risk difference, risk ratio, or odds ratio) may not accurately reflect the true value. Finally, as in case-control studies, ascertainment of reliable exposure information for each individual in the sample may be difficult. However, this consideration does not apply when the exposure is a particular genotype, because genotype information would presumably be available for all individuals in the sample. The cross-sectional study is discussed in more detail in epidemiology texts (for example, see ref. 2, pages 108–12, and ref. 1, pages 75–6).

6 Interpretation of epidemiological associations

The various measures of association discussed in the previous sections are summarized in *Table 8*. For an infectious disease, a positive association between the presence of a particular genotype and occurrence of the outcome suggests that the genetic exposure forms part of a *sufficient cause* of the outcome (see ref. 1, pages 7–28). As noted above, genetic factors cannot alone cause infectious disease, since development of the disease is contingent on the presence of the infecting organism. Nonetheless, if genotype is strongly associated with the risk of developing an outcome, it is possible that genotype directly influences risk for the outcome. Alleles of a gene may increase or decrease outcome risk through the variant proteins that they encode or through regulation of protein synthesis. In extreme cases, the allele of interest might make an individual completely susceptible or immune to infection or disease caused by the associated microorganism. Nonetheless, not every strong association is causal in nature; criteria that are useful in determining which associations are causal are discussed below. It is especially important to consider the possibility of confounding or chance in assessing whether a specific genetic makeup actually affects the risk of infectious disease.

Conclusions regarding the association between exposure and outcome in epidemiological studies are necessarily based on information provided by the finite study sample from the larger population. Investigators attempt to obtain their study sample in a way that increases the likelihood that it is representative of the population, for instance, by taking a random sample of cases from a hospital log or enrolling a consecutive group of individuals presenting to a clinic. Selection of a representative sample of subjects is one necessary component of study design to ensure that estimates of association are free of *systematic* error, or bias. Eliminating systematic error is needed to guarantee that the conclusions based on the study sample can be expected, at least on average, to reflect accurately the reality in the population.

Table 8 Summary of measures of association

Measure of association	Description	Type of study where calculable	Comments	Text references
Risk ratio (relative risk)	Proportion of subjects with the event (cumulative incidence) among the exposed, divided by the proportion of subjects with the event among the unexposed.	Cohort, cross-sectional	Subjects should all be followed over comparable time periods. Provides simple measure of relative difference in risk.	Sections 3.1, 5
Risk difference	Proportion of subjects with the event (cumulative incidence) among the exposed, minus the proportion of subjects with the event among the unexposed.	Cohort, cross-sectional	Subjects should all be followed over comparable time periods. Provides simple measure of absolute difference in risk.	Sections 3.1, 5
Odds ratio	Odds of event among the exposed, divided by odds of the event among the unexposed.	Cohort, case-control, cross-sectional	Only measure calculable for case-control studies. When the event is rare, the odds ratio approximates the risk ratio.	Sections 3.1, 4, 5
Incidence rate ratio	Incidence (events per person-time interval) in exposed, divided by incidence in the unexposed.	Cohort	Incorporates information about different follow-up durations among subjects.	Section 3.2
Relative hazard (hazard ratio)	Instantaneous risk in exposed, divided by instantaneous risk in unexposed.	Cohort	Derived from a Cox proportional hazards regression.	Section 3.2
Per cent attributable risk	In relative terms, excess risk present among exposed subjects compared to unexposed subjects.	Cohort, cross-sectional	Provides a method for quantifying the impact of the exposure on risk.	Section 3.4

7 Confounding

An important source of systematic error in epidemiological studies is *confounding*. Confounding occurs when the measured association between exposure and outcome does not reflect the true association because of mixing in the study sample of two or more groups of individuals. The mixed groups are each defined by a different level of a characteristic that is itself related to both the exposure and the outcome of interest. As an example, consider a cohort study in which the outcome of interest is infection, and the exposure of interest is one of two levels of an exposure A (A_1 or A_2). Further, assume that there is another exposure B, with levels B_1 and B_2. *Table 9*, which shows a hypothetical study sample in which individuals have been classified according to exposures (A and B) and infection status, illustrates a situation in which confounding occurs.

Notice that A_1 is not associated with an elevation in infection risk *within* either of the two groups defined by levels of B (relative risk 1.0 for persons with B_1 or B_2). However, in the *combined* group (which includes individuals with both B_1 and B_2), A_1 appears to be associated with a doubling of infection risk (relative risk 2.0). In this situation, B is said to *confound* (distort) the relationship between A and infection. These data could lead to the inaccurate conclusion that A_1 increases infection risk. Confounding occurs here because B is related both to A (notice that 17% of individuals with A_1 have B_1, whereas only 6% of individuals with A_2 have B_1) and to infection (individuals with B_1 have a 25% infection risk, compared with individuals with B_2 who have a 1% infection risk).

To make the preceding discussion more concrete, consider AIDS as the outcome of interest. Before the discovery of HIV, the cause of AIDS was unknown, but among homosexual men a strong association was noted between use of amyl nitrate (a recreational drug taken in the form of 'poppers') and AIDS. However, amyl nitrate use does not cause AIDS, and the apparent association turned out to be the result of confounding. Amyl nitrate use was most common among men who engaged in risky sexual behaviours. Because HIV can be acquired sexually, it was the risky sexual behaviour that was the truly relevant exposure. In the terminology of *Table 9*, the infection outcome is AIDS, A is amyl nitrate exposure (A_1 is use, A_2 is no use), and B is risky sexual activity (B_1 is activity, B_2 is no activity). The risk ratio of 2.0 for AIDS found with amyl nitrate use (A_1) is seen to be due to confounding: there is a relatively high prevalence of risky sexual behaviour among those who use amyl nitrate (17% of those with A_1 have B_1), and

Table 9 Example of confounding

	Individuals with B_1		Individuals with B_2		All individuals combined		
	Infected	Uninfected	Infected	Uninfected	Infected	Uninfected	Per cent with B_1
A_1	5	15	1	99	6	114	17%
A_2	5	15	3	297	8	312	6%
Risk ratio	$(5/20) / (5/20) = 1$		$(1/100) / (3/300) = 1$		$(6/120) / (8/320) = 2.0$		

there is relatively high risk of AIDS among those with risky sexual activity (25% of those with B_1 have the infection AIDS).

The confounding factor (B in the above example) can be any type of exposure, whether environmental or genetic. In particular, one can view *linkage disequilibrium* as a type of confounding. Linkage disequilibrium occurs when two genetic loci lie so closely together on a chromosome that crossover between the loci occurs either never or only very rarely. As a result, in linkage disequilibrium one allele at one of the loci (e.g. A_1 at A) is associated with one allele at the other locus (e.g. B_1 at B) more commonly than expected by chance alone. For genetic loci A and B in linkage disequilibrium, it may be that it is the allele of B that affects risk for the outcome. If the investigator examines the relationship between A and the outcome, he or she may be misled by the association between A and the outcome that is induced by the relationship between A and B.

Confounding alters the apparent relationship between the exposure of interest and the outcome. Without data on potential confounding factors, it is impossible to control for confounding completely. However, if data on potential confounders are available, there are several methods for controlling for confounding. One may utilize *stratification* to examine the relationship between exposure and outcome at each of several levels of the potential confounder. In the example above, B is a confounder of the relationship between A and infection status. By examining the relationship between A and infection status separately for individuals with B_1 and for individuals with B_2, one can observe the relationship between A and infection *independent* of B. The levels of B form strata, and an estimate of the effect of A on infection risk can be obtained by averaging the stratum-specific measures of the relationship between A and infection risk. The Mantel-Haenszel odds ratio statistic is one method of averaging effects across strata (see ref. 1, pages 253–79).

An alternative technique for dealing with confounding is *regression analysis*. In general, regression techniques allow one to identify independent effects of various variables on the outcome. When the measure of association is the odds ratio, *logistic regression* provides a way to quantify the relationship between exposures of interest (such as particular genotypes) and the odds of developing the outcome (12). In cohort studies, in which one may examine the relationship between exposures and the incidence of the outcome, the *Cox proportional hazards regression* model is often used (6, 7).

8 Bradford Hill's criteria for causality

The existence of an association between a gene and outcome, even if it is *statistically significant* (see discussion of statistical significance in Section 9), does not prove that the gene plays a *causal* role in determining whether the outcome occurs. In 1965, Austin Bradford Hill proposed nine criteria for determining whether an epidemiological association was causal (13). Bradford Hill's criteria are easily applied when the exposure of interest is a particular genotype. They provide useful grounds for formulating questions to ask in determining whether a causal relationship is present. However, no single criterion or combination of criteria can definitively identify a causal relationship. As Bradford Hill noted, 'What [the criteria] can do, with greater or less strength, is to help us to make up our minds on the fundamental question—is there any other way of explaining the set of facts before us, is there any other answer equally, or more, likely than cause and effect?' (13). Bradford Hill's nine criteria are listed below:

1 *Strength of association.* How large is the measure of association (odds ratio, risk ratio, risk difference, or hazard ratio)? A dramatic difference in risk between individuals with different genotypes suggests that the gene plays a role in susceptibility to infection or disease. Exactly what constitutes a 'dramatic' difference is context-dependent. In many situations where a chronic disease is the outcome, and where exposures can be difficult to measure, a risk ratio or odds ratio of two might be considered evidence of a strong association. In other circumstances, only relative risks of 5–10 or more might be considered strong. Nonetheless, even a strong association can arise because of confounding, such as when the gene of interest is in complete linkage disequilibrium with another gene and the second gene actually mediates risk.

2 *Consistency.* Can the association be demonstrated using a variety of study designs (e.g. case-control and cohort studies) in different populations? Replication leads to reassurance that the apparent association is not just due to chance or unnoticed problems with a single study.

3 *Specificity.* This criterion requires that a single genotype produce a single specific effect, i.e. cause a single disease. As Bradford Hill himself noted, specificity is not an absolute requirement and one should not demand that it be present, as there are many examples in which a single exposure (e.g. tobacco smoking) causes multiple diseases. One also can easily find examples of genotypes that lead to heightened susceptibility to several different types of infections (e.g. deficiency of complement proteins, which are involved in host defence against numerous micro-organisms, especially bacteria).

4 *Temporality.* This criterion requires that the exposure precede the outcome in any causal relationship. Because an individual's genetic constitution is fixed before birth, this criterion is always met for genetic exposures.

5 *Biologic gradient.* This criterion requires that successively larger doses of exposure be accompanied by related increases (or decreases) in the probability of the outcome. For genetic exposures, this requirement is equivalent to a *gene–dose* model, in which the probability of the outcome increases (or decreases) in a monotonic, steady manner for individuals with zero, one, or two copies of the allele of interest.

6 *Plausibility.* Is there a plausible reason to suppose that the gene of interest could exert an effect on infection or disease risk? What is known about the protein for which the gene codes that could lead one to believe that the gene can influence risk? Plausibility is not an absolute requirement, because the epidemiological study under consideration may be the first study to suggest a relationship between the gene and disease susceptibility. Nonetheless, it is usually the case that previous studies will provide some evidence that makes the association more or less plausible.

7 *Coherence*. This criterion requires that the hypothesized causal relationship not conflict with what is already known about disease pathogenesis.

8 *Experimental evidence*. Do laboratory experiments provide supportive evidence for a causal association? Although one cannot alter genotypes in humans, one can study knockout mice, which lack the gene of interest. What is the effect of the gene knockout on susceptibility to infection or disease?

9 *Analogy*. Are there similar examples of association between other genotypes and outcomes that suggest that the relationship of interest is causal? Heterozygosity for one haemoglobin variant, sickle cell anaemia, protects against malaria. By analogy, this makes more plausible as a causal relationship any association between heterozygosity for another variant, such as α-thalassemia, and malaria risk.

9 Statistical considerations

Even for a sample that is obtained in a representative manner from a study population, the sample by chance may not reflect the true proportion of individuals in each exposure or outcome category. The finite nature of the study sample therefore creates potential for another type of error in epidemiological studies, namely *random* error. A further source of random error arises from the lack of precision of laboratory measurements and other quantitative tests. These random errors lead to lack of precision of study results. One way to decrease random error is to increase sample size. However, increasing sample size will not correct *systematic* errors, which arise from structural relationships between components of the study that bias study results away from the true value.

Statistical methods allow quantification of the uncertainty (random error) associated with an observed measure of association, such as the odds ratio. One way of quantifying uncertainty is through calculation of a *confidence interval*. A confidence interval provides information about the range of values for the measure of association that are reasonably consistent with the data obtained in the study. Typically a 95% confidence interval is used, although the choice of confidence intervals is somewhat arbitrary and alternative confidence intervals, such as 90% or 99% confidence intervals, are also informative. As an example, a case-control study may find an odds ratio of 2.0 for the association between a genotype and disease risk, with a 95% confidence interval from 0.5 to 8.0. In simple terms, this implies that we can be '95% confident' that the true odds ratio lies between 0.5 and 8.0 (i.e. that possessing the genotype could reasonably be expected to halve disease risk or increase its likelihood by a factor of 8). Note that the confidence interval in this case implies that we do not have enough information to determine whether the allele really does increase disease risk, even though our best single estimate of the odds ratio (2.0) suggests that it does, because the confidence interval includes values less than 1.0. In general, whenever the 95% confidence interval excludes the *null* value consistent with no association (1 for odds ratios and risk ratios, 0 for risk differences), the observed association is said to be *statistically significant* at the p = 0.05 level. A more technical discussion of confidence intervals and methods for deriving them are provided in biostatistics texts (for example, see ref. 5, pages 82–98, and ref. 14, pages 69–143).

The *p-value* provides information about uncertainty that is formally equivalent to that provided by the confidence interval. The p-value is the probability that one would observe an association as notable as the one that was actually observed if, in reality, there was no relationship between exposure and outcome. As a probability, p lies between 0 and 1, and p-values close to 0 indicate that the observed disease association would have been unlikely to arise by chance alone. When p is less than 0.05, it is often stated that the observed association has reached *statistical significance*. However, the practice of presenting p-values dichotomously (e.g. 'less than 0.05' or 'greater than 0.05') should be discouraged in favour of reporting exact p-values or confidence intervals. Methods for calculating p-values are provided in biostatistics texts (see ref. 5, pages 82–98, and ref. 14, pages 69–143).

We emphasize again that random error is only one type of error that arises in epidemiological studies. A narrow confidence interval excluding the null value or a low p-value merely suggests that the observed association did not arise by chance alone. Of course, systematic (non-random) errors are not excluded by the achievement of statistical significance and can lead to biased estimates of association.

10 Further statistical considerations

In epidemiological studies, as in other types of studies, two types of random errors may arise. The first type of error (termed *type 1 error*) occurs when investigators conclude that an association is present when, in reality, there is no association between exposure and outcome. The second type of error (termed *type 2 error*) arises when investigators conclude that there is no association between exposure and outcome when, in actuality, there is an association. Because these errors are complementary, steps that are taken to minimize the occurrence of one type of error can increase the likelihood of the other type of error. In general, the most direct way to decrease both types of random errors simultaneously is to increase the study sample size.

Type 1 errors are quantified using the p-value, which measures the probability that an observed association could have arisen through chance alone. An important consideration for epidemiological studies involving genetic markers as exposures is the problem of *multiple comparisons*. This issue becomes particularly relevant because recently developed technologies, such as measurement of single nucleotide polymorphisms (SNPs), allow the investigator to examine simultaneously the relationship between many genetic markers and the outcome. While a small p-value provides for each individual association a reassuringly low estimate of the likelihood of a type 1 error, in the setting of multiple independent comparisons done at the same time, there is substantially greater probability that at least one association will be found significant by chance alone. Another setting in which multiple comparisons create a problem arises when HLA polymorphisms are utilized as the genetic exposures of interest; because this system is extremely polymorphic, the likelihood of a chance association between at least one allele and any given outcome is high.

One way to manage the problem of multiple comparisons is to recognize explicitly a difference between *hypothesis-generating* and *hypothesis-confirming* studies. If the investigator has an a priori belief that one of several genes may affect risk for the outcome of interest, then the finding of a significant association between that gene and risk for the outcome confirms a pre-existing hypothesis and might be taken at face value. On the other hand, multiple comparisons usually arise when the investigator has no strongly identified a priori hypothesis and so evaluates multiple associations at the same time. In such cases, the finding of a significant association might best be viewed as generating new hypotheses. The investigator should either seek confirmation of the finding in another study population prior to reporting the finding, or report the finding as preliminary and attempt to confirm the statistically significant association in a subsequent study.

An alternative approach to the problem of multiple comparisons is to utilize statistical methods to increase the stringency of the criteria used to decide whether an association is significant. The simplest of these approaches is the Bonferroni method. Using this method, the investigator determines the number of comparisons that will be made and then adjusts downward, by a corresponding factor, the p-value required for statistical significance. For instance, if the investigator plans to examine the association between each of 20 separate genetic markers and infection risk, then he or she decides in advance that only associations that produce p-values below 0.0025 (i.e. 0.05/20) will be considered statistically significant. The Bonferroni and other methods for statistical adjustment are presented in more detail elsewhere (for example, see ref. 14, page 128). A problem with any method of statistical adjustment for multiple comparisons is that it increases the chance of making a type 2 statistical error.

Type 2 errors arise when a true association between exposure and outcome is present but the study, by chance, fails to detect it. Type 2 errors would be expected to occur most commonly when either the outcome (for cohort studies) or genotype (for case-control studies) is rare. Type 2 errors can be corrected by increasing the study sample size. One attractive way to expand the effective sample size is to use techniques of *meta-analysis* to 'pool together' results of several separate studies. While meta-analyses have gained their broadest application in combining results of randomized controlled trials, meta-analyses of epidemiological studies, including studies of genetic effects on infectious disease (15), have also been conducted. Attention to the quality of studies combined in the meta-analysis is important, because pooling together flawed studies cannot be expected to correct their biases. Nonetheless, meta-analysis offers the opportunity to examine published studies systematically and, if the results of the individual studies are found to vary, to determine how much of this variation can be attributed to characteristics of the individual studies, such as their choice of subjects or their quality. Variation in the strength of association between genotype and outcome across studies, if due to characteristics of the study population such as race, would suggest that other exposures (genetic or environmental) interact with the genotype of interest. When performed well, meta-analyses can produce valid results that are more precise than the separate results from the individual studies. Techniques of meta-analysis are reviewed in several sources (see ref. 16, and ref. 1, pages 643–73).

11 Interaction

Interaction occurs when one exposure affects the strength of the association between another exposure and the outcome of interest. This may occur, for instance, when one exposure increases risk for the outcome to a much greater extent when a second exposure is present than when the second exposure is absent. Consider a case-control study in which there are again two exposures, A and B, and an outcome, infection (Table 10).

If one examined the relationship between A and infection status without attention to B ('all individuals combined') one would identify a moderate-sized effect of A_1 on infection risk (odds ratio 2.3). However, this conclusion would be misleading, because only individuals who also have B_1 as a co-exposure experience increased infection risk in association with A_1, and for these persons the effect of A_1 is quite strong (odds ratio 10). There is no association between A_1 and infection risk among those individuals with B_2 (odds ratio 1).

Interactions are sometimes called examples of *effect modification* because one exposure modifies the effect of the other. *Gene–gene* interactions are examples of this phenomenon, in which the joint effect of two genes on disease risk cannot be predicted simply from their individual effects on disease risk.

In *gene–environment* interactions, environmental exposures influence how much the gene of interest affects risk. An extreme form of gene–environment interaction is seen in considering the effect of a gene on risk for infection and viewing the *exposure to the infectious organism* as the environmental exposure (in

Table 10 Example of interaction

	Individuals with B_1		Individuals with B_2		All individuals combined	
	Infected	**Uninfected**	**Infected**	**Uninfected**	**Infected**	**Uninfected**
A_1	50	10	40	60	90	70
A_2	10	20	10	15	20	35
Odds ratio	$(50 \times 20)/(10 \times 10) = 10$		$(40 \times 15)/(10 \times 60) = 1$		$(90 \times 35)/(20 \times 70) = 2.3$	

Table 10, A would be the gene and B would be exposure to the micro-organism). When individuals are exposed to the micro-organism (B_1) then A may have a strong effect on infection risk. However, when individuals are not exposed to the micro-organism (B_2), the effect of A on infection risk is negligible or not measurable, since no individuals develop infection. If the status of exposure to the micro-organism B could not be determined, then all study subjects would be grouped in the 'all individuals combined' category in Table 10. In that case, the estimated relationship between A and infection status would be biased because it would not reflect the true relationship for the subset of individuals who are actually exposed to the micro-organism.

Interactions between two exposures can be identified by stratifying observations based on levels of one of the exposures. Variation in the magnitude of the association between one exposure and the outcome, across strata defined by the second exposure, suggests that there is an interaction between the two exposures. If substantial variation in the relationship between exposure and outcome across strata is apparent, averaging the effect across strata would be inappropriate. When an interaction is present, one should explore reasons for the variation in effect across the strata. Regression techniques allow one to quantify interactions and test for their statistical significance.

12 Identifying candidate genes for epidemiological studies

We have discussed at length epidemiological methods for evaluating relationships between genetic exposures and infectious disease risk, without discussing how one might identify candidate genetic exposures of interest for these studies. In fact, there are several methods for identifying such candidates. Epidemiologists can use observations made in complementary types of investigation to generate hypotheses regarding which genetic polymorphisms might affect outcome risk and thus be fruitful subjects for an epidemiological study.

Laboratory studies of the host response to infection provide hints for many possible avenues of investigation for epidemiological studies. Individuals may respond to micro-organisms in different ways, and some of the genes that influence this response, through the proteins that the genes encode, have been extensively characterized in the laboratory. Well-studied systems that show diversity among individuals, and which therefore might demonstrate variation among individuals in concert with their risk for infection or disease, include the highly polymorphic HLA system, the complement system, and the system of chemokines and their receptors. This synergy between laboratory and epidemiological studies can also work in the opposite direction. Well-conducted epidemiological studies demonstrating a link between infectious diseases and particular genotypes or their associated phenotypes provide a strong impetus for further laboratory investigations to characterize the implicated genes.

Ecological studies can suggest the need for more formal analytical epidemiological studies. In an ecological study, observations about geographical variation in disease risk are related to geographical variation in exposures. While a correlation between geographically defined population rates of disease and exposure can suggest a causal relationship, this type of study is not definitive, because it provides no information about exposure and outcome among individuals (17). Nonetheless, ecological studies can help frame useful hypotheses. The high rates of sickle cell anaemia and β-thalassemia in regions where malaria is highly endemic led to the hypothesis that the geographical distribution of haemoglobinopathies was due to the reduced risk of severe malaria found among heterozygous carriers of these polymorphic genes. Epidemiological studies in malarious regions subsequently confirmed that individual sickle cell carriers were less likely than non-carriers to develop severe malaria (18). This protection arises, at least in part, because variant haemoglobins inhibit the growth of *Plasmodium falciparum* parasites.

Segregation analysis and *linkage analysis* are classical genetic methods for identifying genes that influence disease. These study designs can provide valuable information regarding the mode of inheritance and chromosomal location of genes involved in susceptibility to infectious diseases through information collected on individuals who are sampled in large *families* from the population of interest. Segregation and linkage analysis have been applied to identify genetic influences on risk for several infections or infectious diseases, including human T cell lymphotropic virus type I infection (19), malaria (20), schistosomiasis (21), and AIDS (22). However, for many infectious diseases, these types of studies are difficult to implement, because they require that most individuals in the families be exposed to or infected with the micro-organism that causes the disease or that extensive information be available on exposure risk for each family member. If few family members are exposed or infected with the micro-organism, then the family can provide little information on risk for the outcome of interest. Because of the limitations of applying linkage and segregation analyses to the study of infectious diseases, these study types are not discussed further in this chapter. The interested reader is referred to an excellent text for additional information (3).

13 The future of genetic epidemiology

The Human Genome Project and related activities in the commercial sector promise to vastly increase the tools and data available to genetic epidemiologists (23). Of particular interest is the possibility of performing *whole-genome association studies* of common disorders (24). Although the human genome is very large (about 30 000 genes), there are relatively few common variants for each gene, and it is anticipated that all of these variants will eventually be identified. Once a sufficient number of common variants are identified, investigators will be able to screen the genome systematically for associations between genetic polymorphisms and a disease of interest.

Whole-genome association studies may be either *direct* or *indirect* (25). Direct whole-genome studies will look for associations between a given infection or disease and either functional variants that lie within genes or polymorphisms (such as microsatellite polymorphisms) that lie near these genes and are in linkage disequilibrium with functional variants. Such studies will require detailed maps of coding region polymorphisms and are, therefore, less feasible in the near future than indirect whole-genome studies. Indirect association studies could make use of the dense, but incomplete, single nucleotide polymorphisms (SNPs) maps that are currently being developed (26). SNPs are diallelic variants that occur about once in every 1000 base pairs of the human genome. Most SNPs are unlikely to directly influence disease risk, either because they exist in non-coding regions of the genome or because they exist as synonymous mutations that do not affect protein coding (27,28). However, SNPs that do not directly affect disease risk may be in linkage disequilibrium with loci that themselves affect disease risk. Therefore, indirect whole-genome association studies would help investigators locate specific areas of the genome that contain important functional variants.

Whole-genome studies will, obviously, entail a large number of statistical comparisons. Therefore, type 1 statistical errors will be an important consideration in the interpretation of these studies. In fact, finding an association between a SNP and a disease will be only an initial step in a process that will entail replicating the initial finding in other populations and determining the function of the genetic variant under study.

References

1. Rothman, K. J. and Greenland, S (eds.) (1998). *Modern epidemiology* 2nd edn. Philadelphia: Lippincott-Raven.
2. Hennekens, C. H. and Buring, J. E. (1987). *Epidemiology in medicine*. Boston: Little, Brown.
3. Khoury, M. J., Beaty, T. H., and Cohen, B. H. (1993). *Fundamentals of genetic epidemiology*. New York: Oxford University Press.
4. Dean, M., Carrington, M., Winkler, C., Huttley, G. A., Smith, M. W., Allikmets, R., *et al.* (1996). *Science*, **273**, 1856.
5. Dawson-Saunders, B. and Trapp, R. G. (1994). *Basic and clinical biostatistics*, 2nd edn. Norwalk, CT: Appleton and Lange.
6. Kleinbaum, D. G. (1999). *Survival analysis: a self-learning text*. New York: Springer–Verlag.
7. Klein, J. P. and Moeschberger, M. L. (1997). *Survival analysis. Techniques for censored and truncated data*. New York: Springer.
8. Smith, M. W., Dean, M., Carrington, M., Winkler, C., Huttley, G. A., Lomb, D. A., *et al.* (1997). *Science*, **277**, 959.
9. Bellamy, R., Ruwende, C., Corrah, T., McAdam, K. P. W. J., Whittle, H. C., and Hill, A. V. S. (1998). *N. Engl. J. Med.*, **338**, 640.
10. Wacholder, S., McLaughlin, J. K., Silverman, D. T., and Mandel, J. S. (1992). *Am. J. Epidemiol.*, **135**, 1019.
11. Nadel, S., Newport, M. J., Booy, R., and Levin, M. (1996). *J. Infect. Dis.*, **174**, 878.
12. Hosmer, Jr. D. W. and Lemshow, S. (1989). *Applied logistic regression*. New York: Wiley and Sons.
13. Hill, A. B. (1965). *Proc. R. Soc. Med.*, volume 58, 295.
14. Shott, S. (1990). *Statistics for health professionals*. Philadelphia: Saunders.

15. Ioannidis, J. P., O'Brien, T. R., Rosenberg, P. S., Contopoulos-Ioannidis, D. G., and Goedert, J. J. (1998). *Nature Med.*, **4**, 536.

16. Petitti, D. B. (1994). *Meta-analysis, decision analysis, and cost-effectiveness analysis. Methods for quantitative synthesis in medicine.* New York: Oxford University Press.

17. Greenland, S. and Robins, J. (1994). *Am. J. Epidemiol.*, **139**, 747.

18. Allison, A. C. (1954). *Br. Med. J.*, **1**, 290.

19. Plancoulaine, S., Gessain, A., Joubert, M., Tortevoye, P., Jeanne, I., Talarmin, A., *et al.* (2000). *J. Infect. Dis.*, **182**, 405.

20. Abel, L., Cot, M., Mulder, L., Carnevale, P., and Feingold, J. (1992). *Am. J. Hum. Genet.*, **50**, 1308.

21. Marquet, S., Abel, L., Hillaire, D., Dessein, H., Kalil, J., Feingold, J., *et al.* (1996). *Nature Genet.*, **14**, 181.

22. Kroner, B. L., Goedert, J. J., Blattner, W. A., Wilson, S. E., Carrington, M. N., and Mann, D. L. (1995). *AIDS*, **9**, 275.

23. Ellsworth, D. L., Hallman, D. M., and Boerwinkle, E. (1997). *Epidemiol. Rev.*, **19**, 3.

24. Lander, E. S. (1996). *Science*, **274**, 536.

25. Collins, F. S., Guyer, M. S., and Chakravarti, A. (1997). *Science*, **278**, 1580.

26. Wang, D. G., Fan, J. B., Siao, C. J., Berno, A., Young, P., Sapolsky, R., *et al.* (1998). *Science*, **280**, 1077.

27. Halushka, M. K., Fan, J. B., Bentley, K., Hsie, L., Shen, N., Weder, A., *et al.* (1999). *Nature Genet.*, **22**, 239.

28. Cargill, M., Altshuler, D., Ireland, J., Sklar, P., Ardlie, K., Patil, N., *et al.* (1999). *Nature Genet.*, **22**, 231.

Chapter 2

Molecular differentiation of bacterial strains

Eric W. Brown

Department of Biological Sciences, Loyola University of Chicago, Chicago, Illinois 60626

1 Introduction

Understanding the epidemiological principles that govern bacterial populations has become paramount in the fields of medical, environmental, and agricultural microbiology (1). The introduction of bacterial strains which exhibit more aggressive and deadly pathological phenotypes, development of multi-drug antibiotic resistance, and acquisition of novel modes of transmission between host organisms has placed a renewed pressure on researchers to be able to identify and monitor the origins and dissemination of destructive genetic variants (strains) within a species. It has become apparent that the best approaches to characterizing individual strains are founded in the practical application of molecular biology. Molecular genetic techniques such as polymerase chain reaction (PCR), nucleic acid fingerprinting, and DNA sequence analysis of the bacterial chromosome have allowed for remarkable advances in bacterial identification as in many other areas of microbiology (2). Whether the need for molecular typing involves the tracking of nosocomial (hospital-borne) outbreaks, identifying the reservoirs of food-borne infections, or the discrimination of plant pathogenic strains in the field, the isolation of a specific genotype in conjunction with a specific bacteria often allows for a larger understanding of the epidemiological principles that govern the evolution and spread of many bacterial diseases.

Since the age of Pasteur, epidemiological approaches involving the typing and discrimination of bacteria have relied heavily on phenotypic or biotypic methods (2–5). These methods were forged in answer to a call from the fledgling discipline of bacterial systematics, which strived, often in vain, to identify and catalogue bacterial species into a logical Linnaean hierarchy (6). Early bacterial discrimination and classification methods were further confounded by the nature of bacterial taxonomy, itself. Classical 'species' concepts seemed inapplicable to the classification of bacteria from the outset, with the 'species' paradigm persisting as a significant caveat to the taxonomic classification of bacteria through most of the 20th century. More recently, classical or morphological species definitions have been displaced entirely by 16S rDNA nucleotide sequence comparisons, which are considered the benchmark for delineating bacterial species. Strains are often denoted in the context of subspecific nucleotide diversity in association with some prominent or unique phenotype (e.g. pathogenicity traits). None-theless, phenotypic approaches remain a bastion of the microbiology laboratory. Several of these methods currently include the metabolic fingerprinting of nutritional requirements, analysis of differences in fatty acid composition, and structural variation in discrete morphological characters found on the surface of a bacteria (4, 5). Indeed, the Gram stain itself was originally introduced as a way to identify and discriminate one bacterium from another. However, there are a number of caveats associated with these types of classical typing methods that have historically made them at the very least, controversial, and more often, simply unreliable (6). Subtle changes in culture conditions, relative shortages in the number of phenotypic characters available, and evolutionary convergence among these characters may jeopardize conclusions regarding the epidemiology of a specific outbreak (7). The recalcitrance of phenotypic characters to recon-struct the origins and modes of dissemination of many strains has actually been noted for some time and has only served to further open the door to more re-liable genotypic characterization methods.

Molecular typing methods that focus on the identification of unique genotypes among bacterial strains have revolutionized the way we study strain diversity and monitor infectious outbreaks. These techniques offer several benefits over classical typing methods such as avoiding the need for stable monocultures of bacterial cells, increased assay sensitivity/stability, and significantly faster reaction times (2). Finally, a molecular type which stems from a DNA fingerprint or nucleotide sequence will inherently contain more information about a given strain. For example, a repetitive fingerprint analysis employing ERIC, REP, and BOX probes can yield dozens of informative amplicons (amplified fragments) about an individual strain while a single ompA gene sequence can offer hundreds of potentially polymorphic characters in the form of nucleotide substitutions (see below).

By convention, strain identification methods can be broken down into three basic strategies:

(a) Fingerprint analysis of the chromosome using oligonucleotide primed ampli-fication techniques.

(b) Restriction endonuclease fragmentation of the bacterial chromosome.

(c) Enzymatic amplification of single gene sequences and subsequent sequence analysis of successfully generated PCR products (8–10).

There are a number of experimental modifications that coincide with each of these three basic types of identification methods. For instance, PCR-based finger-print methods can exploit several different families of repetitive oligonucleotide primers including repetitive extragenic palindromic sequences (REPs), rRNA inter-genic spacer sequences, and randomly amplified polymorphic DNA sequences (RAPDs). Restriction fragment length polymorphism (RFLP) strategies can simply be analysed on ethidium bromide stained agarose gels or can be blotted and hybridized with labelled DNA probes. Finally, single target PCR amplification and sequence analysis can vary in which gene is chosen to be examined, the extent of sequence information obtained from the gene of choice, and whether analysis of the corresponding computer-translated amino acid sequences are useful in the evaluation of a particular strain.

Undoubtedly, the greatest advances in bacterial typing have occurred among techniques which employ PCR to amplify multiple segments of bacterial DNA. Multilocus oligonucleotide primers are now available that target several families of conserved repeat elements distributed around the bacterial chromosome (11). These techniques are non-radioactive and can be easily performed using a thermal cycler and a modest horizontal gel apparatus. One of the biggest advantages of PCR-based typing approaches relates to the flexibility that they allow in quantity and quality of input genomic DNA preparations (see Chapter 3). Preparations can be as simple as the addition of whole cells directly into the reaction mixture, or conversely, a variety of commercial and non-commercial rapid DNA extraction protocols are now available that allow for the recovery of nucleic acids in a matter of minutes. PCR-based fingerprinting techniques currently being exploited in strain discrimination include repetitive PCR fingerprinting (REP-PCR), rDNA PCR of the 16S–23S intergenic spacer region ('ribotyping'), and randomly amplified polymorphic DNA PCR (RAPD-PCR).

Strain evaluation directly from nucleotide sequences has become equally powerful in the resolution of a specific bacterium, and when coupled with single target genomic PCR strategies and automated sequencing techniques, can yield rapid and detailed genotypic information about a strain. The greatest achievements spawned by the analysis of nucleotide sequences have come in the sub-disciplines of microbial taxonomy and systematics (6). The ribosomal DNA sequences have proven useful in discerning the phylogenies of distantly related families of eubacteria (12). Small subunit rRNA sequences, in particular, have proven to be very powerful in resolving the evolutionary relationships within the phylum, purple bacteria (6). However, the extraordinarily slow substitution rates within rRNA genes preclude their use in resolving more closely related taxa (e.g. species and strains) (13, 14). For this reason, a number of bacterial protein coding genes have been examined for their phylogenetic utility in resolving closely related strains of bacterial taxa (15). The discriminatory efficiency of genes used for the nucleotide-based typing of various strains is often determined empirically within a specific bacterial system. In some cases, several different loci may be used in conjunction with each other in order to increase the accuracy of strain identification and increase resolution between strains (16). These types of approaches have been most effective in typing enterobacterial strains. For example, *gap*DH and *omp*A nucleotides simultaneously demonstrated that current isolates of *Escherichia vulneris* do not have a monophyletic origin, as previously thought, and should not be considered strains within a single species (7). In general, there are several factors within bacterial coding genes which may lend to their recognition as generally useful molecular markers for strain differentiation:

(a) Levels of nucleotide sequence variation that far surpass conventional small and large subunit rDNA sequences (17).

(b) The encoding of a functionally conserved protein across several enteric genera, suggesting that the gene will be intact in its entirety in distantly related species (7).

(c) A physical location of the gene on the bacterial chromosome that reveals chromosomal synteny between disparate bacterial taxa (18).

In conjunction with the recent advances made in techniques for the molecular typing of bacterial strains, breakthrough in the analysis of molecular data have also greatly enhanced our current ability to answer basic epidemiological questions about the origins, directions, and diversity of bacterial pathogens (19). Over the past decade, major bioinformatic advances have been made on several fronts but, arguably, most dramatically in the areas of storage, assembly, and systematic evaluation of DNA and protein sequence data. Phylogenetic algorithms are now capable of handling larger numbers of taxa and longer gene segments than ever before (ref. 20; also see Chapter 8). The 'co-evolution' of analytical and computational power along with the development of more sensitive molecular typing techniques has allowed for novel insight into the evolutionary properties that govern strain relatedness in bacteria. Phylogenetic trees can now be constructed from molecular data that often yield answers to epidemiological questions that are frequently asked when tracking bacterial outbreaks. Issues involving host transmission, infection reservoirs, and geographical origination of strains are more easily understood when examined in light of the phylogenetic evidence that can be readily collected about a specific bacteria and its relatives. When coupled with phylogenetic reconstruction, 'ribotyping', in particular, has yielded valuable insight into the origins and diversity of nosocomial infections induced by strains of *Pseudomonas cepacia*, *P. aeruginosa*, and *Staphylococcus aureus* to name just a few (21).

While molecular genetic approaches do offer themselves as the most powerful analytical tools available to identify and track bacterial strains, they are not without fault. Deficiencies associated with the use of molecular probes and various chromosomal loci to successfully delineate bacterial genotypes can and do arise. Genes that often work in the discrimination of one species may lack the sequence variation necessary to differentiate strains in another unrelated species. The empirical determination of the efficacy of a typing method for a specific bacterial taxa can sometimes be a cost-intensive and time-consuming process. For instance, small subunit rDNA sequences are effective in differentiating *Pseudomonas* species but often lack the substitutions necessary to resolve closely related enterobacterial species such as a few *Escherichia* species and strains of necrogenic *Erwinia* species (2, 22). Further, the ultrasensitive nature of most molecular typing techniques, particularly those involving PCR analysis, often adds a level of caution to the resultant genotypic assessment of a given strain, and great care must be taken in avoiding the contamination of reactions (2).

With the recent advances that have been made in DNA sequence analysis and hybridization techniques, most approaches are now performed completely free of radioactive labels. A number of protocols now provide efficient, economical, and safe identification and discrimination of bacterial strains in the veterinary, medical, or agricultural microbiological laboratory. In this chapter, a summary of the currently available and most-widely employed procedures for bacterial genotyping and strain discrimination is provided. Non-radioactive methods which incorporate restriction endonuclease digestion, polymerase chain reaction-based fingerprints, and single locus PCR of macromolecular coding genes located on the bacterial chromosome are presented. Procedures and discussions are included for the isolation of genomic DNA, restriction enzyme digestion, PCR oligonucleotide selection, electrophoresis, DNA sequencing, and data interpretation currently employed in the evaluation of bacterial strain identification and diversity.

2 PCR-based fingerprinting of the bacterial chromosome

Several methods exist for the enzymatic amplification-based fingerprinting of bacterial genomes. Repetitive PCR fingerprint analysis, simply called REP-PCR, focuses on several conserved families of DNA repeat elements distributed on the bacterial chromosome (23). Similar to VNTR analysis in eukaryotes, the oligonucleotides employed in REP-PCR detect size polymorphisms by amplifying chromosomal regions between the repetitive motifs. In this way, the amplification fragment pattern is a function of the physical location of the repeat element on the chromosome. PCR analysis of the 16S–23S rRNA intergenic spacer region, 'ribotyping', also yields genotypic information about a strain in the form of size polymorphism (21). Oligonucleotide primers designed from the 3' end of the 16S rDNA gene and the 5' end of the 23S rDNA gene flank the intergenic spacer (IGS) that lies between the two rRNA subunits. The third approach, known as randomly amplified polymorphic DNA (RAPD-PCR) analysis, involves the enzymatic amplification of anonymous sections of genomic DNA, directed by one or more short arbitrary oligonucleotide primers (24). Agarose gel evaluation produces a characteristic spectrum of amplicons which are frequently unique to a specific bacterial strain. Finally, amplification fragment length polymorphism (AFLP) is yet another effective PCR-based method used in discriminating closely related bacteria (25). AFLP involves DNA amplification following cleavage with restriction endonucleases. Briefly, bacterial DNA is first digested with restriction enzymes (e.g. *Eco*RI and *Mse*I). This yields a swarm of DNA fragments of various lengths. Specific double-stranded adapter oligonucleotides are then ligated to the ends of these DNA fragments. Adapter-specific primers with various selective 3' nucleotides are then used to amplify subsets of fragments out of the pool. AFLP differs from RAPD-PCR in that the amplification step is not completely random and from REP-PCR in that it does not rely on a known bacterial consensus sequence. Rather, AFLP relies on the selective amplification of a portion of the fragments that share sequence homology with the PCR primer (25).

2.1 Preparation of genomic DNA from Gram negative and Gram positive eubacterial species

There are several rapid and straightforward approaches for the preparation of genomic DNA for PCR-based fingerprint procedures (1, 8, 26). Genomic DNA samples employed for PCR do not require the same levels of purity as do other conventional molecular applications. This often makes the extraction of DNA for amplification-based studies a quick and inexpensive process. A variety of commercially available products are now available that allow for the rapid preparation of genomic DNA from Gram negative bacteria: Instagene (Bio-Rad), Wizard (Promega), and DNeasy (Qiagen), just to name a few. These products usually employ purification resins that irreversibly bind to cellular proteins and other components that may inhibit an amplification reaction. DNA from Gram positive strains can also be prepared using several commercially available extraction kits such as Puregene (Gentra Systems) and Isoquick (Orca Research). However, it is often unnecessary to employ commercial methods as there are now a number of simplified strategies that allow for the preparation of both Gram negative and Gram positive cells for PCR (8, 16). Gram negative bacteria can be prepared using a strategy that simply lyses the cells and allows the contents to be released into solution. *Protocol 1* is a simple cell lysis procedure for use with Gram negative cells that employs physical processes to lyse the cells such as boiling and sonication. Gram positive bacteria may require substantially more physical disruption to ensure lysis. *Protocol 2* uses a freeze–fracture technique to disrupt the bacterial cell wall. This technique has been particularly effective for use with *Bacillus* species (26). While these rapid extraction techniques work well for most species and strains, several species do exist that may require the application of more traditional DNA purification methods for the yield of high quality chromosomal DNA (e.g. certain *Streptococcus* and *Staphylococcus* strains). *Protocol 3* is a modification of the Marmur technique (27) and presents an approach for the extraction of high quality chromosomal DNA. The protocol is presented in this chapter for use primarily with RFLP and PFGE analyses. This technique, while time-consuming and more laborious, can be used for PCR fingerprinting of more refractory species.

Protocol 1

Rapid preparation of cell lysates from Gram negative bacteria

Reagents

- TE: 10 mM Tris–HCl pH 7.5, 1 mM EDTA pH 8.0
- TLE: 10 mM Tris–HCl pH 7.5, 0.1 mM EDTA pH 8.0
- 1 M NaCl
- Sterile ddH_2O

Method

1 An inoculation loop (1 µl size) full of cells are scraped from a 24 h culture plate, suspended in 1 ml of 1 M NaCl, and pelleted in a 1.5 ml microcentrifuge tube at 18 000 g (high speed in a microcentrifuge) for 5 min.

2 Resuspend the pellet in 1 ml of TE, vortex for 10 sec, and centrifuge again as above.

3 Resuspend the cells in 1 ml of TLE, vortex for 10 sec, and place tubes into a floating rack for sonication.

4 Sonicate the tubes in a 25 °C tap-water-bath for 10 min at 40 watts.

5 Centrifuge again as above and resuspend the cell preparation in 1 ml of sterile ddH$_2$O (vortex vigorously).

6 Incubate the suspension at 65 °C for 25–30 min in a water-bath or heat block.

7 Boil the suspension for 10 min, vortex one last time, and 2 µl of suspension are added to each PCR reaction. The remainder can be stored at −20 °C until needed.

Protocol 2

Rapid freeze–fracture preparation of cell lysates from Gram positive bacteria

Reagents

- 1 M NaCl
- Activated carbon powder (Sigma, C-3345)
- Sterile ddH$_2$O
- 95% EtOH

Method

1 An inoculation loop (1 µl size) full of cells are scraped from a 24 h culture plate, washed once in 1 ml of 1 M NaCl, and pelleted in a 1.5 ml microcentrifuge tube at 18 000 g for 5 min.

2 Resuspend the cells in 100 µl of ddH$_2$O and a loop full of activated carbon powder.

3 Place the cells in a handled rack and freeze in an ethanol/dry ice bath for 2 min.

4 Immediately submerge the tubes in a boiling water-bath for 2 min.

5 Repeat steps 3 and 4 five more times alternating back and forth between freezing and thawing stages.

6 After the last thaw cycle, cell debris is removed by centrifugation at 18 000 g for 3–5 min and 2 µl of the remaining supernatant is used per PCR reaction. Suspensions can be stored at −20 °C until needed.

Protocol 3

Preparation of high quality chromosomal DNA for restriction endonuclease analyses and other applications where high quality DNA is needed

Reagents

- Minimal salts solution: 0.2% $(NH_4)SO_4$, 1.4% K_2HPO_4, 0.6% KH_2PO_4, 0.1% Na-citrate, 0.02% $MgSO_4$

- 50% glucose

- CAYE: 2% casamino acids, 10% yeast extract

- Minimal medium: 2% minimal salts solution plus 0.01 vol. (w/v) of glucose and CAYE

- Lysis buffer: 0.15 M NaCl, 0.1 M EDTA pH 8.0, 0.5 mg/ml lysozyme (added immediately before use)

- 10% SDS

- 5 M $NaClO_4$

- 1:1 phenol (TE saturated)/chloroform[a]

- Chloroform/octanol: 24:1 mixture chloroform and octanol

- 100% EtOH

- 70% EtOH

- TEN buffer: 10 mM Tris–HCl pH 7.5, 1 mM EDTA pH 8.0, 10 mM NaCl

- TE buffer: 10 mM Tris–HCl pH 7.5, 1 mM EDTA pH 8.0

- RNase buffer: 10 mg/ml ribonuclease A in 0.1 M Na-acetate pH 4.8, 0.3 mM EDTA pH 8.0 (pre-heated to 90 °C for 10 min and stored at −20 °C)

- Pronase (Type XIV bacterial protease, Sigma, P-5147): 2 mg/ml in TEN buffer, stored at −20 °C

Method

1 Add a single bacterial colony (24 h old) to 200 ml of minimal medium and incubate/shake the culture at 37 °C for 18 h.

2 Centrifuge the culture fluid at 15 000 g for 10 min at 4 °C.

3 Resuspend the pellet in 10 ml of lysis solution and gently swirl the culture on a rotating platform for 1 h. (Note: lysis solution without the lysozyme can be made up in advance and stored at −20 °C until needed.)

4 Mix the following reagents to the lysis solution in the following sequence: 1 ml of 10% SDS, 4 ml of 5 M $NaClO_4$, and 20 ml of chloroform/octanol (24:1). Mix thoroughly between each addition.

5 Incubate/shake the entire mixture at 50–75 r.p.m. at 25 °C for 15 min.

6 Centrifuge the solution at 15 000 g for 20 min and transfer the viscous aqueous phase to a clean tube.

7 Add 2 vol. of cold 100% EtOH to the tube, gently mix for 5–10 min, and spin at 15 000 g for 20 min.

8 Save the supernatant in a clean tube, add 5 ml of cold 70% EtOH to the DNA pellet, and centrifuge once again at 15 000 g for 20 min.

Protocol 3 continued

9 Decant the EtOH wash and let the pellet air dry for 5 min.

10 Resuspend the DNA pellet in 5 ml of TEN. Resuspension may require gentle agitation at room temperature for about an hour.

11 Add 20 μl of RNase buffer to the solution and incubate at 37 °C for 1 h. At the and of 1 h, add 50 μl of pronase and repeat the incubation for an additional hour.

12 Extract the solution by adding 5 ml of phenol/chloroform, mix thoroughly, centrifuging the tube for 5 min at 15 000 g, and transferring the aqueous (upper) phase into a clean tube.

13 DNA is recovered by repeating steps 7–9 and pellets are resuspended in 1.5 ml of TE.

14 DNA concentrations and qualities are calculated using A_{260} and A_{280} spectrophotometric measurements. Adjust to a final concentration of 0.5 μg/μl using the calculation:

$$50 \times 200 \times OD_{260} = \text{DNA concentration (μg/ml)},$$

where '50' is the correction coefficient for double-stranded DNA, '200' is the dilution factor (1:200), and OD_{260} is the observed reading at 260 nm. DNAs are stored at 4 °C until needed.

[a] Saturated phenol is prepared by mixing pure phenol with two volumes of TE buffer in a separatory funnel. The mixture is shaken vigorously and allowed to stand until the layers separate. The lower phenol layer is drained off. This process should be repeated several times with fresh buffer to neutralize the phenol. The resulting saturated phenol is stored at −20 °C. TE saturation of phenol inhibits loss of volume in the aqueous layer during DNA extraction.

2.2 Reaction conditions

Many of the reaction conditions invoked for repetitive PCR fingerprinting are applicable to any of the three techniques described above. *Protocol 4* is a general PCR set-up strategy for initiating 'ribotype', REP-PCR, or RAPD-PCR reactions. An optimal set up volume for most reactions is 50 μl. This amount prevents the usage of excessive amounts of costly PCR reagents while allowing for a large enough volume to be easily analysed in agarose gels. Generally, oligomers in the amount of 50 pmol are sufficient to prime most reactions. In reactions where only a single primer is employed (e.g. BOXA1, GTG5, MBO1, and the RAPD primers) that amount is increased to 100 pmol. A PCR reaction buffer with a $MgCl_2$ concentration of 1.5 mM appears to work consistently well in the generation of a spectrum of amplicons for each of the three techniques. Commercial reaction buffers are readily available with 1.5 mM $MgCl_2$ from Perkin Elmer, Promega, and other suppliers of *Taq* polymerase. $MgCl_2$ concentrations may need to be adjusted accordingly between 1.5 mM and 4 mM in the optimization of some RAPD fingerprints. If necessary, this should be determined empirically and is easily done by preparing your own reaction buffer (see *Protocol 4*).

Protocol 4

A general PCR set-up strategy for amplification-based DNA fingerprinting

Reagents

- 10 × PCR buffer: 15 mM MgCl$_2$, 100 mM Tris–HCl pH 8.4, 500 mM KCl, 1 mg/ml gelatin
- 2 mM dNTPs: dATP (2 mM), dGTP (2 mM), dCTP (2 mM), and dTTP (2 mM)
- Sterile ddH$_2$O
- *Taq* polymerase

- Oligonucleotide primers: 50 pmol of each primer from 10 μM stock solutions, 100 pmol of BOXA1R, MBOREP1, and GTG5 (see *Table 1*)
- Template genomic DNA from cell lysates (*Protocols 1* and *2*)
- Light white mineral oil

Method

1 For a 50 μl reaction, add 5 μl of 10 × PCR buffer, 5 μl of 2 mM dNTP solution, 2.6 μl of each primer (5.2 μl of the single BOXA1R primer), and ddH$_2$O to a final volume of 50 μl into a 0.5 ml microcentrifuge tube.

2 Mix in 0.5 μl (2.5 units) of *Taq* polymerase to the reaction mixture.

3 Add 2 μl of genomic DNA solution (cell lysate solution from *Protocols 1* or *2*) to the reaction mixture, and give the tube a pulse of centrifugation to ensure reaction components are in the tube bottom. (Note: if using a thermal cycler without a heated lid, it is important to overlay the reaction with 30 μl of mineral oil.)

4 Insert tubes into a thermal cycler pre-heated to 94°C. (Note: to ensure rapid and even heating, one drop of mineral oil should be added into each well in the heat block of Perkin Elmer 480 or older thermal cyclers that lack a heated lid.)

2.3 The 'ribotype' method

As previously mentioned, the rRNA genes have been useful for detecting genetic differences between higher taxa of bacteria (28). Recently, the more variable intergenic spacer (IGS) region which lies between the 16S and 23S rRNA transcription units, was targeted for differentiation of bacterial species (21). As a result of relaxed selection constraints on this intergenic region, the rRNA IGS has evolved numerous size polymorphisms that can be exploited to differentiate closely related microbes. The 'ribotyping' method was originally exploited in an effort to track epidemic outbreaks in clinical settings due to its universal applicability to all eubacterial strains and its highly stable and reproducible banding patterns (29). However, this technique is also powerful for the differentiation of many other enterobacterial species and strains (*Figure 1*). Banding patterns shown in *Figure 1* reveal two important aspects. First, each of the five plant pathogenic species depicted in the gel possess distinct banding patterns (lanes 1–3, *Erwinia*

Table 1 Oligonucleotides and related cycling conditions often employed in PCR-based fingerprint analyses of bacteria

Oligo name / sequence (5'–3')	Method	Annealing temp (°C)	Extension temp (°C)	Extension time (min)	Number of cycles
1. 16SF / TTGTACACACCGCCCTCA 23SR / GGTACCTTAGATGTTTCAGT	'Ribotyping'	55	72	1.5	35
2. REP1R-I / IIIICGICGICATCIGGC REP2-I / ICGICTTATCIGGCCTAC	Repetitive PCR	40	65	8.0	35
3. ERIC1R / ATGTAAGCTCCTGGGGATTCAC ERIC2 / AAGTAAGTGACTGGGGTGAGCG	Repetitive PCR	52	65	8.0	35
4. BOXA1R / CTACGGCAAGCGACGCTGACG	Repetitive PCR	52	65	8.0	35
5. MBO1 / CCGCCGTTGCCGCCGTTGCCGCCG	Repetitive PCR	54	65	8.0	35
6. GTG5 / GTGGTGGTGGTGGTG	Repetitive PCR	40	65	8.0	35
7. OPA-1 / CAGGCCCTTC	RAPD-PCR	35	72	2.0	35
8. Bc3 / CCGGCGGCG	RAPD-PCR	35	72	2.0	35
9. Bc4 / CGGCCCCTGT	RAPD-PCR	35	72	2.0	35
10. Bc5 / CGGCCACTGT	RAPD-PCR	30	72.	2.0	35

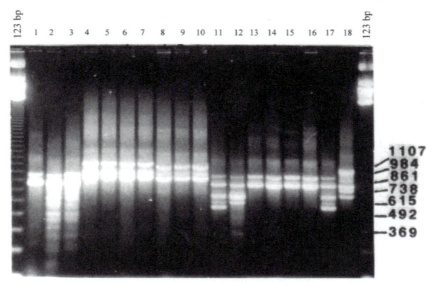

Figure 1 Specific rDNA IGS ('ribotype') banding patterns for select *Erwinia* species as revealed by agarose gel electrophoresis. Lanes are designated as follows: lanes 1–3, *E. lupinicola* strains 3l31, 346, 348, respectively; lanes 4–7, *E. psidii* strains 49406, 8427, 8428, Ep8429; lanes 8–10, *E. mallotivora* strains 29573, 8646, 8645; lanes 11–17, *E. quercina* strains 29281, 27622, 1919, 29282, 1846, 1845, 11d32; lane 18, *E. alni* strain pvf20. The fragments were generated as a result of polymorphism in the length of the IGS region in rDNA operons on the bacterial chromosome thus resulting in amplification fragment length polymorphisms. The relative sizes in bp are given to the far right of the gel for the 123 bp DNA size standard shown in the first and last lanes of the gel.

lupinicola; lanes 4–7, *Erwinia psidii*; lanes 8–10, *Erwinia mallotivora*; lanes 11–17, *Erwinia quercina*; and lane 18, *Erwinia alni*. Secondly, genetic variation among strains can be detected in two of the species shown (e.g. *E. lupinicola* and *E. quercina*). The technique has been applied to a number of bacterial pathogens of both clinical and agricultural significance (30). A single primer pair is currently available to fingerprint the intergenic rDNA spacer (IGS) region (21). Their respective nucleotide sequences, optimal annealing temperatures, and suggested extension temperatures/times are given in *Table 1*. The forward 'ribotype' primer, 16SF, anneals to the 3′ end of the 16S subunit gene while the reverse primer, 23SF, binds to the 5′ terminus of the 23S subunit gene. Together, these primers span the IGS detecting size variations within and between strains. 'Ribotype' amplicons generally range in size from 200 bp to 2 kb in size and comprise highly stable banding patterns even when DNA quality is relatively poor.

2.4 Repetitive PCR fingerprinting

Several families of repetitive DNA sequences have recently been characterized in a number of eubacterial species (31). The first repeat sequences to be isolated were known as REPs (repetitive extragenic palindromes) and were first described as possible regulatory sequences within untranslated regions of bacterial operons (32). More recently, a second class of repetitive element has been characterized from the genomes of *E. coli* and *Salmonella spp.* These enterobacterial repetitive intergenic consensus (ERIC) sequences are also present in untranslated regions of the enterobacterial chromosome, and, like the REP sequences described above, consist of conserved and repeated segments of DNA. These ERIC elements possess no sequence homology to the shorter REP motifs (33). The most recent family of repeats to be elucidated are the BOX elements, isolated from the Gram positive species, *Streptococcus pneumoniae.* BOX's are modular in nature and consist of three subunits, BOX-A, -B, and -C (8). BOX-A appears to be highly conserved and present in multiple copies throughout the entire spectrum of Gram negative organisms. The evolutionary origin of these motifs around the bacterial chromosome remains unclear though its mosaic structure has been noted (33). Regardless of the lack of knowledge regarding the origins and functions of these loci, the repetitive family of bacterial DNA elements have proven quite useful for the differentiation of enteric species and the development of strain-specific fingerprints (34). PCR-based fingerprints of repetitive sequences have allowed for the genetic distinction between a number of closely related bacterial species and strains (*Figure 2*), and species-specific fingerprints of a number of human and plant pathogenic microbial genomes have now been reported (35). REP primers were initially designed from the left and right sides of a conserved palindromic sequence and oriented in opposite directions such that extension moves outwardly in a 3' direction away from the palindrome. In this way, amplicons are formed between repetitive palindromic islands (ranging in size from 200 bp up to 4 kb) resulting in a total chromosomal fingerprint for a given strain. In the case of several repetitive primers, inosine was added to increase both degeneracy and sensitivity in the reaction (8). This leads to the production of a greater number of bands and a more accurate discrimination of isolates. Some repetitive PCR reactions yield highly strain-specific fingerprints using only single oligomers, such as BOXA1, GTG5, and MBO1 and crude DNA preparations (8). A list of these primers is provided in *Table 1*.

2.5 RAPD-PCR

RAPD (randomly amplified polymorphic DNA) PCR (36) has become a popular method for the typing of closely related genomes and has demonstrated utility in a variety of organisms for different applications. For instance, RAPD analysis has been instrumental in the genetic mapping of the plant genome and is key to understanding the divergence of races among fungal pathogens (24). RAPD-PCR holds its greatest promise in the genetic differentiation of bacterial strains and has been employed to differentiate both Gram negative and Gram positive organisms (26). Using a single, short arbitrary primer, segments of the bacterial genome are preferentially amplified depending on the level of sequence complementarity shared between the oligonucleotide primer and the bacterial chromosome. In this way, strains differing by only a few nucleotide substitutions can be discriminated based on the presence or absence of specific amplicons. That is,

41

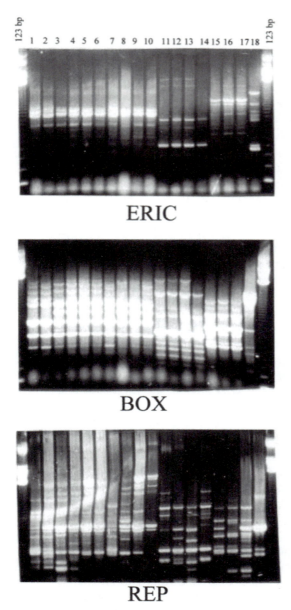

Figure 2 DNA fingerprint gels of *Erwinia* species and strains as revealed by several repetitive PCR fingerprint primers. Each lane denotes a specific band pattern for each isolate analysed. Lanes are designated as follows: lanes 1–10, *E. amylovora* strains 178, 179, 1232, 1804, 1539, 1540, 1108, 1004, 1829, 1450, respectively; lanes 11–14, *E. psidii* strains 49406, 8427, 8428, 8429; lanes 15–17, *E. mallotivora* strains 29573, 8645, and 8646; lane 18, *E. alni* strain Ealpvf20. This order is also applicable to the BOX and REP gels. The name of each agarose gel corresponds to the PCR-based genetic probe used to fingerprint the *Erwinia* species shown. Strains within each species are clearly shown to group together based on band-sharing identities. A 123 bp DNA size standard is shown in the first and last lane of each gel.

because of the inherent variation in DNA, the number and sizes of PCR products (intervening sequences) will vary among different strains. Because of its marked sensitivity, the technique has been particularly useful for fingerprinting micro-organisms as part of epidemiological investigations into nosocomial and food-borne outbreaks (26). One caveat associated with the technique relates to the ability to reliably and accurately reproduce stable banding patterns using RAPD oligomers. Several factors have been reported to affect the reproducibility of RAPD fingerprints including: DNA quality and concentration, the type of *Taq* DNA polymerase employed, and $MgCl_2$ concentration in the reaction buffer (37). Care must be taken to maintain the greatest consistency in reagent selection and experimental design when performing RAPD-PCR experiments. Specifically, DNA yields should be of the highest purity. Protocol 3 is an acceptable method for obtaining high quality DNA. Additionally, a number of commercial DNA extraction techniques also perform equally as well (e.g. Puregene, Gentra Systems; Isoquick, ORCA). *Taq* polymerase from Perkin Elmer has been shown to yield highly stable RAPD fingerprints in conjunction with a final concentration of 2.5 mM $MgCl_2$.

RAPD-PCR reactions require the addition of a single oligomer usually between 8–10 bp in length (36). These primers are synthetic and do not represent any known primary sequence structure on the bacterial chromosome. Most primers are designed with a GC content between 70% and 100% and, because of their short length, often require very low annealing temperatures (*Table 1*). RAPD primers tend to work with varying degrees of success depending on the bacterial species being analysed, and, often, several different primers will be assessed against the same template DNA in order to determine which primers yield the greatest number of polymorphic products. OPA-1 works well for eubacterial genomes in general while the *Bc* series primers have been reported to yield consistent and polymorphic fingerprints for the genus *Bacillus* and other Gram positive taxa (26).

2.6 Gel electrophoresis of amplicons

For the rapid visualization of DNA fingerprint patterns resulting from 'ribotype', REP-PCR, or RAPD-PCR analysis, products should be separated on 1.5% agarose gels constructed from DNA-typing grade agarose and at least 7.5 cm × 10 cm in size. For a more rigorous analysis and comparison of REP-PCR and RAPD products, larger gels should be used that are 20 cm × 24 cm in size. Gels should be run in TAE buffer at about 5 V/cm. For post-electrophoretic staining, gels are submerged in a Tupperware container containing ethidium bromide solution (0.5 μg/ml) and TAE for 30 min–1 h and are destained for 1–2 h in TAE alone. Gels are photographed under UV light and an orange filter with a Polaroid type 55 or 57 land film. For purposes of clarity, it is strongly suggested that 5 × 7 photographic prints be made from Polaroid negatives before scoring and interpretations are initiated (8). Alternatively, laboratories possessing digital image enhancement equipment can also produce high quality gel reproductions on thermal paper or computer screens.

2.7 Analysis and interpretation of PCR fingerprint data

Molecular epidemiological interpretations can be made readily from photographs of the gel data. A genotype can be 'scored' by simply sizing each band in a single lane of the gel against several molecular weight markers. Using several different molecular weight ladders allows for a more accurate assessment of the size in base pairs of each band. Since most of these PCR approaches yield bands in the 0.2–2 kb range, ladders which resolve shorter bands are often employed. Ladders such as the 123 bp, the 1 kb, and the 100 bp (Gibco BRL) are optimal for sizing each band in the resultant agarose gel. The epidemiological monitoring of bacterial strains through their genotype is an efficient and reliable approach for tracking the dissemination of bacterial pathogens (38). These genotypes are stable and readily reproducible given controlled reaction conditions. This has been observed empirically for several strains following continued passage and reisolation from host tissues. *Figure 3* illustrates the continuity of genotypes generated from ribotyping (*Figure 3A*) and BOX PCR analysis (*Figure 3B*) for several plant pathogenic strains following repeated passage through host tissues. Lanes 2–4 represent three separate passages of *Erwinia mallotivora* strain 8645, all of which yielded identical genotypes. This trend held true for *E. mallotivora* 29573 (lanes 5–7) and *E. lupinicola* (lanes 8–10), both of which were also passaged three times through host tissues (*Figure 3A* and *3B*). Each of the above methods is capable of strain-specific identification for most species; however, certain bacteria tend to be more genetically homogeneous and may demand the application of all three techniques in order to obtain the necessary genotypic variation sufficient to discriminate between strains.

In addition to tracking individual strains with the use of PCR fingerprints, these types of data can also be employed in the genetic and phylogenetic differentiation of multiple strains. Binary (0,1) matrices can be constructed from the gels based on the presence or absence of a band at a specific site. This matrix can then be used to calculate pairwise genetic distances between strains using a number of algorithms designed to convert fingerprint data into quantitative distance measurements (e.g. the Nei–Li distance formula) (24). Further, binary matrices are directly amenable to cladistic analysis (39). Provided sufficient variation exists between fingerprints, entire phylogenies of multiple strains, populations, or species can be constructed using programs such as PAUP v.3.11 (39), PAUP* betaversion (40), and DNAPARS, available in PHYLIP (41). A great number of phylogenies have been reported for Proteobacterial strains and species by coupling PCR fingerprinting techniques with cladistic and other tree-building methodologies (42). Chapter 8 of this book provides a detailed description of phylogenetic reconstruction.

3 RFLP analysis of the bacterial chromosome

Genomic DNA restriction analysis or restriction fragment length polymorphism (RFLP) analysis and heterologous probing has been applied to variable alleles in

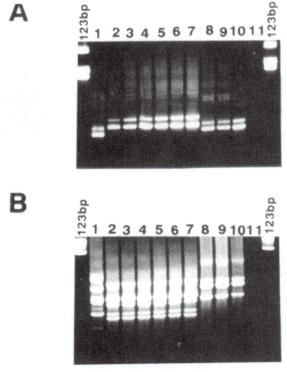

Figure 3 Ethidium bromide stained DNA agarose gel depicting the continuity of repetitive PCR genotypes following repeated passage of strains through host organisms. (A) 'Ribotype' analysis of select *Erwinia mallotivora* and *E. lupinicola* strains. (B) BOX repetitive PCR fingerprint analysis the same *E. mallotivora* and *E. lupinicola* strains. Lanes are designated as follows: 1, *E. amylovora* 581; 2–4, *E. mallotivora* 8645 passaged through Bartlett pear trees once, twice, and thrice, respectively; 5–7, *E. mallotivora* 29573 passaged three times through pear tissues as described above; and 8–10, *E. lupinicola* 346 passaged three times through pear tissues as described above.

the mammalian genome, for example, in order to discriminate individuals and populations (43). More recently, enzymatic restriction of the entire bacterial chromosome lends itself as a highly reproducible and sensitive method for the detection of DNA sequence variation and for the differentiation of bacterial strains (44). This differentiation technique is based on the premise that DNA from two different bacterial strains will have a different nucleotide sequence, thus following restriction with the same enzyme, different mixtures of fragments may be produced. Because the bacterial genome is roughly 1/1000th the size of the human genome, it is possible to restrict the entire chromosome in single reactions and electrophoretically resolve the resultant fragments without the need for radioactively or enzymatically labelled probes that only highlight specific subregions of the genome. This method is highly sensitive to sequence variation and has been able to identify individual clonal lines of eubacteria in species such as *Erwinia*, *Agrobacterium*, *Pseudomonas*, and *Xanthomonas* (10).

3.1 General considerations

The method reported here allows for restriction of the entire bacterial genome followed by separation of the resultant fragments using standard gel staining techniques rather than relying on hybridization approaches and probe construction. This protocol offers several advantages over more conventional hybridization techniques. First, this approach avoids the need to clone and identify DNA sequences as is required when hypervariable probes are employed. Secondly, the presence of repetitive DNA is not a factor since probes are not required that may potentially span these highly conserved regions in the genome. Next, hybridization analyses are often not easily repeated in other laboratories. That is, for a separate laboratory to independently evaluate an analysis, the same probe must be used. This is often problematic given the potential commercial significance of most diagnostic markers. Finally, material and supply costs are kept at a minimum as costly isotopic or luminescent probe detection systems can be avoided using this technique (10).

Certain strains of bacteria possess episomal elements or segments of DNA not located on the major chromosome and not part of the nuclear DNA component. This DNA can be found inside of the cell usually in the form of plasmids and/or lysogenic bacteriophages (45). Strains carrying extra chromosomal DNA may yield subtly different RFLP patterns when compared to the same strain lacking these extra DNA elements. As expected, strains possessing extra DNA exhibit one or two extra fragments on the gel, and this fragment does not usually appear equal in intensity to authentic chromosomal bands. This latter observation results from a disproportionate molarity between chromosomal fragments and episomal fragments (10). If this is the case, the strain carrying the extra fragment(s) should be screened for the presence of unknown plasmids or viruses.

3.2 Preparation of genomic DNA for RFLP analysis

The quality of genomic DNA required for endonuclease restriction must be substantially higher than for uses involving PCR or other rapid fingerprinting assays. As discussed in Section 2.1, a variety of commercial kits exist for the preparation of high quality genomic DNA from bacteria with or without extensive cell walls. Each of these protocols focuses on a different strategy for purification including: 'salting-out' methods (Puregene, Gentra Systems; Isoquick, ORCA); column purification (QiaAmp, Qiagen; Wizard, Promega); and organic extraction (Oncor, Appligene-Oncor). However, as in the case of rapid-throughput DNA preparations, there are several reliable protocols readily available in the literature that yield DNA of high enough quality for genomic restriction. Protocol 3 is an organic extraction method capable of purifying DNA from Gram negative or Gram positive species. While unnecessary for Gram negative strains, the addition of lysozyme to the lysis buffer allows for digestion of cell wall proteins and the efficient release of intracellular contents from most eubacterial species.

3.3 Enzymes

The decision of which specific restriction endonuclease will be used to digest the bacterial chromosome is strain-dependent and remains largely an empirical process. There are several factors that must be considered when selecting a restriction enzyme for analysis including: the strain or species of interest, the specific chromosome size, %GC composition of the chromosome, and cost of the enzyme. There is a great deal of variation in the price range of various restriction enzymes, and often, the least costly enzymes can be found to yield the most optimal results. Strains in the family *Pseudomonadaceae*, which includes a variety of fluorescent and non-fluorescent Pseudomonads, Aeromonads, and Xanthomonads, have elevated GC levels, and *Hae*III and *Msp*I tend to yield useful data for these taxa. Both of these enzymes recognize unique GC motifs four nucleotides in length. Conversely, the family *Enterobacteriaceae*, comprising the vast majority of nosocomial and food-borne pathogens, contains many species and strains that have a larger genome size but lower GC content (about 50–55%). *Hin*fI cleaves at GANTC and has been found to be effective in yielding discriminating fragment patterns for several enterobacterial species (10).

Once an enzyme has been selected, digestions can be set up as detailed in *Protocol 5* (10). This protocol contains an organic extraction phase which is used to terminate digestion, allowing for long-term storage of the reaction before it is resolved on an acrylamide gel. Again, it should be stressed that only through empirical observation can the most useful enzyme for a particular analysis be found. In some cases, it may be necessary to digest a genomic DNA sample with two or more enzymes simultaneously in order to generate polymorphic banding patterns and unique genotypic markers for a given strain. If this is the case, enzymes should be chosen that require the same reaction buffer. This allows for the digestion to be carried out in a single tube simultaneously.

Protocol 5

Digestion of DNA for RFLP analysis

Reagents

- BSA (molecular biology grade): 1 mg/ml
- 10 × enzyme reaction buffer (as provided by supplier)
- 5 μg genomic DNA (see *Protocol 3*)
- ddH$_2$O (molecular biology grade)
- 4 bp sequence recognition restriction enzyme (8–10 U/μl)
- Phenol (molecular biology grade)/chloroform/isoamyl alcohol (25:24:1)

Method

1 Gently agitate the genomic DNA sample by pipetting the solution up and down in the stock tube. This ensures total suspension of DNA following storage.

2   For one reaction, add the following reagents to a 1.5 ml microcentrifuge tube: 73 μl of ddH₂O, 2 μl of BSA, 10 μl (10–20 U) of 10 × enzyme reaction buffer, 5 μl of the restriction enzyme, and 10 μl of genomic DNA solution from a 0.5 μg/μl stock (Protocol 3) for a total volume of 100 μl.

3   Gently vortex the reaction mixture for a few seconds to ensure an even distribution for the dense enzyme/glycerol solution.

4   Briefly spin the tube in a microcentrifuge.

5   Incubate the mixture in a 37 °C water-bath for 4 h.

6   Cool the tubes to room temperature and add 50 μl of the phenol/chloroform/ isoamyl alcohol mixture.

7   Vortex the tube vigorously for several seconds and centrifuge for 5 min at top speed.

8   The organic phase can now be removed taking care not to remove any of the reaction mix. Reactions can then be stored at −20 °C until needed.

3.4 Polyacrylamide gel electrophoresis (PAGE)

Polyacrylamide gels (5%) are employed to resolve the digestion reactions generated in *Protocol 5*. Polyacrylamide offers several advantages over agarose for electrophoresing genomic restriction digests. First, the amount of restricted DNA that can be loaded onto polyacrylamide gels is greater than can be loaded onto agarose gels, making the identification of fragments much easier. Secondly, the staining of polyacrylamide gel allows for higher visual contrast and greater ease in scoring of the RFLP patterns; and thirdly, the resolving power of PAGE far exceeds that of agarose gel analysis. PAGE gels are capable of resolving single nucleotide size differences while DNA-typing grade agarose gels are not (10). The optimal resolving power of PAGE gels is in the range of about 40–4000 bp. Since this range encompasses the sizes of most fragments generated in restriction digests, PAGE is the logical choice for electrophoresis (10).

Protocol 6 presents a method for the casting, loading, and running of 5% polyacrylamide gels (10). The procedure is drafted for use with a Pharmacia GE 2/4 electrophoresis unit but can be easily adapted to any other PAGE system from manufacturers such as Bio-Rad or Hoefer. An ethidium bromide gel staining procedure is also detailed in *Protocol 6*. Additionally, Gelstar (FMC Bioproducts, Cat. No. 50535) is a highly sensitive fluorescent stain that works optimally well for staining DNA in polyacrylamide gels. Gels are also amenable to silver staining techniques which often yield the highest quality and contrast for genotypic scoring. Silver staining kits are available from Promega. Also, where available, gel imaging and enhancement systems can yield high contract thermal prints of gels.

Protocol 6

Polyacrylamide gel electrophoresis of restriction digests

Reagents

- 30% acrylamide: 30 g acrylamide, 1 g N,N'-methylenebisacrylamide (filter through Whatman 3MM filter paper)
- 3% ammonium persulfate (must be made fresh)
- 20 × TAE pH 7.2: 800 mM Tris–acetate pH 7.4, 20 mM EDTA pH 8.0, titrate with concentrated glacial acetic acid
- TEMED
- TAE loading dye: 5 × TAE pH 7.2, 100 mM EDTA pH 8.0, 50% sucrose, 0.01% bromophenol blue
- Ethidium bromide: 10 mg/ml
- ddH$_2$O (molecular biology grade)

Method

1   In a sterile flask, add 50 ml of 30% acrylamide, 15 ml of 20 × TAE, 6.3 ml of ammonium persulfate, and 228.7 ml of ddH$_2$O. Mix thoroughly.

2   To the flask, gently mix 90 µl of TEMED into the gel solution and pour the entire mixture into the casting apparatus (Note: this makes enough gel solution for the 8-gel cassette system. Volumes can be scaled up or down accordingly depending on the number of gels your system is designed to handle.)

3   Allow the gel to polymerize for 1–2 h, rinse the cassettes and wells with ddH$_2$O, wrap the gels in plastic wrap, and store the gels at 4 °C until needed (gels will keep for about one week).

4   Load the gels into the upper electrophoretic chamber of the gel apparatus that you are using.

5   Fill the gel apparatus with 1 × TAE and replace the upper chamber (with gels in place) into the unit.

6   Initiate recirculation cooling through all upper and lower electrophoretic chambers and apply power to the gel (generally 60–70 volts and 20–25 mA per gel). Pre-electrophorese for 30–60 min.

7   To prepare digested samples: thaw from freezer, vortex briefly, and spin briefly at top speed to concentrate the sample in the bottom of the tube. In a clean 0.5 ml microcentrifuge tube, add 30 µl of the digest to 8 µl of TAE loading. Mix the sample by gently pipetting up and down several times.

8   Load the samples into the wells of the gel with the left and right far outside wells of each gel receiving a standard molecular weight marker (i.e. Life Technology's 123 bp or 1 kb ladders).

9   Electrophorese for 16 h at room temperature. This will retain all fragments roughly greater than or equal to 500 bp in size.

10 After 16 h, turn power supply off, remove the gels from the upper chamber, and pry the glass plates apart under running water. (Note: the blue tracking dye should be visible at or near the end of the gel.)

Protocol 6 continued

11 For ethidium bromide (EtBr) staining of the gel, gently immerse the gel in a flat container containing 200 ml of used electrophoresis buffer and add 20 μl of 10 mg/ml EtBr and disperse by shaking.

12 Stain on an orbital shaker for 1 h and destain, if necessary, in clean electrophoresis buffer.

13 Photograph the gel on a UV box containing a Polaroid camera equipped with an orange filter (Polaroid Type 55 film gives the highest quality and contrast for this application, exposure is usually 15–30 sec at an F stop of 8). Alternatively, gel imaging software also yields high quality prints.

3.5 Analysis and interpretation of genomic restriction data

In the same way as PCR-based amplicon data, restriction fragments can also be scored based on size variation and as presence or absence at a particular site. As before, 100 bp, 123 bp, and 1 kb DNA ladders are necessary for the accurate sizing of the gel fragments. Unlike the highly variable repetitive PCR fingerprint patterns, chromosomal variation discerned by restriction fragmentation is often much less polymorphic, and many strains within the same species will share identical restriction patterns, owing to the clonal population structures exuded by many Proteobacterial species. For this reason, a number of different enzymes should be screened until a polymorphic and stable genotype is found for the strain of interest. *Figure* 4 is a polyacrylamide gel containing the restricted entire chromosomes of 16 different *Azospirillum* species (44). While several polymorphisms are identifiable between lanes, the gel is a vivid representation of the homogeneous genetic structure of many bacterial species and strains. Although restriction analysis of the entire chromosome may require a more rigorous effort in the laboratory, the end-result will be a highly repetitive and undisputed genotype from which to base many epidemiological studies and allow for the molecular tracking of the strain in a variety of settings. Also, as previously mentioned in Section 2.7, these binary data can be used to calculate genetic distances between isolates and can be used as input into cladistic algorithms for the construction of phylogenetic trees (39).

4 PFGE analysis of the bacterial chromosome

Pulsed field gel electrophoresis (PFGE) is an electrophoretic technique designed to separate pieces of linear DNA up to 10 Mb in length (1). This DNA is usually in the form of fragments resulting from enzymatic digestion with diagnostic restriction endonucleases. PFGE, coupled with certain rare cutting restriction enzymes, enables a researcher to scan the entire bacterial chromosome for sequence polymorphisms based on the presence or absence of rare restriction sites (46). Like RFLP analysis described in *Protocols* 5 and 6, PFGE relies on genomic

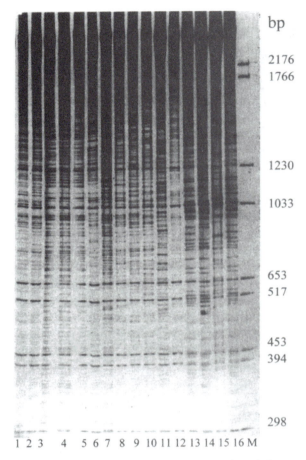

bp

2176
1766

1230

1033

653
517

453
394

298

1 2 3   4   5 6 7   8   9 10 11 12 13 14 15 16 M

Figure 4 Polyacrylamide gel depicting the genetic variation present in 16 total DNA restriction digests of *Azospirillum* species. The gel shown was obtained using the restriction endonuclease *Bgl*II. Lane M contains the molecular weight marker, and the bands of this marker are also present in each of the sample lanes (lanes 1–16) (printed with permission from Humana Press, Totowa, NJ).

digestions as input to be loaded onto the gels. However, this similarity does not extend to the separation properties of PFGE and polyacrylamide gels as these two different analytical procedures possess very different resolving capabilities. PFGE can successfully resolve significantly larger fragments than conventional electrophoresis by requiring the DNA fragments to alter their direction of migration through the gel. This, in turn, maintains a linear configuration of the DNA, allowing it to pass through the gel matrix in a constant and uniform fashion. This unique property of the technique has made it useful for a number of applications including large scale physical mapping of the bacterial genome, investigations into the size and shape of chromosomes, and epidemiological approaches based on chromosomal digests (1, 42). *Figure 5* depicts a PFGE analysis of the

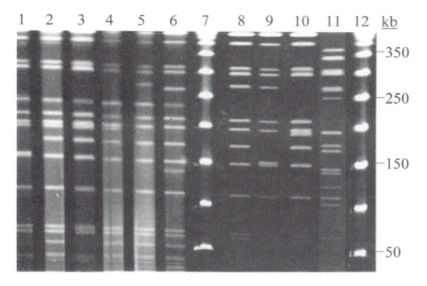

Figure 5 PFGE analysis of *Shigella flexneri* isolates from a single outbreak (lanes 1–6 and 8–10). Lane 11 depicts strain 2457T, an unrelated control strain of *S. flexneri*. The outbreak isolates are highly similar when compared to each other but markedly different from the control strain (lane 11). Several of the outbreak strains differ by a few bands, demonstrating the sensitivity of PFGE for the differentiation of closely related strains (figure kindly provided by Dr Farukh Khambaty, Center for Food Safety and Applied Nutrition, US Food and Drug Administration, Washington, DC).

macrorestricted chromosome of ten strains of *Shigella flexneri* and demonstrates the resolving capabilities of PFGE even among strains originating from a single outbreak (46). The following section focuses upon the use of PFGE to resolve linear chromosomal fragments for the discrimination of pathogenic strains of bacteria.

4.1 General considerations

A number of intrinsic and extrinsic factors are known to alter the resolution of DNA fragments when performing PFGE. Variation in migration properties has been associated with running temperature, the angle that the electric field is applied, pulse time (interval between reorientation of the electric field), and primary and secondary DNA structures, among other things. One of the most significant extrinsic factors is the agarose concentration in the gel. As agarose concentration increases, fragment mobility decreases, but resolution is enhanced. Concomitantly, the ability to resolve more lengthy fragments sharply decreases as agarose concentration rises. This negates a portion of the discriminatory information that could possibly be gathered about a strain. While agarose concentrations generally fluctuate between 1–1.2%, a final determination on the exact amount should be made after considering the enzyme(s) that was employed to digest the chromosome (47).

4.2 Genomic DNA quality

As in conventional RFLP techniques, the quality of genomic DNA required for PFGE analysis must be high. The rare cutting restriction enzymes employed with PFGE require DNA integrity substantially greater than for use in other enzymatic assays (1). Since each enzyme may cut the chromosome in only several places, it is imperative that the chromosome be intact and free of impurities prior to digestion. The use of low grade or partially degraded DNA preparations may result in the loss of high molecular weight fragment data or the development of smaller 'artefactual' fragments that may undermine genotypic interpretations. A general strategy for the preparation of high quality total chromosomal DNA is given in *Protocol 7*. The technique involves the use of agar plugs which traps and protects large DNA in a solid state (48).

Protocol 7

Preparation of DNA in agarose plugs

Equipment and reagents

- Block moulds: these are supplied as strips with PFGE equipment. It is important to clean these moulds before every use as they must be nuclease-free. Before use, seal the underside with tape and chill the assembly at 4°C. This will allow the gel to set more quickly.
- Chloramphenicol: 4% (w/v) in 95% EtOH; store at −20°C for two months
- Tris/NaCl buffer: 10 mM Tris–HCl pH 7.6, 1 M NaCl
- EC lysis buffer: 6 mM Tris–HCl pH 7.6, 1 M NaCl, 100 mM EDTA pH 7.6, 1% (w/v) N-lauryl sarcosine; store at room temperature (immediately before use add 1 mg/ml lysozyme)

- Agarose: 2% (w/v) low-gelling temperature (e.g. FMC Sea Plaque) in Tris/NaCl buffer
- ES buffer: 500 mM EDTA pH 9.0, 1% (w/v) N-lauryl sarcosine
- ESP buffer: 0.1% (w/v) proteinase K (~ 20 U/mg) in ES buffer
- TE buffer: 10 mM Tris–HCl pH 8.0, 1 mM EDTA pH 8.0
- PMSF (phenylmethylsulfonyl fluoride) 140 mM (25 mg/ml) in 95% EtOH; store up to one year at 4°C; dilute to 1 mM in TE immediately before use (Note: PMSF is poisonous and should be handled with extreme caution)

Method

1. Dilute an overnight culture of cells in a fresh, rich medium and grow to an absorbance (A_{600}) of 0.6.
2. Add chloramphenicol to a final concentration of 100 µg/ml (1:40 dilution of stock) and incubate for another 1 h.
3. Harvest the cells from 1 ml of culture by centrifugation for 30–60 sec in a microcentrifuge at 12 000 g.
4. Resuspend the cells in 1 ml of Tris/NaCl buffer and centrifuge as in step 3.
5. Resuspend the pellet in 300 µl of Tris/NaCl buffer.

6   Raise the temperature of the suspension to 42 °C, add an equal volume of 2% agarose (also at 42 °C), and mix by pipetting up and down at least ten times.

7   Dispense 100 µl of the agarose/cell suspension into each well of the moulds (5 × 2 × 10 mm, supplied by Pharmacia-LKB). (Note: it is important to dispense slowly to avoid the formation of bubbles in the moulds.)

8   Allow the agarose to solidify by placing the moulds on a level shelf at 4 °C.

9   Carefully expel the agarose plugs from the mould into 2 ml of EC lysis buffer, and incubate them overnight at 37 °C.

10 Transfer the plugs to the same volume of ESP buffer and incubate at 37 °C for 72 h.

11 Transfer the plugs to 2 ml of PMSF, incubate at 25 °C for 4 h, and repeat with an additional 2 ml of PMSF for 16 h at 25 °C.

12 Wash the plugs with TE three times (2 h and 20 ml of TE for each wash). Plugs can be stored in TE at 4 °C for up to one month.

4.3 Restriction enzymes employed in PFGE

A number of enzymes have shown promise in the macrorestriction of the genomes of bacterial strains. Most of these restriction endonucleases are 'rare cutters', only cleaving the bacterial chromosome in a few places. This rare cutting property is a function of the length of the specific DNA recognition site. In general, the longer the recognition site, the fewer times the enzyme will be able to restrict the DNA. Enzymes, such as *Bln*I, *Spe*I, *Swa*I, *Xba*I, and *Xho*I have worked well for successfully digesting the chromosomes of several enterobacterial and pseudomonad species (49). Other rare cutting enzymes that have been known to successfully macrorestrict the eubacterial genome include *Dra*I, *Nae*I, *Not*I, *Sfi*I, and *Sma*I. The exact number of cleavage sites recognized by these enzymes will vary depending on the species or strain being analysed, but not all enzymes will yield macrofragments on every species analysed (48). Several researchers have reported suboptimal results for certain enzyme–template combinations such as partial digestion, too small fragments, or diffuse banding patterns. For this reason, an empirical determination of efficacy must be made for each enzyme and for each strain in question. Protocol 8 illustrates a general set up strategy for a macrorestriction digest using one of the above enzymes and the agar DNA plugs (see *Protocol 7*).

Protocol 8

Digestion of bacterial DNA for PFGE analysis

Reagents

- Rare cutting restriction endonucleases
- Agarose plugs containing DNA from *Protocol 7*
- 10 × enzyme reaction buffers
- TE buffer: 10 mM Tris–HCl pH 8.0, 1 mM EDTA pH 8.0

Protocol 8 continued

Method

1   Wash an agarose plug with TE at 0 °C (two washes × 20 ml for 25 min each).

2   Wash the plug with 1 × enzyme reaction buffer at 0 °C (two washes × 10 ml for 25 min each).

3   Transfer the plug to Parafilm and use a sterile scalpel to cut it in slices (a slice of 1–2 mm thick is adequate for this procedure).

4   Transfer the slice to an autoclaved microcentrifuge tube containing 10–20 U of restriction endonuclease in 100 μl of 1 × enzyme buffer.

5   Digest the DNA by incubating for a minimum of 3 h at the appropriate temperature (usually 37 °C).

6   Wash the slices in 1.5 ml of TE and store as described in *Protocol 7*.

4.4 Electrophoretic conditions

Protocol 9 outlines a method for the separation of bacterial DNA fragments using PFGE. The method shown specifically enumerates PFGE using a CHEF (contour-clamped homogeneous electric field) electrophoresis system (2) which utilizes multiple electrodes which are ordered in a hexagonal array and clamped to a series of predetermined electrical potentials. These electrical potentials are equal in strength to two electrodes that are arranged in parallel (1). A number of CHEF systems and electrophoretic rigs can be purchased commercially from several sources. The protocol given here is designed for a CHEF-DR III apparatus (Bio-Rad).

Specific electrophoretic conditions will vary depending on the system being used, the size fragments being investigated, and the gel dimensions (1). In general and for the CHEF-DR III apparatus, a field strength of 5–6 V/cm for 16–22 h at a temperature of 15 °C has been reported as optimal (49). In addition, ramped pulse times (varying the pulse times during the run) tend to give optimal resolution of fragments of specific lengths. For instance, genomic fragments in the 8–100 kb range are best resolved with a ramped pulse time of 1–5 sec. DNA fragments ranging in size from 50–240 kb should be run at 1–20 sec, and fragments 200–800 kb are best resolved at 40–80 sec (1).

Protocol 9

Pulsed field gel electrophoresis (PFGE) analysis

Reagents

- Running buffer: 4 mM Hepes pH 6.8; 4 mM Na-acetate pH 5.2, 0.4 mM EDTA pH 8.0

- 1 × TBE pH 8.0: 89 mM Tris–HCl pH 8.0, 89 mM boric acid, 2 mM EDTA pH 8.0, titrated with concentrated glacial acetic acid

- Ultrapure agarose (standard melt)

- Ethidium bromide: 10 mg/ml

- ddH$_2$O (molecular biology grade)

Method

1 When using a Bio-Rad CHEF-DR III PFGE apparatus, follow manufacturer specifications for gel casting and electrophoretic conditions.

2 Cast and insert a 1–1.2% agarose gel (made up in 0.5 × TBE) into the apparatus, fill the chamber with running buffer.

3 Load digested genomic samples (previously prepared in *Protocol 8*) into the gel. This is accomplished by placing a small agarose slice on the flat end of a spatula and inserting it into one of the wells in the gel. (Note: it is important to remove any trapped air from around the slice using a fine gauge needle and syringe.)

4 The two outside wells on each side of the gel should be loaded with a high molecular weight marker such as phage λ DNA (48 kb–1 Mb sized fragments). Fragments must be scored by first determining their size in bp (usually in kb). This is done by comparison of the fragments with known DNA size markers or ladders. High molecular weight fragments should be compared against concatamers of bacteriophage λ DNA or chromosomes of *Saccharomyces cerevisiae* (225 kb − > 2 Mb). Both of these molecular size standards are available commercially.

5 Seal the slices into position in the wells with molten agarose in 0.5 × TBE.

6 Resolve the fragments with linear ramping at 5–6 V/cm for 22 h at 15°C using a circulating coolant apparatus.

7 Linear ramping times may vary based on the enzyme being employed and the genomic sample being examined. Generally, a linear ramped pulse time of 4–35 sec is sufficient.

8 After 22 h, turn power supply off, remove the gel apparatus cover, and place the gel in a flat container already containing 200 ml of 0.5 × TBE.

9 For ethidium bromide (EtBr) staining of the gel, add 20 μl of 10 mg/ml EtBr and disperse by shaking.

10 Stain on an orbital shaker for 1–1.5 h and destain in clean electrophoresis buffer for 2 h to overnight (this destain time should be determined empirically).

11 Photograph the gel on a UV box containing a Polaroid camera equipped with an orange filter (see Protocol 6 for details). Alternatively, gel imaging software also yields high quality prints.

4.5 Analysis and interpretations

Like conventional genome restriction approaches, macrorestriction fragments of the bacterial chromosome can be scored based on size variation and as presence or absence at a particular site. However, DNA-specific size ladders are necessary for the accurate sizing of the larger gel fragments. High molecular weight markers are available in agarose plug form including concatamers of bacteriophage λ DNA (size range 48.5 kb to 1 Mb in increments of 48.5 kb) and chromosomes of *Saccharomyces cerevisiae* (225 kb to 2.2 Mb). Also like RFLP analysis, chromosomal variation discerned by PFGE fragmentation possesses fewer polymorphic sites than many PCR-based fingerprint techniques. If this is the case, a number of different enzymes should be screened until a polymorphic and stable strain-specific genotype is found.

5 DNA sequence analysis of the bacterial *omp*A gene

Indisputably, the most accurate and powerful method for bacterial strain discrimination remains the nucleotide sequence. As has been the case in Metazoan biology for quite some time, DNA sequence analysis of coding loci on the bacterial chromosome has revolutionized what can be learned about bacterial population structure, strain variation, and phylogenetic relationships (7, 16). While nucleotide sequences have been instrumental in discerning evolutionary relationships between disparate lineages of bacteria, DNA sequencing has only recently been applied to discriminate individual genotypes at the strain level (13, 15, 50, 51). However, due to the unusually slow substitution rates of ribosomal genes, other more rapidly evolving genes are now being examined for their utility in discriminating closely related strains.

The outer membrane protein genes have been utilized to discriminate bacteria down to the species and subspecies levels. The *omp*A gene encodes the enterobacterial outer membrane protein 3A (52). Outer membrane proteins are located at the surface of the cell and play a number of critical roles ranging from structural integrity of the bacterial membrane to extracellular transport across the membrane (53). The rapid rate of evolution on this gene makes it an ideal candidate for identifying unique genotypes for pathogenic strains. The utility of *omp*A to differentiate closely related taxa has previously been demonstrated in several pathogenic genera including *Escherichia*, *Vibrio*, and *Chlamydia*, just to name a few (7, 51). *Figure 6* illustrates the genetic diversity uncovered in *omp*A genes from a variety of species and strains in the genus *Erwinia* (50).

While nucleotide sequence analysis can be more costly than enzyme-based approaches, the results offer several advantages over these more conventional fingerprinting methods. First, since every genetic character is taken into consideration, larger numbers of polymorphic sites are usually found to be unique to a given strain. This makes the identification of a particular strain much more determinant and reliable. Secondly, in situations where strains are phenotypically and genetically homogeneous, an examination of nucleotides is likely to reveal enough variation to make a discrimination possible that might have otherwise appeared clonal in nature. Finally, genotypic conclusions drawn from DNA sequence data are unambiguous and do not rely on a secondary measurements such as base pair size to make a determination. This is not always the case for fingerprint data where two bands which appear to be identical in size may not always share the same position on the bacterial chromosome.

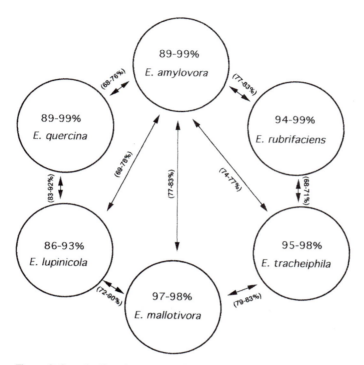

Figure 6 Genetic diversity among select *Erwinia* species based upon *omp*A nucleotide sequences. Genetic similarities were calculated using the Jukes–Cantor distance method (see Chapter 8) and reflect the average similarities of several pairwise strain comparisons. Minimum and maximum sequence similarities within a species are depicted within each circle while mean similarities between species are denoted along the arrows.

5.1 Amplification of the bacterial *omp*A locus

The most straightforward approach to isolating outer membrane genes is by PCR. Several primer pairs have been designed from regions in the gene that show remarkable conservation across the families *Enterobacteriaceae* and *Pasteurellaceae*. While *omp*A sequences have been predominantly reported for enterobacterial species, studies do exist for bacteria in other families (51). The apparent emphasis on characterizing enterobacterial *omp*A genes largely stems from the fact that the family harbours several of the most widely significant and problematic environmental and medical pathogenic species. In addition to enterobacterial isolates, the list of species whose outer membrane molecules have been sequenced and characterized continues to grow, and a substantial number of *omp*A sequences can now be retrieved from GenBank and exploited for species-specific primer design.

5.1.1 *omp*A oligonucleotide sequences

General oligonucleotide primer sequences for amplification of species and strains in the *Enterobacteriaceae* have been available for some time (7). These conserved primers were originally designed from the alignment of cloned *omp*A genes from 17 different species of bacteria in the family and flank regions of sequence heterogeneity across the molecule (7). The sequences for these primers are as follows: [omp280F], 5'-AAAGCTCAGGGCGTTCA-3', and [omp1031R], 5'-GCGGCTGAGTTACAACGTCTT-3'. In conjunction with these oligonucleotides, other primer pairs have been designed for *omp*A gene amplification including: [omp1F], 5'-TGGGTTACCCGATCACTGACGA-3'; [omp2R], 5'-ATGCGGTCGGTG TAGCCCAGAA-3'; [SmompF], 5'-AAAGCTCAGGGCGTTCA-3'; and [SmompR], 5'-GCGGCTGAGTTACAACGTCTTT-3' (50, 54). Primers omp280F/omp1031R yield a 750 bp product and have been used to amplify a number of disparate enterobacterial species. Primer pairs omp1F/omp2R and SmompF/SmompR yield 500 bp and 700 bp products, respectively, and have recently been used to differentiate strains of *Erwinia* as shown in *Figures 4* and *5* (50, 54).

5.1.2 Genomic DNA preparation

Obtaining an amplicon from the outer membrane molecules of most bacterial species relies on a straightforward single copy PCR strategy. Therefore, the quality of genomic DNA is not of serious concern, and rapid strategies for the preparation of bacterial cell lysates (*Protocols 1* and *2*) are generally sufficient for DNA preparation. This is not to say that a more rigorous and high quality DNA extraction protocol (*Protocol 3*) is not acceptable but usually unnecessary.

5.1.3 PCR conditions

As for PCR fingerprint reactions described in *Protocol 4*, a volume of 50 μl is recommended for set up including 50 pmol of each primer. An optimal annealing temperature for primers omp1F/omp2R is 55 °C while omp280F/omp1031R (T_m = 52 °C) and SmompF/SmompR (T_m = 52 °C) both require substantially lower annealing temperatures. Optimal annealing temperatures may fluctuate depending on the primer pairs being used and the particular strains being analysed. The following is a general program for *omp*A amplification: an initial denaturation at 94 °C for 5 min; followed by 94 °C for 1 min, 55 °C for 1 min, and 72 °C for 1.5 min (35 cycles); and ending with an incubation at 72 °C for 10 min. For visualization of *omp*A PCR products, about 10 μl of the reaction should be separated on 1.5% agarose gels constructed from DNA-typing grade agarose (see Section 2.7). A standard mini-gel apparatus will suffice since the purpose of this electrophoresis is to confirm the presence of an *omp*A PCR product for sequencing. Positive PCR products should be purified using Centricon-100 spin columns according to manufacturer's specifications.

5.2 Cloning and DNA sequencing of *omp*A PCR products

In order to obtain the DNA sequences of *omp*A amplicons, several different strategies may be employed including:

(a) Direct automated cycle sequencing of the PCR product (BigDye Terminator Cycle- Sequencing Kit, PE-Applied Biosystems).

(b) Molecular cloning of the PCR product followed by automated cycle sequencing.

(c) Molecular cloning of the product followed by conventional isotopic sequencing.

While specific methodologies involved in sequencing PCR products are beyond the scope of this chapter, these techniques are discussed in detail elsewhere (55). Unless the product is being sequenced directly, a cloning step will be necessary in order to insert the *omp*A gene into a vector amenable to double-stranded cycle sequencing techniques. As these data will likely be used to identify and monitor individual strains, it is highly recommended that both the forward and reverse strands be sequenced before a genotypic determination is made. Plasmids suitable for cloning these products include PCRscript, pBluescript, and pBSK+ (a 'phagemid' vector available from Stratagene). These vectors can easily be modified into TA-cloning cassettes (56), or, alternatively, a TA-vector can now be purchased relatively inexpensively from several different companies. *Protocol 10* provides a rapid and convenient method for the generation of transformation-competent *E. coli* cloning cells (57), and *Protocol 11* is a standard method for cloning PCR products into a TA-vector which relies on ampicillin resistance and blue/white colony formation as the two selections for *omp*A recombinant cells (58, 59).

Protocol 10

A method for the preparation and storage of competent bacterial cells

Reagents

- LB broth pH 6.1: 1% (w/v) tryptone, 0.5% (w/v) yeast extract, 1% NaCl (w/v)

- TSB (transformation and storage buffer): LB broth pH 6.1 containing 10% polyethylene glycol (w/v) (gmw = 3350), 5% DMSO, 10 mM $MgCl_2$, 10 mM $MgSO_4$ (TSB can be stored at $-70\,°C$ for up to one year)

- *E. coli* cloning strain: JM109 (Cat. No. P9751, Promega Corp.) (Note: most cloning strains are acceptable for this procedure; however, strains that are recA⁻ are recommended as these strains lack the ability to recombine episomal DNA with the bacterial chromosome)

Method

1 Grow bacterial cells to an early log phase ($OD_{600} = 0.3$–0.6) in LB broth.

2 Pellet cells by centrifugation (1500 g) for 10 min at 4 °C.

3 Supernatant is discarded and the pellets are resuspended in 1/10th volume of TSB.

4 Incubate the cell suspensions on ice for 10 min and store at $-70\,°C$ for up to three months.

Protocol 11

A strategy for the molecular cloning of PCR products

Equipment and reagents

- LB agar plates: 15% Bacto agar, 10% Bacto tryptone, 5% Bacto yeast extract, 5% NaCl
- LB-amp agar plates: LB agar with 75 µg/ml ampicillin
- ddH$_2$O (molecular biology grade)
- T4 DNA ligase (5 U/µl)
- 5 × T4 DNA ligase buffer: 250 mM Tris–HCl pH 7.6, 50 mM MgCl$_2$, 12.5 mM ATP, 5 mM DTT, 25% (w/v) polyethylene glycol (PEG 8000)
- Purified PCR product (*Protocol 9*)

- TA-cloning vector (TOPO TA-cloning kit, Cat. No. K4500–01, Invitrogen)
- JM109 competent cloning cells (as prepared in *Protocol 10*)
- Super broth: 33% Bacto tryptone, 20% Bacto yeast extract, 7.5% NaCl pH 7.4
- Super broth-ampicillin: super broth with 100 µg/ml ampicillin pH 7.4
- 2% X-Gal (in DMF)
- 100 mM IPTG

A. Ligation

1 To a 1.5 ml tube, add 2 µl of TA-cloning vector (1 µg), 2 µl of 5 × ligase buffer, 1 µl (5 U) of T4 DNA ligase, 5 µl of purified PCR product.

2 Perform a quick spin in a microcentrifuge and incubate the tubes at 14 °C overnight.

B. Transformation

1 Round-bottom 14 ml tubes are placed on ice containing 110 µl of competent *E. coli* cloning cells (JM109 cells from *Protocol 10*) and 7 µl of the ligation reaction (as prepared above). The tubes are incubated on ice for 30 min.

2 The transformation mixture including the cells and ligation is then heat shocked by soaking the tube in a 42 °C water-bath for 1.5 min.

3 Place the tubes on ice again for 2 min.

4 Add 1 ml of super broth (w/o ampicillin) to the tube, cap the top, and incubate at 37 °C for 1 h with gentle rotating (100–150 r.p.m.).

5 While the cells are recovering in super broth, pipette and spread 50 µl of 2% X-Gal and an equal volume of 100 mM IPTG onto a dry LB-amp agar plate. Replace the lid and let the plate dry at 37 °C for 20 min.

6 After 1 h, transfer the cells into a 1.5 ml microcentrifuge tube and spin in a micro-centrifuge for 1 min at 2000 g. Discard the supernatant except for about 60–80 µl which is used to resuspend the pellet thoroughly.

7 Pipette the entire amount of this resuspension onto the LB-amp plates (already containing X-Gal and IPTG). Spread the cells using a sterile glass spreader and place the plates (inverted) in a 37 °C incubator overnight.

8 After an overnight incubation (about 18 h), blue/white selection should have taken place, and white colonies are picked and deposited into 3 ml super broth-ampicillin cultures. These clones are then grown overnight again or until confluent.

9 Harvest the cells by centrifuging the 3 ml culture at 12 000 *g* for 3–5 min. Drain and blot off the supernatant medium and place the pellets at −20°C until they can be mini-prepped and prepared for DNA sequence analysis. Note: a number of inexpensive mini-prep kits are now available that enable rapid and efficient extraction of plasmid DNA. Two that have worked well with this protocol include The Wizard Kit (Promega Corp., Cat. No. A7500) and Qiaprep Spin Kit (Qiagen, Cat. No. 27104).

5.3 Interpretation of *omp*A nucleotide sequence variation

Nucleotide sequence data from the *omp*A region should readily discriminate between closely related strains of bacteria. Nucleotide polymorphisms between closely related strains are frequently identified within outer membrane protein genes. These changes within the *omp*A gene make it possible to reliably identify and discriminate between individual strains. DNA sequence analysis of this gene is an extremely sensitive technique for the differentiation of closely related bacteria and can often yield polymorphisms where other fingerprint-based techniques fail to demonstrate any genetic variability. However, the utility of this gene as an epidemiological tool depends on whether a level of sufficient variation can be ascertained at the nucleotide level. Certainly, one would refrain from making a genotypic identification based on a single nucleotide substitution. Generally, several polymorphisms would be necessary before a reliable and more confident determination could be made. While outer membrane molecules are divergent molecules, a determination of the amount of genetic variation within this gene should be determined for the specific group of strains in question.

In addition to genotyping applications, outer membrane nucleotide data can be examined in a number of time-dependent and phylogenetic comparisons (*Figure 6*). Genetic diversity can be determined between *omp*A alleles using a number of available pairwise distance algorithms designed for DNA sequence data (24). Phylogenetic studies can also be initiated by first subjecting these data to multiple sequence alignment strategies followed by cladistic analysis of the resultant data matrix. *Figure 7* is a phylogenetic tree of *omp*A alleles from 56 strains representing 16 enterobacterial species and serves to emphasize the ability of *omp*A to differentiate closely related strains and species. In this example, every species was resolved in relation to another in the cladogram. The tree was constructed using the maximum parsimony algorithm available in PAUP (Phylogenetic analysis using parsimony) v.3.11 (39, 40). The sequencing of PCR products has made it possible to examine the genotypic diversity of a greater number of strains than ever before, and the protocols presented here serve as a means to this end by coupling the ease and efficiency of PCR with the discriminatory power of automated nucleotide sequence analysis.

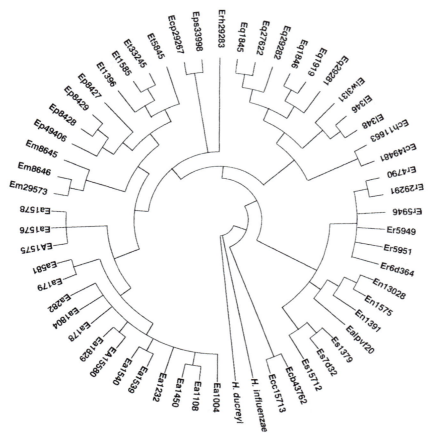

Figure 7 Maximum parsimony phylogenetic trees of *Erwinia* species and strains based on cladistic analysis of 507 nucleotide characters from an *omp*A DNA sequence alignment. The tree shown is a strict consensus cladogram of 18 equally parsimonious topologies and depicts *omp*A nucleotide sequence divergence between *Erwinia* strains and species. The analysis shown resulted from a heuristic parsimony search performed in PAUP v.3.1.1 (40). Abbreviations are as follows: Ea, *Erwinia amylovora*; Em, *E. mallotivora*; Ep, *E. psidii*; Et, *E. tracheiphila*; Ecp, *E. cypripedii*; Eps, *E. psidii*; Erh, *E. rhapontici*; Eq, *E. quercina*; El, *E. lupinicola*; Ech, *E. chrysanthemi*; Ect, *E. cacticida*; Er, *E. rubrifaciens*; En, *E. nigrifluens*; Eal, *E. alni*; Es, *E. salicis*; Ecb, *E. carotovorum* ssp. *betavasculorum*; and Ecc, *E. carotovora* ssp. *carotovora*.

6 Conclusion

The molecular typing of bacterial strains has only reached its developmental outset. As greater amounts of nucleotide sequence data become available from the chromosomes of pathogenic bacterial species and strains, more powerful diagnostic typing probes and protocols should continue to develop for the molecular discrimination of these organisms. As our abilities in molecular sequence analysis continue to improve and as technology continues to consolidate larger regions of the bacterial genome into single screening systems, our ability to not only type strains but to assign these types to meaningful biological properties elicited by a bacterium should be greatly enhanced. The future consolidation of these modifications, along with the standardization of the molecular typing techniques themselves, will aid in making these approaches central to molecular epidemiological strain analysis. Each of the techniques described here is an extremely sensitive measure of genotypic diversity within bacterial populations, while most allow for the rapid and efficient generation of strain-specific bacterial fingerprints. Taken together, these molecular typing methods should offer vast potential in the future characterization of human, animal, and plant pathogenic strains. A wide array of species have already been characterized using these typing strategies (11, 12, 16, 19, 30, 31), and as conditions become more standardized between laboratories, PCR-based typing methods should become commonplace in the molecular epidemiological analysis of bacterial strains.

Acknowledgements

I am indebted to Drs Marc Allard, Jose' Lopez, and Ann Callahan for their useful comments which greatly improved the first draft of this chapter and to the editors of this book for providing a much needed forum for the consolidation of these protocols and techniques. The author would also like to acknowledge Joseph Schluep and Renee Brown for their aid in the development of several figures.

References

1. Howard, J. and Whitcombe, D. M. (ed.) (1995). *Diagnostic bacteriology protocols.* Humana Press, Totowa, New Jersey.
2. Relman, D. A. and Persing, D. H. (1996). In *PCR protocols for emerging infectious diseases* (ed. D. H. Persing), pp. 3–32. ASM Press, Washington, DC.
3. Prescott, L. M., Harley, J. P., and Klein, D. A. (1993). *Microbiology,* 2nd edn. William C. Brown Publ., Dubuque, Iowa.
4. Bochner, B. (1989). *Nature,* **339**, 157.
5. Crichton, P. B. and Old, D. C. (1982). *J. Med. Microbiol.,* **15**, 233.
6. Woese, C. R. (1987). *Microbiol. Rev.,* **51**, 221.
7. Lawrence, J. G., Ochman, H., and Hartl, D. L. (1991). *J. Gen. Microbiol.,* **137**, 1911.
8. Versalovic, J., Schneider, M., DeBruijn, F., and Lupski, J. (1994). *Methods Mol. Cell. Biol.,* **5**, 25.
9. Glassick, T., Giffard, P., and Timms, P. (1996). *Syst. Appl. Microbiol.,* **19**, 457.
10. Gillings, M. (1992). *A manual for the identification of plant pathogenic bacteria using genomic DNA restriction analysis.* Rep. 8th Australasian Plant Path. Soc. Conf. NSW, Australia.
11. Jersek, B., Tcherneva, E., Rijpens, N., and Herman, L. (1996). *Lett. Appl. Microbiol.,* **23**, 55.
12. Ward, N., Rainey, F., Stackebrandt, E., and Schlesner, H. (1995). *Appl. Env. Microbiol.,* **61**, 2270.
13. Lloyd, A. T. and Sharp, P. M. (1993). *J. Mol. Evol.,* **37**, 399.
14. Henderson, I., Duggleby, C. J., and Turnbull, P. C. (1994). *Int. J. Syst. Bacteriol.,* **44**, 99.
15. Ochman, H. and Wilson, A. C. (1988). *J. Mol. Evol.,* **26**, 74.

16. Brown, E. W. (1998). *Ph.D. dissertation.* pp. 11–46. The George Washington University, Washington, DC.
17. Liaud, M. F., Valentin, C., Martin, W., Bouget, F. Y., Kloareg, B., and Cerff, R. (1994). *J. Mol. Evol.*, **38**, 319.
18. Cohan, F. M. (1994). *Trends Ecol. Evol.*, **10**, 192.
19. Harvey, B. S., Koeuth, T., Versalovic, J., Woods, C. R., and Lupski, J. R. (1995). *Infect. Contr. Hosp. Epidemiol.*, **16**, 564.
20. Miller, D. R. and Rossman, A. Y. (1997). In *Biodiversity II: Understanding and protecting our biological resources* (ed. M. L. Reaka-Kurdla, D. E. Wilson, and E. O. Wilson), pp. 217–29. John Henry Press, Washington, DC.
21. Kostman, J. R., Edlind, T. D., Lipuma, J. J., and Stull, T. L. (1992). *J. Clin. Microbiol.*, **30**, 2084.
22. Wilson, K. H., Blitchington, R. B., and Greene, R. C. (1990). *J. Clin. Microbiol.*, **28**, 1942.
23. Versalovic, J., Kapur, V., Koeuth, T., Mazurek, G. H., Whittam, T. S., Musser, J. M., *et al.* (1995). *Arch. Pathol. Lab. Med.*, **119**, 23.
24. Huang, Z. Y., Smalley, E. B., and Guries, R. P. (1995). *Phytopathology*, **85**, 522.
25. Vos, P., Hogers, R., Bleeker, M., Reijans, M., van de Lee, T., Hornes, M., *et al.* (1995). *Nucleic Acids Res.*, **23**, 4407.
26. Nilsson, J., Svensson, B., Ekelund, K., and Christiansson, A. (1998). *Lett. Appl. Microbiol.*, **27**, 168.
27. Marmur, J. (1961). *J. Mol. Biol.*, **3**, 208.
28. Ruiny, R., Breittmayer, V., Elbaze, P., Lafey, B., Bousemarte, O., and Christen, R. (1994). *Int. J. Syst. Bacteriol.*, **44**, 416.
29. Wiedmann, M., Bruce, J. L., Knorr, R., Bodis, M., Cole, E. M., McDowell, C. I., *et al.* (1996). *J. Clin. Microbiol.*, **34**, 1086.
30. Larsen, G. Y., Stull, T., and Burns, J. L. (1993). *J. Clin. Microbiol.*, **31**, 788.
31. Woods, C. R., Versalovic, J., Koeuth, T., and Lupski, J. R. (1993). *J. Clin. Microbiol.*, **31**, 1927.
32. Stern, M. J., Ames, G. F. L., Smith, N. H., Robinson, E. C., and Higgins, C. F. (1984). *Cell*, **7**, 1015.
33. Versalovic, J., Koeuth, T., and Lupski, J. R. (1991). *Nucleic Acids Res.*, **19**, 6823.
34. Sharples, G. J. and Lloyd, R. G. (1990). *Nucleic Acids Res.*, **18**, 6503.
35. De Bruijn, F. J. (1992). *Appl. Env. Microbiol.*, **58**, 2180.
36. Welsh, J. and McClelland, M. (1990). *Nucleic Acids Res.*, **18**, 7213.
37. Hilton, A. C., Banks, J. G., and Penn, C. W. (1997). *Lett. Appl. Microbiol.*, **24**, 243.
38. Traub, W. H., Eiden, A., Leonhard, B., and Bauer, D. (1996). *Zentralblatt fur Bacteriol.*, **284**, 93.
39. Swofford, D. L. and Olsen, G. J. (1990). In *Molecular systematics.* (ed. D. M. Hillis and C. Moritz), pp. 411–501. Sinaur, Sunderland, Massachusetts.
40. Swofford, D. L. (1999). PAUP*, the betaversion. Sinaur, Sunderland, Massachusetts.
41. Felsenstein, J. (1991). PHYLIP: phylogenetic inference package v.3.0. University of Washington, Seattle.
42. Tamplin, M. L., Jackson, J. K., Buchrieser, C., Murphree, R. L., Portier, K. M., Gangar, V., *et al.* (1996). *Appl. Env. Microbiol.*, **62**, 3572.
43. Aquadro, C. F., Noon, W. A., and Begun, D. J. (1992). In *Molecular genetic analysis of populations: a practical approach* (ed. A. R. Hoelzel), pp. 115–57. IRL Press, New York.
44. Giovannetti, L. and Ventura, S. (1995). In *Diagnostic bacteriology protocols* (ed. J. Howard and D. M. Whitcombe), pp. 165–79. Humana Press, Totowa, New Jersey.
45. King, G. J. (1989). *J. Appl. Bacteriol.*, **67**, 489.
46. Khambaty, F. M., Bennett, R. W., and Shah, D. B. (1994). *Epidemiol. Infect.*, **113**, 75.
47. Birren, B. W., Lai, S. M., Clark, L., and Simon, M. I. (1988). *Nucleic Acids Res.*, **16**, 7563.

48. Hillier, A. J. and Davidson, B. E. (1995). *Methods Mol. Microbiol.*, **46**, 149.
49. Zhang, Y. and Geider, K. (1997). *Appl. Env. Microbiol.*, **63**, 4421.
50. Brown, E. W., Janisiewicz, W., and van der Zwet, T. (1996). *Phytopathology*, **86**, 89.
51. Kaltenboeck, B., Kousoulas, K. G., and Storz, J. (1993). *J. Bacteriol.*, **175**, 487.
52. Freudl, R. and Cole, S. T. (1983). *Eur. J. Biochem.*, **134**, 497.
53. Braun, G. and Cole, S. T. (1984). *Mol. Gen. Genet.*, **195**, 321.
54. Brown, E. W. and van der Zwet, T. (1996). *Phytopathology*, **86**, 120.
55. Hoelzel, A. R. and Green, A. (1992). In *Molecular genetic analysis of populations: a practical approach* (ed. A. R. Hoelzel), pp. 159–87. IRL Press, New York.
56. Marchuk, D., Drumm, M., Saulino, A., and Collins, F. S. (1991). *Nucleic Acids Res.*, **19**, 1154.
57. Chung, C. T., Miemela, S. L., and Miller, R. H. (1989). *Proc. Natl. Acad. Sci. USA*, **86**, 2172.
58. Manniatis, T., Fritsch, E., and Sambrook, J. (ed.) (1982). *Molecular cloning: a laboratory manual*. Cold Spring Harbor Press, Cold Spring Harbor, New York.
59. Holton, T. A. and Graham, M. W. (1991). *Nucleic Acids. Res.*, **19**, 234.

Chapter 3

Detection and quantification of heterogeneous viral targets: HIV as a model

Shirley Kwok

Roche Molecular Systems, Inc. 1145 Atlantic Ave, Alameda, CA 94501, USA

1 Introduction

The diversity of the human immunodeficiency virus (HIV) genome presents it as one of the most difficult targets for the development of nucleic acid-based assays. The extensive genetic variability of HIV is primarily due to the high error rates of the viral reverse transcriptase (3.4×10^{-5} per base incorporated) and the absence of proofreading mechanisms (1). HIV-1 and HIV-2 comprise the two groups of viruses that cause AIDS. The HIV-1s are divided into three groups: M (for Major), O (for Outlier), and N (for non-M, non-O). The HIV-1 group M and HIV-2 viruses have been further divided into subtypes A-K and A-G, respectively, based on phylogenetic analysis of proviral sequences (ref. 2; see Chapter 8). The group O viruses are as heterogeneous as the group M viruses and comprise a number of distinct genetic subtypes that remain to be identified and characterized (3). The recently identified, HIV-1 group N viruses are distinct from group M and O (4). Within individuals, HIV-1 undergoes continuous genetic changes; patients usually harbour a swarm of highly related but individually distinguishable viral variants, which are referred to as quasispecies. Genomic recombination between two different HIV-1 populations frequently occurs *in vivo*, which further contributes to HIV genetic variability.

The heterogeneity within and between the virus groups makes it extremely difficult to design a single primer-pair/probe system that efficiently amplifies and detects all variants of HIV-1 (groups M, N, and O) and HIV-2. Consequently, most efforts have focused on designing systems that efficiently amplify each of these viruses separately. The first part of this chapter provides guidelines for designing primers and probes for the amplification and detection of HIV, but the rules can be broadly applied to all heterogeneous targets. Additionally, the parameters for increasing assay sensitivity, specificity, and reducing false positives are applicable to all targets. The second part of the chapter provides protocols for the extraction, amplification, detection, and quantification of HIV RNA and DNA.

2 Impact of sequence heterogeneity on PCR

Efficient detection of viral targets by nucleic acid-based assays depends on the ability of the oligonucleotides to hybridize and form a stable bond to the target. Mismatches between the oligonucleotides and the targeted nucleic acid can affect duplex stability and may compromise the ability of a system to amplify and/or detect the targeted sequence. Mismatches are particularly problematic when assays of high sensitivity are required and/or when quantification of viral load is desired.

The degree to which mismatches affect PCR depends on the:

(a) Number of mismatches.

(b) Types of mismatches.

(c) Position of mismatches.

(d) Length of the oligonucleotides.

(e) Temperature of hybridization.

(f) Presence of co-solvents.

(g) Concentration of oligonucleotides

(h) Concentration of monovalent and divalent cations.

Mismatches at the 3′ terminus of a primer are most detrimental to PCR. However, not all mismatches have the same effect. Using an HIV model system, Kellogg *et al.* demonstrated that while C:C, G:G, and A:A mismatches were most detrimental to PCR, primers with 3′ terminal T were efficiently extended even when mismatched with a C, T, or G (5). Mismatches at the 5′ end of a primer are less detrimental to PCR. It is well known that primers with restriction endonuclease sites added to the 5′ end are readily extended provided that the number of target-specific bases are sufficient to form a stable hybrid between the primer and the template.

Single base mismatches that are 1, 2, or 3 bases from the 3′ terminus had little effect on amplification while multiple internal mismatches had varied effects, depending on the number and location of the mismatches. The presence of multiple mismatches equally distributed throughout a 30 base oligonucleotide was detrimental to PCR, as were multiple mismatches near the 3′ terminus. Christopherson *et al.* observed that two to four mismatches in the primer–template duplexes did not have a significant effect on RT-PCR of the same HIV model system. However, the presence of five and six mismatches within the 28 and 30 base primers reduced PCR product yield by 22- and 100-fold respectively, relative to the homologous template (6).

Mismatches between the template and the reverse transcribing (downstream) primer should affect only the reverse transcription step while mismatches with the upstream primer are expected to affect only the first cycle of amplification. Once a mismatched template is copied, the primers are fully complementary to the PCR products in all subsequent cycles. As heteroduplexes formed between the reverse transcribing primer and RNA templates are more stable than DNA–DNA duplexes, mismatches to the RT primer should be better tolerated.

3 Primer and probe design for HIV

The design of primers and probes that efficiently amplify and detect all HIV subtypes represents one of the major challenges for nucleic acid amplification technologies. While primers and probes can be designed to amplify a large fraction of isolates, the identification of a single primer-pair/probe system that efficiently amplifies all variant isolates is a formidable task. The effort required for primer and probe design for HIV depends on the intended use of the assay. For studies where the sequence of an isolate is known, or where efficient amplification of all isolates is not required, primer design is relatively straightforward. On the other hand, if the primers and probes are to be used in a diagnostic or screening mode, considerable thought is required in designing primers and probes that will provide maximum mismatch tolerance.

3.1 Sequence selection

In designing primers and probes for HIV, several rules have been applied. First and most foremost, is the selection of highly conserved regions that can serve as primer and probe binding sites. As the *env* region of HIV is subjected to extensive genetic variation, regions within the *gag*, *pol*, and LTR are often targeted for amplification. The sequence database for the *gag* region of HIV-1 is quite extensive and is more likely to reflect the diversity of viruses in circulation. By comparison, the number of sequences for the LTR and *pol* regions are relatively few so it remains to be seen whether the currently identified conserved regions will be maintained as more sequences become available. Second, is the design of longer primers. Primers that are 28–30 bases in length are better at accommodating a small number of mutations. Third, is to design primers that amplify a region that is no more than 300 bases in length to ensure efficient reverse transcription and amplification. In general, amplification efficiency is inversely proportional to the length of the PCR product. Fourth, where possible, is to design primers that terminate in a T as 3′ terminal Ts can be extended when hybridized to non-As.

3.1.1 Consensus and degenerate primers

Consensus primers are generally not completely matched with any one isolate but have a sequence in which each base represents the 'consensus' of all the known isolates. The consensus approach can work quite well if the number of mismatches are equally distributed among the variants and kept to a minimum.

Degenerate primers contain a pool of primers where all possible mutations are represented. This approach works best when the degree of degeneracy is relatively low. As the degree of degeneracy increases, the number of sequences that are completely homologous to the target becomes increasingly small. The T_m for the correct primer in such a mixture is reduced due to a lowering of its relative concentration. To compensate for the lower T_m, the hybridization steps need to be carried out at a lower temperature. As a consequence, amplification efficiencies with degenerate primers can be poor and reaction specificity low.

To reduce degeneracy, universal nucleosides such as 3′ nitropyrrole deoxynucleoside have been substituted at ambiguous sites in the DNA (7). These nucleosides lower the T_m of an oligonucleotide but have approximately equal affinity for the four natural deoxynucleotides. Universal purine and pyrimidine bases serve a similar function. Deoxyinosine residues have been erroneously used to compensate for degeneracy in the target sequences. However, it is now known that deoxyinosine is not a neutral base and that it preferentially binds dC (8).

To improve amplification of mismatched templates, several strategies can be implemented to stabilize oligo–template duplexes. Primer–template mismatch tolerance can be increased by either lowering the stringency of the hybridization or by increasing the stability of the primer–template duplexes. Substitution of modified bases such as 5-methyldeoxycytosine or bromodeoxycytosine for cytosine, 2,6-diaminopurine for adenosine, and propynl dU for thymine increases T_m and stabilizes binding of the primer to the template (8).

3.2 Reaction conditions and cycling parameters

Reaction components and thermal cycling parameters can be tailored to favour mismatch tolerance. In addition to longer primers, higher concentrations of enzyme, cations, and/or dNTPs favour mismatch accommodations. Long annealing times coupled with lower annealing temperatures also favour mismatch tolerance, as do longer extension times. To accommodate mutations in the RT primer, a gradual step-up of the RT temperature has been shown to improve mismatch tolerance (6). The gradual temperature increase presumably facilitates the priming and extension of the mismatched duplex. However, it is important to bear in mind that parameters that favour mismatch tolerance also result in decreased specificity, and ultimately sensitivity.

For HIV, the amplification conditions need to be sufficiently relaxed to allow amplification and detection of all divergent isolates, but yet sufficiently stringent to minimize non-specific amplifications. Ideally, optimizations should be performed with a set of isolates with mutations that represent that desired range of detection.

4 Assay sensitivity and specificity

As the number of copies of HIV in a clinical sample is often low, highly efficient amplifications are required to achieve maximum sensitivity. The sensitivity of an assay is highly dependent on the specificity of the reaction, which is largely conferred by the oligonucleotides selected for amplification. Candidate HIV primers and probes should be screened against sequence databases of related organisms, such as HTLV-I, -II, and the human genome to ensure that there are no strong homologies. The most common non-specific products that compromise assay sensitivity are 'primer–dimers'. Primer–dimers are a heterogeneous mix of products that are formed by the two primers alone. Sequencing of these products revealed that primer–dimers may consist of just the two primers alone, or more often a family of random sequences with 1–30 bases inserted between the two primers.

The prevention of primer–dimer formation remains an area of interest. Several methodologies have been introduced to help minimize primer–dimer formation and improve assay specificity (9–13). As non-specific primer extension often occurs during reaction set up, most procedures have focused on either preventing primer extension during reaction set up, or in destroying products formed during PCR set up. The former includes the use of physical barriers such as wax to sequester an essential PCR component (10) or by using DNA polymerases that have been reversibly inactivated through the use of monoclonal antibodies (11) or by chemical modifications, as in AmpliTaq Gold (12). In the latter, dUTP has been used in the amplification and uracil-N-glycosylase (UNG) has been employed to cleave dU-extended products that were made prior to thermal cycling (13). These dU-containing products may consist of both non-specific products as well as extensions of the specific target. Following UNG treatment, the templates are denatured at 95°C and the temperature of the reactions are maintained at or above the annealing temperature. The stringency of these conditions significantly reduces non-specific amplifications. In a different approach, Zangenberg *et al.* showed that using double A-terminated primers can reduce non-specific primer interactions (9).

5 Preventing false positives from PCR carryover

With the ability to amplify a single molecule, cross-contamination of samples during sample preparation or contamination of reactions with PCR products can lead to false positives. Although dUTP and UNG have been instrumental in reducing non-specific amplification, their primary role is to minimize or eliminate false positives through the inactivation of carryover PCR products (14). The principle of dUTP/UNG inactivation is to replace dTTP with dUTP in the amplifications and to treat all subsequent fully assembled reactions with UNG. UNG cleaves the uracil base from the phosphodiester backbone of uracil-containing DNA but has no effect on natural thymine-containing DNA. The resulting abasic site blocks replication by DNA polymerases, and is highly susceptible to alkaline hydrolysis at elevated temperatures, and subsequent strand scission. The slightly alkaline pH and high temperature conditions of PCR are sufficient to render the templates unsuitable for amplification. Aside from adding dUTP and UNG to the reactions, this inactivation approach is virtually invisible to the user. An equal molar substitution of dUTP for dTTP is generally sufficient. However, some slight modifications may be required to improve overall amplification efficiency. In some systems, doubling the dUTP concentration with a concomitant increase in $MgCl_2$ or MnOAc may be required. For

A:T-rich templates such as HIV, a mixture of dUTP/dTTP (10:1) resulted in more reproducible amplifications. Each reaction is initiated with a 2 min incubation at 45–50°C, to facilitate UNG cleavage. The amount of UNG required to cleave and inactivate PCR products varies from system to system and may be affected by the A:T content of the amplicon. In general, two units of UNG are sufficient to cleave a million copies of dU-containing product.

The use of dUTP and UNG, however, should not replace good laboratory practices (15). Separate areas for pre- and post-PCR activities are highly recommended. Dead air boxes work extremely well for setting up amplification reactions. In addition to providing a confined work area, most are equipped with UV lights that can be activated after use to destroy any contaminating nucleic acids which may have been inadvertently transferred into the work area. Special precaution must also be taken to ensure that reagents and supplies are prepared, processed, and stored in 'clean' areas that are free of target or amplified products. The use of positive displacement pipettes or plugged tips have had a significant impact in reducing false positives.

In contrast to the pre-amplification product inactivation strategy of dUTP/UNG, post-amplification inactivation of PCR products has also been described. Post-amplification inactivation of PCR products can be accomplished with photochemical reagents such as psoralens and isopsoralens (13). These furocoumarins contain two reactive double bonds, which, when excited with UV light, covalently bind to the nucleic acid polymers by forming cyclobutane adducts with pyrimidine bases. These modified products are refractory to PCR as the furocoumarin–pyrimidine adducts block the template-dependent extensions by *Taq* DNA polymerase. Copper phenantholine has also been employed to cleave double-stranded DNA post-amplification (16).

6 Amplification target: DNA vs. RNA

HIV is an RNA virus that replicates through a DNA intermediate. Upon entering the cell, the virus uncoats its envelope and the RNA is reversed transcribed to single-stranded DNA. Following second strand synthesis, the resulting linear double-stranded DNA product either remains unintegrated or is integrated into the host genome to give proviral DNA. Either RNA or DNA can serve as targets for amplification; the RNA assays target free virus in the plasma while the DNA assays target unintegrated and integrated proviral DNA in the peripheral blood mononuclear cells (PBMCs). The DNA assays are generally used to screen for HIV infections in babies born to infected mothers, whereas the RNA assays are used to measure response to antiviral therapy. Virus in the plasma is indicative of active viral replication whereas viral DNA is present in both actively replicating and latently infected cells. The simplicity of the DNA extraction protocol and the less stringent sample storage requirement for cells, makes DNA a particularly attractive target, especially in developing countries.

Qualitative and quantitative assays have been developed for both HIV RNA and DNA. The protocols described in this chapter were developed for qualitative amplification and detection of HIV-1 DNA in PBMCs and for quantitative amplification and detection of HIV-1 RNA in plasma.

7 Qualitative vs. quantitative assays

While qualitative assays provide a sensitive means to detect the infectious agents, quantitative assays provide a means to directly measure the amount of pathogen in a given specimen. In recent years, the development of a quantitative PCR assay for plasma HIV RNA has played a major role in assessing therapeutic efficacy. The qualitative and quantitative assays differ in many aspects. For a quantitative assay, extra precautions are required to ensure that the samples are properly handled and sample integrity maintained (see Chapter 6 for further discussion of low copy DNA amplification). The efficiency of virus recovery, nucleic acid extraction, amplification, and detection must be reproducible so that results from one sample can be directly compared to another.

8 Importance of internal controls and quantitation standards

Nucleic acids extracted from clinical specimens are generally of reasonable quality to allow efficient amplification. However, on occasion, a clinical specimen may contain impurities that inhibit amplification. Unless inhibition can be successfully ruled out, negative amplification results do not necessarily indicate the absence of infection. Two approaches have been described to monitor inhibition. One approach is to amplify a normal cellular sequence that is present in all samples (17). This approach has the advantage of monitoring the integrity of the nucleic acid in the sample. A negative result with the endogenous sequence indicates improper sample collection, storage, processing, or the presence of an inhibitor. Disadvantages to the use of a cellular sequence are:

(a) A different primer set is required.

(b) The cellular sequences are often present at a much higher copy number than the target.

The disparity in copy number between a cellular sequence and the target sequence can lead to differential amplification efficiencies. Additionally, the higher copy cellular sequence may be less sensitive to reaction variability than the lower copy viral target.

A second approach is to amplify a synthetic internal control (IC) (18). The IC can be either DNA or RNA, but should be the same nucleic acid as the target molecule. The IC is designed to have the same primer binding sites as the target and to generate a product of the same size and base composition. The intervening sequences are scrambled allowing the IC product to be detected with a different probe. While this strategy will not address sample integrity, it overcomes the disadvantages of the endogenous sequences. The commercially available PCR-based assays use this approach.

The ICs used in the qualitative assays can also serve as quantitation standards (QS) for the quantitative assays. To quantify HIV RNA in plasma, a known copy number of a QS RNA transcript is added to the lysed specimen and carried through extraction, amplification, and detection. The final recovery of the QS is indicative of the combined efficiency at each step.

In order for the IC to qualify as a QS, it must fulfil several performance criteria. First, the QS must be recovered at the same efficiency as the target during sample preparation. Secondly, the QS must be reverse transcribed and amplified with the same efficiency as the target. Thirdly, perturbations to the reactions must affect amplification of the QS and HIV similarly. Finally, the HIV and QS probes must capture their respective products with the same efficiency.

The QS is a critical and necessary component to the quantitative assays as slight decreases in amplification efficiency lead to large differences in the final copy number determinations. For example, a 10% decrease in amplification efficiency at each cycle results in about a 5-fold decrease in product yield after 30 cycles of amplification; a 20% decrease in efficiency results in about a 25-fold decrease in product yield. Unless systems can be developed that reproducibly extract, amplify, and detect every sample with the same efficiency each time, the QS will be essential for accurate quantification.

8.1 Construction of the IC/QS

The IC/QS can be constructed by ligating overlapping oligonucleotides that are about 40 bases in length. The oligonucleotides used to construct the 5′ and 3′ termini of the QS contain restriction endonuclease sites. Following ligation, the fragment is cleaved with the respective restriction enzymes and cloned into a vector, restricted with the same enzymes. The vector of choice will depend on the application. If the fragments are cloned into a transcription vector such as pSP64 with poly(A), both plasmid DNA and RNA transcripts can be generated. Further selection of full-length RNA transcripts could be achieved with an oligo(dT) column.

8.2 Quantitation of the QS

Since the QS is used to determine the copy number of the target, an accurate copy number assignment for the QS is essential. The copy number of the QS/IC is determined by spectrophotometric readings at OD_{260}. A working stock concentration of about 10^4 copies/ml is prepared and then serially diluted to the single copy level. At least 100 reactions at the single copy level are amplified and the number determined by Poisson analysis. This number is then used to back calculate the copy number of the intermediate stocks. An input copy number of about 100 copies QS/PCR is typically used for the quantitative assays; 20 copies are used for the qualitative assays to maximize sensitivity to reaction variability.

9 Evaluation of assay performance

To adequately evaluate the performance of the quantitative assays, well-characterized samples of known copy numbers are essential. The copy number of the sample should ideally be determined with a procedure that is different from the test methodology. For HIV, electron microscopy has been used to quantify the number of virus particles in each cultured virus stock. Viral stocks are diluted to a predetermined copy number and then amplified with the target primers.

As clinical isolates or culture stocks for the variant isolates are not always available, synthetic RNA provides a good alternative. In this approach, a region containing the mutations of interest is constructed by ligation of overlapping oligonucleotides (similar to the construction of the quantitation standards) and cloned into a transcription vector. RNA transcripts from these clones can be quantified as described above and then used in amplification reactions.

10 Qualitative HIV DNA assay

The protocols that follow were developed using many of the guidelines described above for increasing assay specificity and maximizing mismatch tolerance.

10.1 Sample collection for HIV DNA amplification

Blood should be collected in either acid citrate dextrose (yellow top) or in EDTA (lavender top) vacutainers. Heparinized (green top) blood has not been validated with this procedure.

The specimens should be transported and stored at 2–25°C. PBMCs should be separated from whole blood within four days of collection. PBMCs can be separated from whole blood either by differentially lysing the red blood cells with saponin or by Ficoll-Hypaque gradient centrifugation. Specimens should not be frozen prior to separation of PBMCs.

Protocol 1

Preparation of cell pellets from whole blood for HIV DNA PCR

Equipment and reagents

- Microcentrifuge (max RCF 16 000 g) Eppendorf 5415C
- Sarstedt 2 ml screw-cap tubes, sterile (72.693.005 or 72.694.005)
- Sterile gauze strips
- Micropipetters
- Micropipettes with plugged tips
- Vortex mixer
- Specimen wash buffer (Roche Molecular Systems)

Method

1 Draw blood into EDTA or ACD tube and process as soon as possible.

2 To each Sarstedt tube, add 1 ml specimen wash buffer using disposable sterile pipettes.

3 Gently mix whole blood specimen in vacutainer vial, surround cap with gauze strip to avoid splashing of blood, and carefully remove cap. Using a sterile pipette, carefully transfer 0.5 ml of whole blood to each Sarstedt tube containing specimen wash buffer.

4 Replace cap on Sarstedt tube and seal tightly. Mix blood with specimen wash buffer by inverting tubes five to ten times. Let samples stand at room temperature for 5 min and mix again by inversion. Let samples stand for an additional 5 min at room temperature.

5 Centrifuge samples for 3 min at room temperature in a tabletop microcentrifuge at 12 000–15 000 g force.

6 Locate pellet in tube. Aspirate supernatant being careful not to disturb pellet. To the pellet, add 1 ml specimen wash buffer, vortex such that pellet is resuspended, and centrifuge as in step 5.

7 Repeat step 6. Aspirate supernatant being careful not to disturb pellet. Pellet should appear clear or light coloured with no red blood cell contamination. Pellets can be extracted directly (*Protocol 3*) or stored at −20 °C until ready for extraction.

Protocol 2

Preparation of Ficoll-Hypaque separated cells for DNA PCR

Equipment and reagents

- Centrifuge with swinging-bucket rotor
- Microcentrifuge
- Ficoll-Hypaque solution
- Sterile transfer pipette
- Sarstedt tubes
- Phosphate-buffered saline (PBS)

Method

1 Collect patient whole blood in EDTA or ACD tubes.

2 Pipette 3 ml of Ficoll-Hypaque into the bottom of a conical centrifuge tube. Carefully layer 3 ml of whole blood on top of the Ficoll-Hypaque solution.

3 Centrifuge the tube at 20–24 °C for 30 min at 400 g in a swinging-bucket rotor.

4 The layer of mononuclear leukocytes will appear as an opaque band between the Ficoll-Hypaque solution and the plasma. Remove with a sterile transfer pipette, the upper layer to within 0.5 cm of the opaque interface. Discard the upper layer.

Protocol 2 continued

5 Carefully transfer the mononuclear layer with a sterile transfer pipette and place it in a new conical centrifuge tube.

6 Add 10 ml of PBS, mix with gentle aspiration with a sterile transfer pipette.

7 Centrifuge at 250 g for 10 min at 20–24 °C to pellet the cells.

8 Aspirate the supernatant and discard.

9 Resuspend the cell pellet with 5 ml PBS and mix by gentle aspiration with a sterile transfer pipette.

10 Centrifuge at 2500 g.

11 Repeat steps 8–10 and resuspend the cell pellet in 0.5 ml PBS.

12 Enumerate the cells and adjust the sample with sterile PBS to achieve a concentration of 1×10^6 PBMC/ml. Dispense into 1 ml aliquots into Sarstedt tubes. If enumeration cannot be performed, resuspend the pellet in 2.5 ml of PBS and dispense into two 1 ml aliquots.

13 Centrifuge for 3 min at the highest speed in a microcentrifuge (about 12 000 g). Aspirate the supernatant without disturbing the pellet.

14 Store the pellet at −70 °C until ready for extraction.

10.2 DNA extraction from cells

HIV DNA can be extracted directly from PBMC pellets (Protocol 1) or after separation by Ficoll-Hypaque gradient centrifugation (Protocol 2). The cells are extracted with a solution containing proteinase K and detergent. After inactivation of proteinase K, the sample can be amplified directly by PCR. PBMCs that have been separated on a Ficoll-Hypaque gradient and stored in RPMI with DMSO, can be washed with PBS and processed in the identical manner.

Protocol 3

Extraction of DNA from PBMCs

Equipment and reagents

- Microcentrifuge
- Dry heat blocks (60 °C ± 2 °C and 100 °C ± 2 °C containing sand)
- Lysis reagent: 10 mM Tris–HCl pH 8.3, 50 mM KCl, 2.5 mM $MgCl_2$, 1% Tween 20, 1% NP-40, 120 µg/ml proteinase K
- Vortex
- Specimen wash solution (Roche Molecular Systems)
- Phosphate-buffered saline (PBS)
- Internal control at 50 copies/µl

Method

1 Thaw specimens at room temperature.

Protocol 3 continued

2 Prepare the working extraction reagent by adding the internal control (IC). Determine the number of samples to be extracted. Use 200 μl of extraction reagent for each extraction. Calculate the amount of IC to add to the lysis buffer to give 120 copies/ 200 μl of lysis buffer.

3 Add 200 μl extraction buffer to the cell pellets. (Note: for cells that are stored in DMSO, pellet the cells by spinning in a microcentrifuge for 3 min at maximum speed. Remove supernatant. Add 1 ml of specimen wash solution to each tube, re-cap, and vortex to resuspend the pellet; microcentrifuge the tubes for 3 min at maximum speed. Remove supernatant. Repeat once more for a total of two washes. Add 200 μl lysis reagent.)

4 Incubate all tubes for 30 min at 60 °C (± 2 °C) in a dry heat block (containing sand to provide for more even heating).

5 Incubate all tubes for 30 min at 100 °C (± 2 °C) in a dry heat block (containing sand).

6 Vortex samples briefly.

7 Microcentrifuge samples for 3 sec.

8 The specimens are now ready for amplification.

10.3 Preparation of DNA from dried blood spots

The testing of dried blood spots (DBSs) for the presence of HIV has proven to be particularly valuable in developing countries and isolated rural regions (19). The ease and economy of DBS sampling, the minute volumes required, and the unexpected stability of the nucleic acid suggest that DBSs will be particularly valuable for small volume neonatal samples and large, population-based studies.

Protocol 4

Dried blood spot extraction

Equipment and reagents

- Hole puncher
- Alcohol and flame
- Vacuum aspirator
- Forceps
- P200 and P1000 micropipetters
- P200 and P1000 micropipettes with plugged tips
- Vortex

- Shaker
- Stir plate
- Magnetic stir bar
- Sarstedt tubes
- Heat block at 100 °C
- Chelex extraction reagent (Perkin Elmer)
- Specimen wash solution (Roche Molecular Systems)

Method

1 Aliquot 1 ml specimen wash solution to the required number of 1.5 ml Sarstedt tubes.

Protocol 4 continued

2   For each dried blood spot sample, dip the hole punch in alcohol and flame sterilize. Excise a ¼″ circle onto a fresh paper towel using the flamed punch, then place in the specimen wash solution using flamed forceps and re-cap the tube.

3   Vortex for 10 sec to wet the filters thoroughly.

4   Incubate the samples for 60 min at room temperature on a shaker set at approximately 1000 r.p.m.

5   Centrifuge the samples for 1 min at high speed to remove the wash solution from the caps and bring the spot to the bottom of the tube.

6   Uncap the tubes and remove the red-tinged specimen wash solution using a vacuum aspirator fitted with fresh pipette tip for each sample. Make sure the tube is as dry as possible by removing any specimen wash solution trapped between the spot and the wall of the tube.

7   Add 200 μl DNA extraction solution to each sample making sure that the sample is thoroughly saturated. Use P1000 tips as the resin particles are too large to be pipetted accurately with the smaller bore tips. (Note: the DNA extraction solution must be stirred constantly at moderate speed on the stir plate during pipetting in order to keep the resin completely suspended. Decreased resin concentration in the sample may lower the extraction efficiency.)

8   Vortex the samples vigorously for 10 sec.

9   Place the samples in a heat block set at 100°C, making sure each filter circle is immersed in the liquid at the bottom of the tube; incubate for 30 min.

10 Vortex the samples vigorously for 10 sec making sure that the filter papers are immersed in the liquid.

11 Incubate the samples for an additional 30 min at 100°C.

12 Vortex the samples vigorously for 10 sec.

13 Centrifuge the specimens for 3 min at high speed to pellet the resin.

14 Using a P200 pipettor with plugged tips and being careful to avoid the resin at the bottom of the tube, transfer the supernatant to a clean tube. The extracted DNA is now ready for amplification.

10.4 DNA amplification

Numerous primers for HIV have been described in the literature. Two commonly used primer-pairs are SK38–SK39 (20) and SK462–SK431 (6). The latter is used in the commercially available AMPLICOR® HIV-1 and AMPLICOR HIV-1 MONITOR™ tests (Roche Molecular Systems). Both of these primer sets amplify conserved regions of the *gag* gene. The region defined by primers SK462 and SK431 was among the most conserved between HIV-1 and HIV-2ROD. However, as the database expanded, it became apparent that this conservation did not extend to other isolates of HIV-2. Even more disconcerting was the discovery that some divergent non-subtype B isolates were also not efficiently amplified. As a consequence, an HIV-1 specific primer-pair, SK145–SKCC1B, was developed to accommodate these variants (21). SK145 has two base changes relative to SK462 and is highly homologous to the majority of HIV-1 isolates. SKCC1B overlaps with SK431 and was designed to reduce the number of mismatches across all subtypes, particularly subtype G. This primer-pair, which was subsequently incorporated into the AMPLICOR HIV-1 MONITOR™ version 1.5 Test, amplifies a 155 bp sequence in the p24 region of *gag* (see Table 1).

Table 1 Primers and probe for HIV-1 group M amplification and detection

Oligonucleotide	Function	Sequence (5′–3′)
SK145	Primer	AGTGGGGGGACATCAAGCAGCCATGCAAAT
SKCC1B	Primer	TACTAGTAGTTCCTGCTATGTCACTTCC
SK102	Probe	GAGACCATCAATGAGGAAGCTGCAGAATGGGAT

The following protocol has worked well for several HIV primer-pairs, including SK38–39 and SK462–431. Other primer-pair systems may require optimization of MgCl$_2$, enzyme concentrations, and thermal cycling parameters. Amplifications are performed with biotinylated primers and the products are detected colorimetrically on microwell plates.

Protocol 5

DNA amplification

Equipment and reagents

- Pipettors, 50 µl to 1000 µl volume capability
- Aerosol-resistant pipettor tips
- Eppendorf repeat pipettor
- 1.25 ml sterile Eppendorf repeater tips
- 500 µl microcentrifuge tubes
- 1.5 ml microcentrifuge tubes
- MicroAmp® reaction tubes and caps
- MicroAmp® tray, retainers, and base (for Perkin Elmer GeneAmp® PCR System 9600)

- Thermal cycler (Perkin Elmer GeneAmp® PCR System 9600; other thermal cycles can be used, but conditions such as cycling temperatures may need to be adjusted)
- Mastermix, recipe for 2 × reaction mixture (for one reaction): 20 mM Tris–HCl pH 8.3, 100 mM KCl, 5 mM MgCl$_2$, 400 µM each dATP, dUTP, dCTP, and dGTP, 20 µM dTTP, 2 U AmpliTaq® DNA polymerase (Perkin Elmer), 2 U UNG (Perkin Elmer), glass distilled water: q.s. to 50 µl

Method

1 Prepare master mix for the desired number of reactions.

2 Place reaction tubes in MicroAmp™ tray and lock tubes in position with tube retainer.

3 Dispense 50 µl of mastermix into MicroAmp reaction tubes.

4   Add 50 µl extracted DNA (Protocols 3 or 4) into each tube. Cap tubes.

5   Place the sample tray into the thermal cycler sample block.

6   Program the thermal cycler as follows:

   (a) 2 min at 50 °C (for UNG inactivation).

   (b) 10 sec 95 °C, 10 sec 55 °C, 10 sec 72 °C, for 4 cycles.

   (c) 10 sec 90 °C, 10 sec 60 °C, 10 sec 72 °C, for 30 cycles.

   (d) 15 min 72 °C.

7   Carefully remove caps from the reaction tube to avoid aerosolizing the amplicons. Immediately pipette 100 µl of denaturation solution (0.4 M NaOH) into each tube using a multichannel pipettor and plugged tips to inactivate any residual UNG activity. Mix by pipetting up and down five times. The amplified products are ready for detection. The denatured amplification reaction mixtures can be stored at 2–8 °C for up to one week.

10.5 Colorimetric microwell plate detection

The qualitative and quantitative assays described in this chapter use a microwell plate detection format. Following amplification, the biotinylated amplification products are denatured with NaOH, and then captured on microwell plates coated with either the HIV or the IC/QS probe.

Protocol 6

Preparation of coated microwell plates

Equipment and reagents

- Microwell plates with cover
- Incubator
- 1 M ammonium acetate
- Desiccant pouch
- Sealed bag (Zip-Loc or Seal-a-Meal)

- HIV and IC Probe
- Wash buffer: 2.68 mM KCl, 137 mM NaCl, 1.47 mM KH_2PO_4, 8.03 mM Na_2HPO_4, 1 mM EDTA

Method

1   Prepare 1 M ammonium acetate (must be made fresh as the reagent is unstable) containing the probe. (In general, probe concentrations of 50–200 ng/100 µl have worked well, but the optimal concentration needs to be determined empirically for each system.)

2   Coat one plate with 100 µl of the IC probe, and one with 100 µl of the HIV probe.

3   Cover plate with microwell cover.

Protocol 6 continued

4 Incubate plate at 37°C for 10–20 h and then wash each well twice with 300 μl of wash buffer.

5 Remove all excess wash buffer. Pat plates dry.

6 Air dry plates for at least 2 h at room temperature. Store plates at 4°C in a sealed bag containing a desiccant pouch (SORB-IT®, Belen, NM).

7 Plates are stable when stored dry at 4°C for at least one month.

Protocol 7

Colorimetric microwell plate detection for the qualitative DNA assay

Equipment and reagents

- Pipettors, 50 μl to 1000 μl volume capability
- Multichannel pipette
- Aerosol-resistant pipettor tips
- Retainer tray holder
- 10 ml pipettes
- Disposable reagent reservoirs
- Tabletop microcentrifuge
- Microwell plate washer (optional)
- Microwell plate reader
- Incubator 37°C ± 2°C
- Graduated vessels
- HIV microwell plates

- IC microwell plates
- Denaturation solution: 0.4 M NaOH
- 10 × wash solution (Roche Molecular Systems)
- Hybridization buffer (Roche Molecular Systems)
- Avidin–horseradish peroxidase conjugate
- Substrate A: 0.001% H_2O_2
- Substrate B: 0.01% 3,3′,5,5′-tetramethylbenzidine in 40% dimethylformamide
- Stop reagent: 1 M sulfuric acid

Method

1 Warm all reagents to room temperature. Remove the appropriate number of microwell strips from their packages and set into the microwell plate frame. Two detection microwells are needed for each amplification reaction: one for the HIV and one for the internal control.

2 Add 100 μl hybridization buffer to each well to be tested using a multichannel pipettor.

3 Using plugged tips, pipette 25 μl of each denatured sample to the appropriate well of each of the two probes. Pipette up and down to thoroughly mix. (Note: if the amplification samples were stored at 2–8°C, incubate them at 37°C for 2–4 min to reduce viscosity.)

4 Cover the microwell plate and incubate for 1 h at 37°C ± 2°C.

5 Prepare working wash solution by diluting 1 vol. of 10 × wash solution with 9 vol. of distilled water. Mix well.

6 After incubation, wash the microwell plate five times with the working wash solution using an automated MWP washer or manually as follows:

(a) Aspirate contents of wells.

(b) Fill each well to top with working wash solution (400–450 μl), soak for 30 sec. Aspirate dry.

(c) Repeat step (b) four additional times. Tap the plate dry.

7 Add 100 μl avidin–HRP conjugate to each well. Cover the microwell plate and incubate for 15 min at 37 °C ± 2 °C.

8 Wash the microwell plate as described in step 6.

9 Prepare the working substrate by mixing 4 parts of substrate A with 1 part of substrate B. (Note: protect working substrate from direct light. Working substrate must be at room temperature and used within 3 h of preparation.)

10 Pipette 100 μl working substrate solution into each well. Allow colour to develop for 10 min at room temperature in the dark.

11 Add 100 μl stop reagent to each well.

12 Measure the optical density of the microwell plates at 450 nm within 1 h of adding stop reagent.

10.6 Interpretation of results

The OD cut-off varies with each assay and must be established for each system separately. For HIV-1, several hundred low risk, seronegative specimens were analysed along with over a hundred seropositive specimens to establish the cut-off. For the DNA assay, absorbances ≥ 0.35 are considered positive; absorbances < 0.35 are considered negative/undetectable.

Detectable HIV, normal IC	Data valid; HIV positive.
Detectable HIV, low IC	Data valid; suboptimal conditions, but HIV positive.
No detectable IC	Data invalid; poor recovery, amplification/detection.
No HIV, normal IC	Data valid; sample either negative or below detection limit of assay.

11 Quantitative HIV RNA assay

11.1 Sample collection for plasma HIV RNA amplification

Numerous studies have been performed to determine the effects of specimen collection and handling procedures on quantitative measurement of HIV-1 RNA. A comparison of different anticoagulants and sample processing times indicated that HIV RNA was most stable in EDTA tubes and was least stable in heparinized (green top) blood (22). Heparinized samples should be avoided, especially if the GuSCN isopropanol extraction protocol is used, as heparin is inhibitory to PCR. In situations where only heparinized samples are available, the heparin can be removed from the plasma with heparinase. However, this treatment results in lower HIV copy number. Alternatively, the RNA can be extracted using silica beads. The plasma should be separated from whole blood within the first 6 h of collection and stored at –70°C for optimal titre determination. Samples held for longer than 6 h prior to separation, yielded lower HIV copy number.

Protocol 8
Processing plasma for HIV RNA PCR

Equipment
- Centrifuge with swing-bucket rotor
- Sarstedt tubes
- Sterile transfer pipettes
- –70°C freezer

Method
1 Collect blood in EDTA or ACD tubes.
2 Centrifuge tubes at 1200 g for 10 min to separate cells and plasma.
3 Remove plasma, avoiding the cell layer, into a Sarstedt tube.
4 Centrifuge again at 1200 g for 10 min to remove any contaminating cells and platelets.
5 Pipette plasma into Sarstedt tubes.
6 Freeze at −70°C until ready for processing.

11.2 Extraction of viral RNA with GuSCN

Two procedures are described below for the extraction of HIV RNA from plasma. In the standard protocol, 200 µl of plasma are processed of which the equivalent of 25 µl is amplified in a reaction. This protocol yields a detection sensitivity of 400 copies HIV RNA/ml of plasma. The ultrasensitive method processes 500 µl of plasma, of which the equivalent of 250 µl is amplified in a reaction. The higher sample input increases the assay sensitivity to 50 copies/ml.

The extraction protocols for the two methods are similar. For the ultra-sensitive assay, virions from 500 µl plasma are pelleted by high speed centrifugation at 23 000 g and the plasma removed. The samples are then treated according to the standard protocol in which guanidium thiocyanate is used to lyse the virions and to inactivate RNases. Following lysis, viral nucleic acids are precipitated with alcohol. The final pellet for the ultrasensitive assay is resuspended in a smaller volume.

Protocol 9

Extraction of RNA from plasma: standard method

Equipment and reagents

- Sarstedt tubes
- Micropipetters
- Micropipette with plugged tips
- Microcentrifuge
- Sterile transfer pipettes
- Vortex
- Lysis buffer: 5.75 M guanidium thiocyanate, 50 mM Tris pH 7.5, 100 mM 2-mercaptoethanol, 1 µg/ml poly(rA)

- 70% ethanol
- 100% isopropanol
- DEPC-treated water
- Distilled water
- Quantitation standard at about 100 copies/µl
- Positive control(s) of known copy number
- Negative control

Method

1 Prepare the working lysis buffer for the desired number of extractions by adding the QS to the lysis buffer. Prepare 600 µl lysis buffer per extraction. Add 1000 copies of QS per ml of lysis buffer. (This will result in about 75 copies of QS per reaction.)

2 Pipette 600 µl lysis buffer into Sarstedt tube.

3 Add 200 µl sample to tube containing the working lysis buffer. Immediately cap and vortex 3–5 sec.

4 Incubate tubes for 10 min at room temperature.

5 Remove cap and add 800 µl of 100% isopropanol to each tube. Vortex for 3–5 sec.

6 Put an orientation mark on each tube and place tubes into the microcentrifuge with the mark facing outward so that after centrifugation, the pellet will align with the orientation mark. Centrifuge samples at 12 000 g for 15 min at room temperature.

7 Using a fine-tip, disposable transfer pipette, slide the pipette down the side opposite the pellet while drawing off the liquid. The pellet may not be visible at this point. Maintain a continuous negative pressure with the pipette as you draw off the liquid. Take special care to remove as much liquid as possible without disturbing the pellet.

8 Add 1.0 ml of 70% ethanol to each tube, re-cap, and vortex 3–5 sec.

9 Place tubes into the centrifuge with the orientation mark again facing to the outside so that the pellet will align with the orientation mark. Centrifuge samples at 12 500 g for 5 min at room temperature.

10 Carefully remove the supernatant as before without disturbing the pellet. Remove as much of the supernatant as possible as residual ethanol can inhibit the amplification.

11 Add 400 µl of DEPC-treated water.

12 Vortex vigorously for 10 sec to resuspend the extracted RNA. Note that insoluble material often remains.

13 Amplify the processed specimens within 2 h or store at −20°C or colder until ready for amplification.

Protocol 10

Extraction of RNA from plasma: ultrasensitive method

Equipment and reagents

- See *Protocol 9*

- High speed tabletop centrifuge (Heraeus Contifuge 17RS, Biofuge 22R, or Biofuge 28RS centrifuge)

Method

1 Pre-cool high speed centrifuge and rotor to 2–8 °C.

2 Prepare 70% ethanol. Allow 1.25 ml of 70% ethanol for each sample processed.

3 Prepare the working lysis reagent by adding the quantitation standard (QS) to the lysis reagent to yield 250 copies/ml (or 75 copies/PCR). Allow 600 μl lysis reagent per extraction.

4 Label one 1.5 ml screw-cap microcentrifuge tube for each specimen and control.

5 Thaw samples at room temperature and vortex for 3–5 sec. Spin tube briefly to bring specimen to bottom of tube.

6 Pipette 500 μl of sample into an appropriately labelled sample tube containing the lysis reagent. Re-cap the tubes.

7 Put an orientation mark on each tube and place the tubes into the centrifuge with the orientation marks facing outward, so that the pellet will align with the orientation marks. Centrifuge samples and controls at 17 000 r.p.m. in a high speed centrifuge for 60 min at 2–8 °C. The pellet will form on the outer wall.

8 Remove the tubes from the centrifuge and loosen the caps. Using a fine-tip, sterile transfer pipette, carefully draw off the supernatant without disturbing the pellet. Maintain a continuous negative pressure with the transfer pipette as you draw off any liquid. Up to 25 μl of the supernatant can remain in the tube without affecting the performance of the test.

9 Add 600 μl working lysis reagent into each tube. Cap the tubes and vortex for 5–10 sec.

10 Incubate all tubes for 10 min at room temperature.

11 Add 600 μl of 100% isopropanol to each tube. Mix well by vortexing for 3–5 sec.

12 Follow Protocol 9, steps 6–10.

13 Add 100 μl DEPC-treated H_2O to each tube. Re-cap the tubes and vortex vigorously for 10 sec to resuspend the extracted RNA. Note that some insoluble material may remain.

14 Amplify the processed specimens within 2 h of preparation or store the processed specimens frozen at –20 °C or colder for up to one week.

11.3 RNA amplification

Amplification of RNA has conventionally been performed with two enzymes, one specific for reverse transcription, and one for DNA polymerization. In 1991, Myers and Gelfand described a DNA polymerase that exhibited both reverse transcriptase and polymerase activities (23). This enzyme, rTth DNA polymerase, has facilitated the development of RT-PCR assays for the RNA viruses (18, 24). In contrast to conventional reverse transcriptases, rTth DNA polymerase is thermostable and thermoactive, allowing reverse transcription to occur at elevated temperatures. The higher temperature reduces non-specific priming events and facilitates amplification through GC-rich regions with stable secondary structure. This feature has been particularly useful in amplifying HCV. An additional advantage of the thermostable polymerase is that UNG can be readily incorporated into the reactions. Incorporation of UNG with conventional reverse transcriptases has been problematic since their thermal activity profiles are similar to that of UNG. As temperatures that inactivate UNG also inactivate the reverse transcriptases, methods to sequester UNG from the reverse transcriptases would be required if this carryover prevention strategy were to be employed. With rTth DNA polymerase, the 94°C UNG inactivation step does not affect the enzyme's activity. All components of the assay are added together, making it possible to perform a single step RT-PCR in a single buffer system.

The following protocols were designed for amplification and quantitative detection of plasma HIV RNA. There are two major differences between the qualitative and quantitative assays. First, amplifications for quantification are performed for fewer cycles to ensure that the products are still within the dynamic range of the microwell plate assay. Secondly, since the dynamic range of the microwell plate itself is limited, serial dilutions of the amplified products are required.

Protocol 11

Amplification of HIV RNA for quantitative assay

Equipment and reagents

- See *Protocol 5*
- Mastermix, recipe for 2 × reaction mixture (for one reaction): 20 mM Tris pH 8.3, 180 mM KCl, 300 μM each dATP, dCTP, dGTP,

dTTP, 400 μM dUTP, 1.8 mM MnCl$_2$, 20 pmoles each primer, 30% glycerol, 10 U rTth DNA polymerase, 2 U UNG

Method

1 Prepare mastermix for the desired number of reactions.

2 Place reaction tubes in MicroAmp™ tray and lock tubes in position with tube retainer.

3 Pipette 50 μl of working master mix into each reaction tube using a micropipettor with a plugged tip or a repeat pipettor.

Protocol 11 continued

4   Add 50 μl of the extracted RNA into each tube. Program the thermal cycler as follows:

   - 2 min at 50 °C
   - 30 min at 60 °C
   - 10 sec at 95 °C, 10 sec at 55 °C, 10 sec at 72 °C for 4 cycles
   - 10 sec at 90 °C, 10 sec at 60 °C, 10 sec at 72 °C for 26 cycles
   - 15 min at 72 °C

5   Remove the tray from the thermal cycler at any time during the final 72 °C hold. Do not extend the final program beyond 15 min.

6   Remove the caps from the reaction tubes and immediately pipette 100 μl of denaturation solution into each reaction tube using a multichannel pipettor and mix by pipetting up and down five times.

7   The denatured amplicon can be held at room temperature no more than 2 h before proceeding to the detection reaction. If the detection reaction can not be performed within 2 h, re-cap the tubes and store the denatured amplicon at 2–8 °C for up to one week.

11.4 Quantification of amplified products

Serial fivefold dilutions of the amplicon are required to obtain a 3-log detection range. For the quantitative assay, the HIV and QS wells are on the same plate. Rows A through F of the microwell plates are coated with the HIV probe; rows G and H with the QS-specific oligonucleotide probe. Only two wells are used for the QS as the 100 copies of QS should be within the detection range of the two wells.

The detection range of the microwell needs to be determined for each assay. For the assay described below, the detection range is 0.2–2.0 OD units. The background, in the absence of target, was determined to be 0.07 OD units. Again, this needs to be determined for each individual assay.

Protocol 12

Colorimetric detection of amplified products for the quantitative assays

Equipment and reagents

- See *Protocol 7*

Method

1   Warm all reagents, including microwell plates to room temperature.

2   Prepare 1 × working wash solution by diluting 10 × wash solution with distilled water. Mix well.

3 Add 100 µl of the hybridization buffer to each well to be tested using a multi-channel pipettor.

4 Add 25 µl of the denatured amplicon to the HIV wells in row A of the microwell plate, and mix up and down ten times with a 12-channel pipettor with plugged tips. Make serial fivefold dilutions in the HIV wells in rows B through F as follows. Transfer 25 µl from row A to row B and mix as before. Continue through row F. Mix row F as before, then remove and discard 25 µl. Discard pipette tips.

5 Add 25 µl of the denatured amplicon to the QS wells in row G of the microwell plate and mix up and down ten times with a 12-channel pipettor with plugged tips. Using a 12-channel pipettor with plugged tips, pipette 25 µl of denatured amplicon into row G of the microwell plate and mix by pipetting up and down ten times. Transfer 25 µl from row G to row H. Mix as before, then remove 25 µl from row H and discard.

6 Cover the microwell plate and incubate for 1 h at $37\,°C \pm 2\,°C$.

7 Follow *Protocol 7*, steps 7–12.

Protocol 13

Results calculation for the quantitative RNA assay

Calculate the HIV-1 RNA level as follows:

1 Choose the appropriate HIV well as follows:

(a) The HIV wells in rows A through F represent neat and 1:5, 1:25, 1:125, 1:625, and 1:3125 serial dilutions, respectively, of the HIV-1 amplicon. The absorbance values should decrease with the serial dilutions (see results interpretation for exceptions).

(b) Choose the well with the lowest OD_{450} that is ≥ 0.20 and ≤ 2.00 OD units.

2 Subtract background from the selected HIV OD value (background = 0.07 OD units).

3 Calculate the Total HIV OD by multiplying the background-corrected OD value of the selected HIV well by the dilution factor associated with that well.

4 Choose the appropriate QS well as follows:

(a) The QS wells in rows G and H represent neat and 1:5 dilutions, respectively, of the QS amplicon. The absorbance value in row G should be greater than the value in row H.

(b) Choose the well with the lowest OD_{450} that is ≥ 0.30 and ≤ 2.00 OD units.

5 Subtract background from the selected QS OD values (background = 0.07 OD units).

6 Calculate the *Total QS OD* by multiplying the *background-corrected OD* value of the selected QS well by the dilution factor associated with that well.

Protocol 13 continued

7   Calculate *HIV-1 RNA copies/ml plasma* as follows:

(a) For the standard assay :

$$\text{HIV RNA copies/ml} = \frac{\text{Total HIV OD}}{\text{Total QS OD}} \times \text{Input QS copies/PCR} \times 40$$

(b) For the ultrasensitive assay:

$$\text{HIV RNA copies/ml} = \frac{\text{Total HIV OD}}{\text{Total QS OD}} \times \text{Input QS copies/PCR} \times 4$$

Where: 40 is a factor to convert copies per PCR to copies per ml of plasma for the standard assay; 4 is a factor to convert copies per PCR to copies per ml for the ultra-sensitive assay.

Note: the linear range of each assay system needs to be established. The upper range of quantification for the test protocols described here are 750 000 copies/ml for the standard assay and 75 000 copies/ml for the ultrasensitive assay. Quantitative results above the established level of each test are less accurate.

11.5 Interpretation of results

1 *All HIV OD values are less than established OD cut-off, but QS wells have expected values.* Report the result as 'No HIV-1 RNA detected, less than 'X' where 'X' is the copies/ml calculated with cut-off OD in row A'.

2 *All HIV OD values > 2.0.* If all HIV-1 wells have OD values greater than 2.0, the HIV-1 copy number is above the linear range of the assay. Prepare a 1:50 dilution of the original specimen with HIV negative human plasma and repeat the test. Calculate the HIV-1 result as above, but change the conversion factor to reflect the difference in the dilution factor.

3 *HIV OD values out of sequence.* HIV wells should follow the general pattern of decreasing OD values from well A to well F. There are two exceptions to this pattern. In reactions containing high HIV-1 RNA copies per ml, wells A, B, and C can become saturated and will not dilute out appropriately. These wells may turn a greenish-brown colour prior to the addition of stop solution. In reactions containing low HIV-1 RNA copies/ml wells B through F may only contain background OD values. In both situations, the results are valid even though the HIV wells do not have decreasing OD values from well A through well F. Otherwise, an error has occurred and the entire test procedure for that specimen (including specimen preparation) should be repeated.

4 *Both QS OD values < 0.30.* If both QS wells have OD values less than 0.30 then either the processed specimen was inhibitory to the amplification or the RNA was not recovered during specimen processing. The specimen should be re-processed and the amplification/detection repeated.

5 *Both QS OD values > 2.0.* If both QS wells have OD values greater than 2.0, an error occurred.

6 *QS OD values out of sequence.* QS OD values out of sequence. If the absorbance of well H is greater than the absorbance in well G, then an error occurred.

11.6 Controls

A HIV negative control, a HIV high (+) control, and a HIV low (+) should be included with each test run. All control and test samples should yield OD values for the QS that meet the established criteria, demonstrating that the specimen processing, reverse transcription, amplification, and detection steps were performed correctly.

The expected range for the user prepared HIV high (+) and HIV low (+) controls should be established by the user. For valid assays, the HIV-1 RNA copy number/ml for the HIV (+) controls should fall within the expected range. The negative control should give OD values < 0.20 or the lower limit of detection established for the specific assay.

12 Quantitative DNA assay

A quantitative DNA assay has been developed to follow patients whose viral RNA levels have been successfully reduced to below the detection limit of the ultra-sensitive assays. This assay uses PBMCs as the specimen. PBMCs were selected as the specimen of choice, based on its accessibility and on studies that showed that viral burden in the peripheral blood is representative of the total body population. This assay provides a new tool to monitor patients with undetectable RNA levels, and may prove useful in evaluating new therapies that target the integrated virus.

The DNA assay uses:

(a) The sample preparation method described for the qualitative DNA assay (Protocol 2).

(b) A plasmid DNA rather than an RNA transcript as the quantitation standard.

(c) The amplification protocol and cycling parameters described for the quantitative RNA assay in Protocol 11 but minus the reverse transcription step.

(d) The same detection format as the quantitative HIV RNA assay. The results calculation for the DNA assay is similar to the RNA assay, but differs in that the viral load is normalized to total cellular input (see Protocol 15).

12.1 Quantification of total genomic DNA

For the quantitative DNA assay, we have chosen to normalize the HIV copy number to total genomic input. Conventionally, HIV DNA are reported as either copies/10^6 cells or as copies/μg DNA. Cell counts are typically performed using a haemocytometer or a Coulter counter. The accuracy of the haemocytometer counts is affected by the density of the cell suspension, the number of cells counted per field, and the number of fields counted. DNA concentrations are determined by spectrophotometric measurements. However, as the accuracy of the spectrophotometric determinations depends on the purity of the nucleic acids, organic extractions are generally required. We have assessed an alternate method for quantifying genomic DNA that is simple, accurate, and can be performed on crude cell lysates. The DNA released by the extraction process is quantified using Hoechst dye (bisbenzimide) which binds to the minor groove of DNA. When 365 nm light excites the bound dye, its fluorescence at 458 nm can be measured and quantified. This procedure circumvents the need to perform cell counts and does not assume 100% recovery and lysis of the PBMCs.

Protocol 14

Total DNA determination

Equipment and reagents

- DyNA Quant 200 fluorometer (Pharmacia, 80-6226-49)
- Hoechst dye 33258 (Pharmacia, 80-6226-87) at 1 mg/ml
- 10 × TNE buffer: 100 mM Tris–HCl, 10 mM EDTA, 2.0 M NaCl pH 7.4
- Calf thymus DNA

Method

1 Turn on fluorometer 15 min before use.

2 Prepare 100 μg/ml calf thymus standard.

3 Prepare 1 × TNE buffer by diluting 1 vol. of 10 × TNE in 9 vol. of distilled water.

4 Prepare a 1 × working dye buffer by diluting 10 μl Hoechst dye stock (1 mg/ml) into 100 ml 1 × TNE buffer.

5 Add 2 ml of working dye buffer to the cuvette. Adjust the fluorometer to zero. Add 2 μl of the DNA standard to the cuvette. (Note: it is recommended by the manufacturer to use a pipette that ranges from 0.5–10 μl to insure accuracy.) Mix the sample well (by pipette or inverting with a cover). Adjust the reading on the fluorometer to read 100. The machine is now normalized and ready for use with the samples.

6 For each unknown, add 2 μl of sample to 2 ml of working dye buffer. Record reading. This number corresponds to the DNA concentration of the original sample in μg/ml.

7 If the DNA extraction protocol renders the DNA single-stranded, the DNA concentration should be multiplied by two to account for the twofold difference in Hoechst dye binding. The proteinase K extraction protocol used in Protocol 3 generates single-stranded DNA.

12.2 Quantification of HIV DNA

Protocol 15

Quantification of HIV DNA

1 Follow the same instructions for the quantitative HIV-1 RNA assay to select the appropriate HIV and QS ODs (Protocol 13).

2 Calculate for HIV-1 DNA copies/ml of lysate using the following equation:

$$\frac{\text{Total HIV OD}}{\text{Total QS OD units}} \times \text{Input QS copies/PCR} \times 20 = \text{HIV DNA copies/ml}$$

where 20 is a factor to convert copies per 50 µl to copies per 1 ml.

3 Calculate the HIV-1 DNA copies/µg genomic DNA:

$$\frac{\text{HIV-1 DNA copies/ml}}{\text{Total DNA µg/ml}} = \frac{\text{HIV-1 DNA copies}}{\text{µg total DNA}}$$

where µg/ml DNA is determined using Protocol 14.

13 Real time detection formats

Over the last few years, significant interest has been generated in adapting real time detection to PCR amplification. The two most frequently described real time assays use dye intercalation (25) or TaqMan® (26) as the detection format. The advantages of these procedures are multi-fold. First, amplification and detection occurs simultaneously in a single tube; no post-PCR manipulations are required. Secondly, a 6–7 log detection range can be obtained in a single reaction. Thirdly, amplification and detection are carried out in a closed system that minimizes risks of contamination. Fourthly, the elimination of post-PCR manipulations results in a faster time to result, higher throughput, and use of fewer disposables.

13.1 TaqMan® technology

The TaqMan® assay takes advantage of the inherent $5' \rightarrow 3'$ exonuclease activity of DNA polymerases. A fluorophore, labelled with two different fluorophores is added into the amplification reaction. One probe serves as the reporter molecule and the second as the quencher. In its intact form, the fluorescence of the reporter molecule is 'quenched' by the second fluorophore. During amplification, the probe is cleaved by the DNA polymerase, which releases the reporter molecule from the quencher. The increase in fluorescence signal of the reporter molecule is directly proportional to the amount of amplified product and is used to quantify the initial sample input.

While the TaqMan® assay has been used in quantitative determinations, very few studies have incorporated a QS into the amplifications. As addressed in an earlier section, the QS serves an important role in tracking the entire process, from extraction to detection. In contrast to the end-point detection assays, the incorporation of a QS into the TaqMan® assay significantly complicates the amplification and the data reduction. To differentiate the QS from the target, a second probe, with minimally a different reporter group is required. Since the QS uses the same primers as the target, competition between the QS and target amplifications is often observed in the TaqMan® assays. This competition results from the fact that a large number of cycles is required before signals from the TaqMan® assay can be detected. These competitions were not observed in the microwell detection format, where the signal amplification in the detection step provided more sensitive detection and required fewer cycles of amplification. Whereas amplification and detection of a single target can easily achieve a 6–7 log detection range, a co-amplification of the QS and target can limit the range to 4-log due to competition between the two. Using different primers for the QS can eliminate this competition. However, this approach is less attractive as it will not monitor the efficiency of amplification with the same primers.

13.1.1 Effects of sequence heterogeneity on probe cleavage

In the TaqMan® assay, the probe must efficiently bind to the target to allow cleavage by the polymerase during the anneal phase of PCR. While a 30 second anneal phase at 60°C is sufficient to allow efficient hybridization and cleavage when the probe is perfectly matched to the templates, these conditions are suboptimal for mismatched templates. Studies indicated that the presence of as few as two mismatches reduced cleavage efficiency and resulted in an under-estimation of the true copy number by two- to fourfold (27). The presence of four or more mismatches resulted in a significant underestimation of the copy number. Consequently, strategies to increase mismatch tolerance will be required before the assay can be broadly used to quantify and detect heterogeneous targets such as HIV. Mismatches in the probe binding region have not signifi-cantly affected detection by the microwell plate assays as the hybridization conditions used readily accommodated as many as five mutations within the 33 base probe.

13.2 Dye intercalation

In the dye intercalation approach, ethidium bromide or SYBR Green is added to the amplification and the fluorescence generated by the intercalation of these dyes into the newly synthesized DNA is measured. This approach is simple to use, inexpensive, and does not require a probe. A major advantage in using this approach for HIV is that only mismatches at the primer binding sites need to be considered; mismatches in the probe binding site are irrelevant. However, there are two major drawbacks in using this approach for HIV. First, the assay must have exquisite specificity as it cannot discriminate non-specific products from true target. Detection of low copies becomes a major challenge. An additional drawback is that a QS cannot be incorporated into the assays unless some other strategies are employed to differentiate the QS from the target. Although the dye intercalation procedure has been successfully used in numerous research applications, its use in quantifying HIV and other low copy pathogens will require further development.

Acknowledgements

I thank my present and former colleagues at Roche Molecular Systems whose research have contributed to a better understanding of the PCR technology and whose efforts have resulted in the development of these protocols. I especially thank the HIV team for their tireless effort in working with this challenging target.

References

1. Steinhauer, D. A. and Holland, J. J. (1986). *Annu. Rev. Microbiol.*, **41**, 409.
2. Korber, B., Kuiken, C., Foley, B., Hahn, B., McCutchan, F., Mellors, J., *et al.* (1998). *Human retroviruses and AIDS*, pp. 1–18. Los Alamos National Laboratory, Los Alamos, NM.
3. Gurtler, L., Hauser, P. H., Eberle, J., von Bruan, A., Knaps, S., ZeKing, L., *et al.* (1994). *J. Virol.*, **68**, 1581.
4. Simon, F., Mauclere, P., Roques, P., Loussert-Ajaka, I., Muller-Trutwin, M., Saragosti, S., *et al.* (1998). *Nature Med.*, **4**, 1032.
5. Kwok, S., Kellogg, D. E., McKinney, N., Spasic, D., Goda, L., Levenson, C., *et al.* (1990). *Nucleic Acids Res.*, **18**, 999.
6. Christopherson, C., Sninsky, J. J., and Kwok, S. (1997). *Nucleic Acids Res.*, **25**, 654.
7. Nichols, R., Andrews, P. C., Zhang, P., and Bergstrom, D. E. (1994). *Nature*, **369**, 492.
8. Wetmur, J. G. and Sninsky, J. J. (1995). *PCR strategies* (ed. M. A. Innis, D. H. Gelfand, and J. Sninsky), p. 69. Academic Press, Inc.
9. Zangenberg, G., Saiki, R., and Reynolds, R. (1999). *PCR applications: protocols for functional genomics* (ed. M. A. Innis, D. H. Gelfand, and J. J. Sninsky) p. 73. Academic Press, Inc.
10. Chou, Q., Russell, M., Birch, D., Raymond, J., and Bloch, W. (1992). *Nucleic Acids Res.*, **20**, 1717.
11. Kellogg, D. E., Rybalkin, I., Chen, S., Mukhamedova, N., Vlasik, T., Siebert, P. D., *et al.* (1994). *Biotechniques*, **16** (6), 1134.
12. Birch, D. E., Kolmodin, L., Laird, W. J., McKinney, N., Wong, J., Young , K., *et al.* (1996). *Nature*, **381**, 445.
13. Persing, D. H. and Cimino, G. D. (1993). *Diagnostic molecular microbiology principles and applications* (ed. D. H. Persing, T. F. Smith, F. C. Tenover, and T. J. White), p. 105. American Society for Microbiology.
14. Longo, M. C., Berninger, M. S., and Hartley, J. L. (1990). *Gene*, **93**, 125.
15. Kwok, S. and Higuchi, R. (1989). *Nature*, **339**, 237.
16. Hu, H. Y., Burczak, J. D., Leckie, G. W., Ray, K. A., Muldoon, S., and Lee, H. H. (1996). *Diag. Microbiol. Infect. Dis.*, **24**, 71.
17. Kellogg, D. E., Sninsky, J. J., and Kwok, S. (1990). *Anal. Biochem.*, **189** (2), 202.
18. Mulder, J., McKinney, N., Christopherson, C., Sninsky, J. J., Greenfield, L., and Kwok, S. (1994). *J. Clin. Microbiol.*, **32**, 292.
19. Comeau, A. M., Hsu, H. W., Schwerzler, M., Mushinsky, G., Walter, E., Hofman, L., *et al.* (1993). *J. Pediatr.*, **123**, 252.
20. Ou, C. Y., Kwok, S., Mitchell, S. W., Mack, D. H., Sninsky, J. J., Krebs, J. W., *et al.* (1988). *Science*, **238**, 295.

21. Triques, K., Coste, J., Perret, L., Segarra, C., Mpoundi, E., Reynes, J., *et al.* (1999). *J. Clin. Microbiol.*, **37**, 110.

22. Dickover, R. E., Herman, S. A., Saddiq, K., Wafer, D., Dillon, M., and Bryson, Y. J. (1998). *J. Clin. Microbiol.*, **36**, 1070.

23. Meyers, T. W. and Gelfand, D. H. (1991). *Biochemistry*, **30**, 7661.

24. Young, K. K., Resnick, R. M., and Myers, T. W. (1993). *J. Clin. Microbiol.*, **4**, 882.

25. Higuchi, R., Fockler, C., Dolllinger, G., and Watson, R. (1993). *Bio/Technology*, **11**, 1026.

26. Holland, P. M., Abramson, R. D., Watson, R., and Gelfand, D. H. (1991). *Proc. Natl. Acad. Sci. USA*, **88**, 7276.

27. Christopherson, C., Lu, S., and Kwok, S. (1998). *Antiviral Ther.*, **3**, 247.

Chapter 4

Mutation detection by single-stranded conformation polymorphism and denaturing high performance liquid chromatography

Michael Dean
Laboratory of Genomic Diversity, National Cancer Institute-Frederick Frederick, MD 21702, USA

Bernard Gerrard
SAIC-Frederick Frederick, MD 21702, USA

Rando Allikmets
Departments of Ophthalmology and Pathology, Columbia University, New York, NY 10032, USA

1 Introduction

Single-stranded conformation polymorphism (SSCP) alone or in combination with heteroduplex analysis (HA) is one of the most widely used and practical manual methods for mutation detection (1). The principal advantage of this method is that it is rapid to perform and can be carried out using equipment available in most molecular biology laboratories. When properly optimized, the method is highly sensitive, and many different mutations within a DNA fragment can often be distinguished on the same gel (2,3). SSCP and HA can be performed on the same gel since, after the denaturation of the sample prior to loading, there is often the re-formation of a significant amount of double-stranded DNA which will appear in a lower position from the single-stranded products on the SSCP gel. Since heteroduplexes can often be resolved from homoduplexes, the appearance of heteroduplexes on the SSCP gel can give additional information on the presence of variants (see Chapter 6 for further discussion and complementary protocols).

Oefner and colleagues have described the use of high performance liquid chromatography (HPLC) employing columns containing non-porous poly-

(styrene/divinylbenzene) beads for the separation of DNA molecules by size (4). DNA binds to the column in a buffer of triethylammonium acetate, and is eluted off with an increasing gradient of acetonitrile. When the column is run at increasing temperatures, partial denaturation of the double-stranded DNA occurs, resulting in a loss of the dependency between retention time and size. Underhill *et al.* (5) reported the use of this denaturing HPLC (DHPLC) for the detection of DNA sequence variants. Heteroduplex molecules formed in heterozygotes typically denature at lower concentrations of acetonitrile and are detected as a peak or peaks with shorter retention times. The column can regenerate within a minute, allowing run lengths of 6–10 min to be achieved. Thus, as many as ten samples per hour can be run on a single column. The DNA is injected into the column directly from the PCR reaction and the cost per reaction in terms of the buffer and column is low. DHPLC is non-radioactive and automatable. The sensitivity of the method is very high, making this method competitive if not superior to most existing scanning methods (6).

2 Single-stranded conformation polymorphism (SSCP) and heteroduplex analysis (HA)

In SSCP/HA analysis the sample is amplified by the polymerase chain reaction (PCR) in the presence of a radiolabelled nucleotide, usually ^{32}P. This product is denatured to generate single-stranded molecules and loaded on a non-denaturing gel. The single-stranded molecules are resolved on the gel, and DNA sequence alterations between the primers appear as fragments of altered mobility due to differential folding of the single strand. The conditions of the gel can be varied by altering the running temperature, the degree of crosslinking in the gel matrix, or by the inclusion of glycerol or sucrose. These variations change the type of conformations seen and can increase the sensitivity of detection (7).

2.1 Optimization of the PCR reaction

Optimum conditions for the PCR are essential to generating easily interpretable SSCP gels (various chapters discuss PCR optimization, e.g. see Chapters 3 and 5). Important variables to consider are the concentration of Mg^{2+} in the reaction and the parameters of the PCR cycles in terms of temperatures and the number of cycles. We have found that a step-down PCR program gives clean product from a number of primers using identical Mg^{2+} concentrations (8). In this procedure, the annealing is initially carried out at a high temperature, often above the T_m of the primers, and gradually lowered. In this program the reaction is initiated at the temperature that is optimum for the fully base paired product. In subsequent cycles at lower temperatures, a sufficient mass of the expected product is generated, outcompeting any unwanted side-reactions. This procedure allows primers to initiate priming at their optimum temperature, eliminating the need for optimization of Mg^{2+} concentrations. An example of this type of program is given in Protocol 1.

Protocol 1

PCR set up and optimization

Equipment and reagents

- PCR machine (P E Biosystems, or MJ Research)
- Small (10–20 cm) acrylamide or agarose gels for visualizing PCR products
- 100–500 V power supply
- UV light box with camera for photographing gels

Method

1. Make a cocktail of all of the following reagents except the DNA. Add the DNA to the PCR tube and then add 24 μl of the cocktail. Spin briefly in a microcentrifuge and place in the PCR machine.

2. 25 μl PCR reaction:
   - 1.0 μl genomic DNA (100 ng)
   - 2.5 μl of 10 × PCR buffer with 15 mM $MgCl_2$ (PE Biosystems)
   - 2.5 μl of 200 μM dATP, dCTP, dGTP, TTP solution (Life Technologies)
   - 1.0 μl primer 1 (1 O D/ml) (Life Technologies)
   - 1.0 μl primer 2
   - 16.8 μl water
   - 0.1 μl *Taq* Gold polymerase (5 U/μl) (PE Biosystems)

3. A standard PCR program is:
   (a) 94 °C 10 min
   (b) Followed by 35 cycles: 94 °C 0.5 min, 55 °C 0.5 min, 72 °C 1.5 min.
   (c) Final extension of 72 °C for 10 min.

4. The step-down program is:
   (a) 94 °C 10 min
   (b) Then two cycles: 94 °C 30 sec, 65 °C 30 sec, 72 °C 1 min
   (c) Then two cycles: 94 °C 30 sec, 64 °C 30 sec, 72 °C 1 min
   (d) Continue stepping down 0.5 °C for the annealing step, two cycles each step, until 59 °C is reached.
   (e) Then 30 cycles: 94 °C 30 sec, 50 °C 30 sec, 72 °C 1 min
   (f) Final extension at 72 °C for 10 min.

5. Following the PCR, run 10 μl of the reaction on an 8% acrylamide gel or a 1.5% agarose gel. The conditions giving the highest yield and cleanest product will be used for SSCP analysis.

2.2 SSCP sample preparation

Once optimum conditions for the PCR are established, a scaled down reaction (10 μl) is performed with the presence of a radiolabelled nucleotide, typically ^{32}P. Other labelled isotopes such as ^{35}S or ^{33}P can be used. Alternatively, the primers can be end-labelled using $\gamma\alpha^{32}$P ATP. (Note that both primers need to be labelled to visualize the two strands, since both strands must be visualized in SSCP analysis because conformers can be observed on either strand.) Amplified samples are then run on a long, thin acrylamide gel.

Protocol 2

Preparing an SSCP/HA gel

Equipment and reagents

- 35 cm sequencing gel box with 0.4 mm spacers and shark's tooth combs
- 2000–3000 volt power supply (Bio-Rad)
- 4 °C cold room
- 40% acrylamide/bis 37.5:1 (2.6% C) solution (Bio-Rad): dissolve 39.5 g acrylamide, and 1.06 g bis-acrylamide in a total volume of 100 ml of distilled water

Method

1. Treat one glass plate with repel silane. This treatment needs to be done only occasionally.

2. Clean a set of plates for a 35 cm, 0.4 mm thick gel.

3. Prepare one of the below listed gel formulations and use to prepare the gel. For 75 ml of gel solution (enough for one 35 cm gel) add 500 μl of 10% ammonium persulfate solution and 50 μl of TEMED. Allow the gel to polymerize for 30 min.

4. Load 3–5 μl of sample and allow to run until the bromophenol blue has reached the bottom.

5. Carefully separate the plates and remove the gel onto a piece of Whatman 3MM filter paper and cover with plastic film. Dry the gel and expose to X-ray film for 2–24 h at -70 °C or at room temperature.

6. Gel formulations.

Final conc.	Stock	250 ml
• 5% acrylamide 1.3% C)	40%	62.5 ml
• 1 × TBE	10 ×	25 ml
• 0.5 × MDE	2 ×	62.5 ml
• 10% glycerol	100%	25 ml
• 1 × TBE	10 ×	25 ml
• 10% acrylamide (1.3% C)	40%	62.5 ml
• 10% sucrose	–	25 g
• 1 × TBE	10 ×	25 ml

All solutions are to made up to final volume (250 ml) with distilled water.

2.3 Optimization of SSCP/HA detection

The conditions of the SSCP gel can be varied to produce gels in which the samples form alternate conformations. The number of possible conformations is so large that there is no theoretical basis for choosing conditions. Clearly, the more conditions run, the greater the sensitivity. The researcher, however, is limited in the number of gels that can be run. A single gel can give 60–90% efficiency of detection and can be used as an initial screening method. Two to four different gels can be employed to reach close to 100% detection. The variables that have been employed are as follows:

(a) Temperature:
   (i)   Room temperature overnight at 20 watts constant power for a total of 7000–9000 volt hours.
   (ii) 70 W 3–5 h in a 4°C cold room.

(b) Crosslinking:
   (i)   19:1 (5% C).
   (ii) 37.5:1 (2.6% C).
   (iii) 75:1 (1.3% C).
   (iv) 0.5 × MDE.

(c) Additives:
   (i)   5–10% glycerol.
   (ii) 10% sucrose.

Each of these variables can alter the conformation of single-stranded molecules. SSCP was initially run on 5% acrylamide gels with 5% bis-acrylamide crosslinker (5% C) at either room temperature or 4°C with or without glycerol. More recently researchers have shown that gels with higher percentage of acrylamide and lower crosslinking can detect more mutations (9). Sucrose has also proven to be a useful additive (7). Table 1 gives gel recipes for several different conditions that produce optimum results (3). Unfortunately, it is not possible to predict how a given change in conditions will affect the mobility of a specific fragment.

The size of the PCR product can also affect sensitivity. In general, the smaller the product, the higher the sensitivity, with the optimum being 200–300 bp. SSCPs have been observed on products as small as 50 bp and as large as 1 kb. Longer products can be cleaved with restriction enzymes to yield a series of bands that can be assayed simultaneously.

2.4 Multiplexing

The following multiplexing methods are useful when a large number of samples are to be analysed. In each case a test gel with known sample sizes and mutations should be run to provide a visual comparison for the expanded project.

(a) Use two primer pairs for each PCR reaction, provided the amplified products differ in size by at least 75 base pairs. Pre-test the combinations since some primer pairs are incompatible with each other.

(b) Amplify fragments that differ in size by at least 75 base pairs or more separately and load both amplifications of the same DNA in the same well. Again, run a test lane of each fragment size separately to obtain a visual comparison.

(c) To screen many DNA samples, amplify two DNAs together, thereby halving the number of gels that need be run. If a lane appears with an alteration, the two DNAs that this lane represents will have to be amplified separately to identify the mutant.

(d) Some PCR machines have a 96-well microtitre plate capability. This is a quick and economical way of amplifying large numbers of samples, particularly if the panel of DNAs are to be analysed with a number of primer pairs. Make a master plate of the DNAs; the amount of DNA per PCR reaction should be diluted to 5 μl with water multiplied by the number of plates that will eventually be run. Use a multichannel pipettor to transfer 5 μl of the diluted DNA from the master plate to the plates that will be used in the PCR machine. Allow these samples to dry in the plates. Add 10 μl of the appropriate PCR reaction mix to each well and proceed with the amplification program. 30 μl of loading dye can be added to each well after cycling, using a multichannel pipettor.

2.5 Interpretation of results

The interpretation of the results of an SSCP gel requires some experience. Controls with known mutations can assist in the analysis. Some double-stranded DNA often re-forms after the denaturation step which will produce bands nearer the bottom of the gel. It is helpful to include a undenatured sample to aid in identifying these bands. Double-stranded heteroduplex molecules formed when a mutant and wild-type strand anneal, can also indicate sequence alterations. These heteroduplexes migrate just above the double-stranded DNA. While heteroduplexes are most prominent in the case of insertions or deletions, they can be seen with some point mutations (10).

Since the exact migration of SSCP conformers can vary from gel to gel, it is useful to include any available control samples at least once on each gel. While it is expected that the two strands will migrate differently, this is not always the case. Similarly, in a heterozygote, not all four strands are always resolved. It is important to note that a mutant sample should give a clearly different pattern from a wild-type sample. In addition, a heterozygote should display approximately equal intensity in all four bands.

Occasionally PCR artefact bands occur that can confuse the interpretation. If a band appears only in samples that amplified better than the rest, it is likely an artefact. In samples that amplify well or are overloaded, alternate conformations can appear. These may be the result of two conformers partially annealing. Diluting the samples will chase the double-stranded DNA into single strands and remove some of these additional bands. Where possible, the confirmation of the segregation of altered bands should be demonstrated within a family. The final proof of the alteration ultimately comes from sequencing.

2.6 Applications

Since the invention of the PCR-SSCP technique in 1989, many applications of the method have been demonstrated. SSCP has been used to identify alterations in tumour DNA samples as well as mutations in human disease genes and their animal counterparts (1, 11–13). SSCP can be applied to RNA or to reverse transcribed RNA (cDNA) either to increase sensitivity or to assay multiple exons simultaneously (14).

SSCP has been applied to complex loci with many alleles, such as the *HLA* locus (15). Since different alleles usually give distinct patterns, five to ten alleles can usually be resolved on the same gel. SSCP can also be readily applied to the mapping of genes in interspecies backcrosses, where differences between the parental species can be easily detected in a 200–500 bp PCR product. SSCP alterations are often found in the 3′ untranslated regions and introns of genes (16, 17). The 3′ untranslated regions are rarely disrupted by introns, and such polymorphic sequence-tagged sites can allow a gene to be mapped genetically in families, as well as physically on yeast artificial chromosome clones and radiation hybrids (18).

2.7 Other methods

SSCP using radiolabelled samples is an excellent method for many applications. However, other methods may be warranted for some applications. A successful 'cold' SSCP method has been developed (19). Denaturing gradient gel electrophoresis (DGGE) involves resolving heteroduplex molecules by running them through an increasing concentration of denaturant (20). This method detects nearly 100% of all mutations and is also performed 'cold' without using radioactive compounds. In the GC-clamped version of this method (21) a special primer is required. Excellent protocols are provided in ref. 22. Other established methods to consider are chemical cleavage and RNase protection (reviewed in ref. 23). Methods to identify unknown mutations relying on enzymatic detection (enzyme mismatch cleavage, mismatch repair enzyme cleavage) (24, 25) have been developed that may prove useful in population-based studies.

3 Denaturing high performance liquid chromatography (DHPLC)

The use of high performance liquid chromatography (HPLC) employing columns containing non-porous poly-(styrene/divinylbenzene) beads for the separation of DNA molecules by size has been described by Oefner and colleagues (4). In this system DNA binds to the column in a buffer of triethylammonium acetate and is eluted off with an increasing gradient of acetonitrile. Triethylammonium acetate is a positively charged alkyl amine ion pairing agent which attaches to the negatively charged DNA molecules covering the DNA with a hydrophobic layer. In this state the DNA can now bind to the hydrophobic surface of the non-porous poly-(styrene/divinylbenzene) beads in the column.

Figure 1 displays a diagram of a typical DHPLC system of a set of pumps to provide the flow of the mobile phase, a mixer to mix the buffers as they are proportioned out, a UV detector to detect the DNA eluted from the column, an oven to maintain the column at a constant temperature, an autosampler to load samples from microtitre plates, and a computer to control the system and analyse the data. Figure 2 displays chromatograms of DNA size markers (pUC18 digested with *Hae*III) demonstrating the size-dependent separation of DNA fragments at non-denaturing temperatures (> 50 °C). A steeper solvent gradient (top panel) allows better separation of smaller fragments whereas a shallower solvent gradient (lower panel) is used to resolve larger DNA fragments.

Mutation detection depends upon the presence of heteroduplex molecules and on the differences in the melting temperatures between these molecules. Thus, DHPLC finds sequence anomalies in heterozygous samples and in order to do so, samples must be denatured and re-annealed to form heterozygous DNA species should they be present (heteroduplex formation). Underhill (5) reported the use of this denaturing HPLC (DHPLC) for the detection of DNA sequence variants, wherein the fact that heterozygous molecules having a different melting temperature than their homozygous counterparts is employed to detect mutations. The ion pairing agent, TEAA causes, in a manner not fully understood, the modified melting domain of the heterozygous molecules to melt at or near the melt temperature of the entire sequence. In addition, the exact temperature for partial denaturation is sequence dependent. Therefore, precise temperature control of the sample in the analytical column allows the differential detection of partially denatured heteroduplex species that are detected by the UV detector and displayed as new chromatographic peaks at a lower retention time. In order to detect heteroduplex formation, the system operating temperature must be carefully optimized to achieve partial denaturation of the heteroduplex species while leaving the homoduplex species intact.

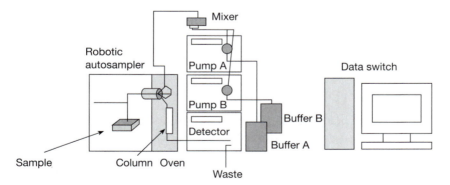

Figure 1 Diagram of a DHPLC system. The arrangements of the components of a DHPLC system are shown including the autosampler to load samples from microtitre plates, an oven to maintain the column at a constant temperature, a set of pumps to provide the flow of the mobile phase, a mixer to mix the gradient in the specified proportion, a UV detector to detect the DNA eluting from the column, and a computer to control the system.

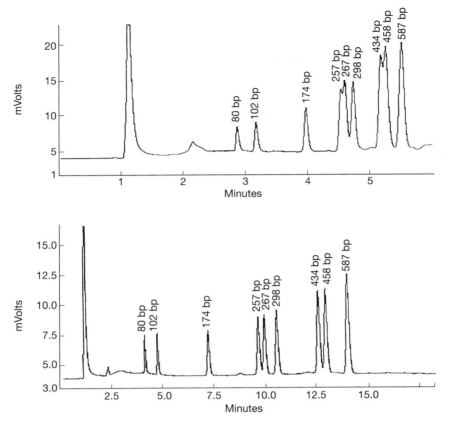

Figure 2 Size separation of molecular weight standards. The separation of a pUC18 *Hae* III digest on the DHPLC system is shown. The top panel shows a short run with a steep gradient to resolve smaller fragments. A longer run using a shallower gradient allows the resolution of larger fragments.

To determine the melting temperature of a PCR product made with specific primers, aliquots of a known wild-type product are run on the equipment at different temperatures. This temperature is determined by running a sample at a high temperature, above any possible product T_M, (70°C) and repeating sample runs with a decrease of 3°C per sample. The time at which the sample elutes when run at 70°C is noted (approximately 2.5 min). The times at which the samples elute when run at lower temperatures are noted until an increase in retention time occurs. At this point additional samples are run to determine a temperature that is approximately 2°C below the temperature at which the DNA first begins its increased retention time. If a sample with a known mutation is available, amplify it as above and run in the HPLC system at the determined melting temperature of the wild-type sample. This should give a peak different from the wild-type. Most mutations can be detected over a several degree range with the peak patterns altered at different temperatures. The temperature at

105

which the most obvious pattern change occurs in the known mutation is subsequently used for extended screenings.

A simpler method of determining the melting temperature of an amplicon of any primer pair can be obtained by calling up the sequence on the Internet (http://www.ncbi.nlm.nih.gov/Entrez/nucleotide.html) and pasting the product sequence into a melt-temperature determining algorithm provided by Stanford University at the following Internet address (http://hardy-weinberg.stanford.edu/dhplc/melt.html). This program has proven a quick and reliable tool to determine the T_m of PCR products.

The DNA is injected into the column without any additional preparation from the PCR/heteroduplexing reaction. The analytical column itself regenerates within a minute giving a sample runtime of 6–10 min, allowing the analysis of as many as ten samples per hour.

A typical DHPLC chromatogram is shown in Figure 3 with an initial peak immediately following the sample injection containing unincorporated nucleotides and primers with the amplicon peak showing at 3–6 min. The position of the sample peak depends on the size and sequence content of the fragment and the characteristics of the solvent gradient. A peak is often seen at 2–3 min composed of primer–dimer products and not to be confused with the true PCR product. Figure 4 displays chromatograms for wild-type (A) and mutant heterozygote (B) samples amplified from a portion of the *CCR5* gene. The wild-type amplicon shows a single sample peak eluting at 5.117 min. The shoulder in front of that peak probably represents DNA fragments that have incorporated errors during PCR. The heterozygous sample displays three different peaks representing the two different heteroduplex products and a homoduplex. However, in most cases heteroduplexes display a single heteroduplex and a single homoduplex peak. These peaks can be typically observed in some form over a temperature range of several degrees. It has been observed that by running samples

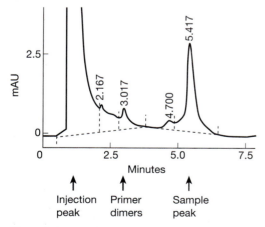

Figure 3 A typical DHPLC chromatogram of an amplicon of wild-type DNA showing the injection peak composed of unincorporated nucleotides, primers, and PCR reagents. A major artefact is a primer–dimer peak (3.017 min).

106

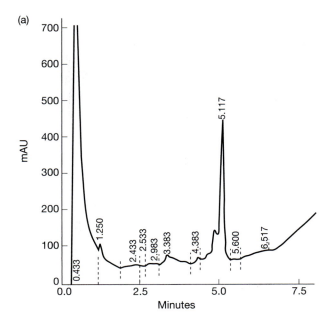

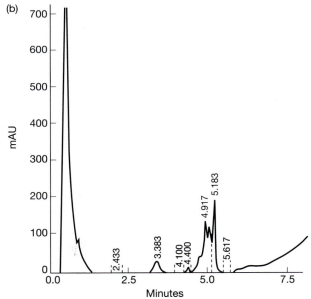

Figure 4 Chromatograms of wild-type and mutant *CCR5* gene products. (A) A DHPLC trace of a 405 bp segment of the *CCR5* gene is shown. Note the single sharp peak at 5.1 min which represents the homoduplex product. (B) A sample heterozygous for a single bp alteration C20S (26). The homoduplex peak is reduced in intensity approximately 50%. Two heteroduplex peaks, with elution times 0.13 and 0.26 min shorter than the homoduplex can be seen.

at 2 °C above the predicted temperature, those few mutants that appeared as barely detectable peak changes will resolve quite clearly resulting in close to 100% identification of all variants.

3.1 Application of DHPLC to mutation detection

In most mutation scanning applications, homozygous mutant individuals are expected to be rare and samples can be directly analysed. In the cases of consanguineous families or haploid genomes, known sample can be included with each known unknown sample. Alternately several samples, up to four, can be pooled in one PCR reaction. Dilution of a mutant sample by pooling actually drives more of the mutant DNA into the formation of heteroduplexes. The individual DNAs in a pool must be amplified and analysed separately should a mutant be detected to determine which single DNA is affected. In the search for rare variants, pooling strategies can result in dramatic increases in efficiency.

3.2 Sensitivity of detection

The principle of DHPLC is quite similar to denaturing gradient gel electrophoresis (DGGE) that has a sensitivity approaching 100%. In certain sequence contexts, when the fragment contains two melting domains that differ substantially in temperature, the samples should be run at temperatures that encompass these domains. The Stanford melting temperature program will provide these alternatives if they are indicated. In our experience we have been able to confirm this sensitivity in a large number of variants, known and unknown, in a variety of sequence contexts in PCR products of 200–425 bp length with GC contents of 38–50%. Some examples are shown in Table 1.

3.3 Conclusions

DHPLC is an efficient method for the analysis of DNA samples with a maximum throughput of less than 144 samples in a 24 hour period. The cost of analysing a sample by DHPLC in terms of the column and buffer is relatively low. This technology does not require the use of radioactive isotopes and is semi-automated. Most importantly, the sensitivity of the method approaches 100%, making this

Table 1 Variants detected by HPLC under different sequence contexts[a]

Gene	Fragment	Size (bp)	%GC	No. variants
CCR5	1	405	45	8
	2	407	46	3
	3	425	50	4
	4	272	38	9
	5	284	38	5
CCR2	1	327	46	4

[a] Portions of the *CCR5* gene coding region, intron, and promoter, and a portion of the *CCR2* coding region were examined by DHPLC to detect variants previously detected by SSCP (26–28).

method both competitive and less labour-intensive than most existing scanning methods.

Protocol 3

DHPLC analysis

Equipment and reagents

- PCR tubes (0.2 ml or PCR microtitre plates)
- Triethylamine acetate solution 2 M (Perkin Elmer)
- HPLC grade acetonitrile (Baker)
- Deionized water (must be free of metal ions, particularly Fe^{2+})

- Analytical column (Transgenomic DNASep or Varian Helix)
- HPLC machine with titanium components, temperature controlled oven, autosampler, UV detector, and computer control with peak analysis software (Varian Helix or Transgenomic Wave)

Method

1. Prepare 20–25 μl heteroduplexed PCR reactions 200–400 bp in length using Taq Gold™ and the step-down PCR program as described (Protocol 1).

2. Prepare the buffers using volumetric flasks and clean, dedicated glassware.

   (a) Buffer A, the aqueous phase, is:

Final concentration	Stock solution	Amount for 1 liter
0.1 M TEAA	2 M	50 ml
0.1 mM EDTA	0.5M	200 μl
0.1% acetonitrile	100%	1 ml (to discourage bacterial growth)

   (b) Buffer B, the organic phase, is:

Final concentration	Stock solution	Amount for 1 liter
25% acetonitrile	100%	250 ml
0.1 M TEAA	2 M	50 ml
0.1 mM EDTA	0.5 M	200 μl

3. A running program for the buffers must be determined. A typical program is:

Time	Flow (ml/min)	%A	%B
0.0	0.9	65	35
1.0	0.9	39	61
5.0	0.9	32	68
6.0	0.9	0	100
7.0	0.9	0	100
8.0	0.9	65	35

   In addition to this gradient profile, a 1.25 min equilibration time is needed between runs. This and the other machine settings are accomplished using the software provided.

Protocol 3 continued

4. Determine the optimum temperature for the analysis using the algorithm available from Stanford (http://hardy-weinberg.stanford.edu/dhplc/melt.html) and generate the running program using the machine software.

5. Run two blank samples to ensure equilibration of the machine before running research samples.

3.4 Interpretation of results

In order to gain experience in the interpretation of the chromatograms generation by DHPLC, known samples of different heterozygous polymorphic DNAs with their wild-type counterparts should be amplified and run. If possible include known point mutations, insertions, and deletions in this testing panel. The profiles of these samples will provide the comparison needed to differentiate between the mutant chromatograph peak and the wild-type peak(s) and to indicate at which position on the chromatograph any spurious PCR product(s) elute. There are often products formed by mismatching during the PCR reaction and these need to be identified in order not to confuse them with the true amplicon. Different amplicons often produce different wild-type peak outlines, thus comparison of a number of known pairs will provide familiarity with this sort of variation. Any suspected polymorphism detected by the screening process must be confirmed and characterized by sequence analysis.

3.5 Genotyping

If genotyping using a characterized mutation is to be undertaken it is advisable to optimize the running conditions to detect that particular polymorphism. Often a one degree difference above or below the predicted melting temperature will yield a more easily read chromatogram.

References

1. Orita, M., Suzuki, Y., Sekiya, T., and Hayashi, K. (1989). *Genomics,* **5**, 874.
2. Glavac, D. and Dean, M. (1995). *Hum. Mutat.,* **6**, 281.
3. Glavac, D. and Dean, M. (1993). *Hum. Mutat.,* **2**, 404.
4. Huber, C. G., Oefner, P. J., and Bonn, G. K. (1993). *Anal. Biochem.,* **212**, 351.
5. Underhill, P. A., Jim, L., Lin, A. A., Mehdi, S. Q., Jenkins, T., Vollrath, D., *et al.* (1997). *Genome Res.,* **7**, 996.
6. Jones, A. C., Austin, J., Hansen, N., Hoogendoorn, B., Oefner, P. J., Cheadle, J. P., *et al.* (1999). *Clin. Chem.,* **45**, 1133.
7. Ravnik-Glavac, M., Glavac, D., and Dean, M. (1994). *Hum. Mol. Genet.,* **3**, 801.
8. Hecker, K. H. and Roux, K. H. (1996). *Biotechniques,* **20**, 478.
9. Ravnik-Glavac, M., Glavac, D., Chernick, M., di Sant'Agnese, P., and Dean, M. (1994). *Hum. Mutat.,* **3**, 231.
10. White, M. B., Carvalho, M., Derse, D., O'Brien, S. J., and Dean, M. (1992). *Genomics,* **12**, 301.

11. Claustres, M., Laussel, M., Desgeorges, M., Giansily, M., Culard, J. F., Razakatsara, G., *et al.* (1993). *Hum. Mol. Genet.*, **2**, 1209.

12. Soto, D. and Sukumar, S. (1992). *PCR Methods Appl.*, **2**, 96.

13. Dean, M., White, M. B., Amos, J., Gerrard, B., Stewart, C., Khaw, K. T., *et al.* (1990). *Cell*, **61**, 863.

14. Danenberg, P. V., Horikoshi, T., Volkenandt, M., Danenberg, K., Lenz, H. J., Shea, L. C., *et al.* (1992). *Nucleic Acids Res.*, **20**, 573.

15. Carrington, M., Miller, T., White, M., Gerrard, B., Stewart, C., Dean, M., *et al.* (1992). *Hum. Immunol.*, **33**, 208.

16. Nielsen, D. A., Dean, M., and Goldman, D. (1992). *Am. J. Hum. Genet.*, **51**, 1366.

17. Glavac, D., Ravnik-Glavac, M., O'Brien, S., and Dean, M. (1994). *Hum. Genet.*, **93**, 694.

18. Poduslo, S. E., Dean, M., Kolch, U., and O'Brien, S. J. (1991). *Am. J. Hum. Genet.*, **49**, 106.

19. Hongyo, T., Buzard, G. S., Calvert, R. J., and Weghorst, C. M. (1993). *Nucleic Acids Res.*, **21**, 3637.

20. Myers, R. M., Maniatis, T., and Lerman, L. S. (1987). In *Methods in enzymology*, Academic Press (ed. R. Wu), vol. 155, p. 501.

21. Sheffield, V. C., Cox, D. R., Lerman, L. S., and Myers, R. M. (1989). *Proc. Natl. Acad. Sci. USA*, **86**, 232.

22. Landegren, U. (1996). *Laboratory protocols for mutation detection*. Oxford University Press, Oxford.

23. Cotton, R. G. H., Edkins, E., and Forrest, S. (1998). *Mutation detection: a practical approach*. IRL Press, Oxford.

24. Youil, R., Kemper, B. W., and Cotton, R. G. (1995). *Proc. Natl. Acad. Sci. USA*, **92**, 87.

25. Mashal, R. D., Koontz, J., and Sklar, J. (1995). *Nature Genet.*, **9**, 177.

26. Carrington, M., Kissner, T., Gerrard, B., Ivanov, S., O'Brien, S. J., and Dean, M. (1997). *Am. J. Hum. Genet*, **61**, 1261.

27. Dean, M., Carrington, M., Winkler, C., Huttley, G. A., Smith, M. W., Allikmets, R., *et al.* (1996). *Science*, **273**, 1856.

28. Smith, M. W., Dean, M., Carrington, M., Winkler, C., Huttley, G. A., Lomb, D. A., *et al.* (1997). *Science*, **277**, 959.

Chapter 5

DNA pooling methods for association mapping of complex disease loci

Lisa F. Barcellos

Department of Neurology, University of California, San Francisco, 513 Parnassus Avenue, S-258, San Francisco, CA 94143-0435, USA.

Soren Germer

Department of Human Genetics, Roche Molecular Systems, 1145 Atlantic Avenue, Alameda, CA 94501, USA.

William Klitz

Children's Hospital Oakland Research Institute, 5700 Martin Luther King Avenue, Oakland, CA 94609, USA.

1 Introduction

The rapid development and application of highly informative microsatellite markers throughout the human genome has greatly facilitated the identification of disease loci in hundreds of rare Mendelian disorders. Utilization of large multigenerational pedigrees with multiple affected individuals is a proven strategy for isolating chromosomal regions containing disease genes using microsatellite markers and traditional lod score linkage analysis. Linkage studies are often followed by association studies to further define the candidate region and to identify the putative disease gene. Linkage disequilibrium, the basis of marker associations, is typically found within a distance of 500 kb, about 0.5 (cM), although, in general, this distance may vary considerably according to population history, across different regions of the genome, and with marker type (1–4). Disease genes mapped to date, however, have shown linkage disequilibrium with markers sufficiently close to the disease gene to guide discovery of the disease locus. Examples of these successes include cystic fibrosis, Huntington disease, Wilson disease, Batten disease, Friedreich ataxia, myotonic dystrophy, torsion dystonia, hereditary haemochromatosis, diastrophic dysplasia, adult on-set polycystic kidney disease, familial breast cancer, and many others.

During the past decade, genetic researchers have turned from positional cloning of Mendelian disease genes to the dissection of complex or multifactorial diseases. These refer to common disorders that do not demonstrate simple patterns of inheritance, but instead are more consistent with contributions from multiple interacting loci of modest effect as well as environmental factors and stochastic influences. Rather than being due to specific and relatively rare mutations, complex diseases may result primarily from genetic variation that is relatively common in the general population. The list of diseases within this category is lengthy, most of which pose significant social and economical burden to society. These include diabetes, bipolar disorder, schizophrenia, alcoholism, Alzheimer disease, cardiovascular and autoimmune diseases, and others. For many of these, large multigenerational pedigrees suitable for linkage analysis may not be available. Therefore, sampling and linkage analysis of nuclear families with pairs of affected siblings is another commonly used, though less powerful, mapping strategy.

Efforts to detect genetic factors in linkage studies for complex diseases have been successful to some extent, but progress has been exceedingly slow, and to date only a few genes and some candidate regions have been identified—most of these await confirmation in independent studies. For example, in type 1 diabetes (insulin-dependent diabetes mellitus or IDDM), a total of seven chromosomal regions have been identified definitely (including the major histocompatibility complex or MHC) and another ten implicated (5–7). In general, failure to both detect and replicate linkages in complex diseases is probably due to heterogeneity among different data sets, and also to the large number of loci involved, each of which might contribute a small overall effect and be caused by common alleles in the general population. Standard linkage approaches are not powerful enough to detect small or even very modest genetic effects.

Allelic association studies have been proposed as a powerful alternative for locating genes of small or modest effect in complex traits (8, 9). Large genome-wide association studies using case-control and/or family-based methods may be much more sensitive than traditional genome screens using affected sib pair linkage analyses (8, 10, 11). In addition to utility in fine mapping susceptibility loci as part of positional cloning strategies, association screening may also be applied to zero in on disease genes that are initially localized to chromosomal regions by family linkage analysis. Although the careful matching of cases and controls likely eliminates potential problems of population stratification that might result in the detection of false associations, the use of family-based data removes these concerns. Ideally, a study design that incorporates both case-control and family data will be the most effective (11).

Association studies of this magnitude will require very dense and integrated marker maps, both microsatellite and single nucleotide polymorphisms (or SNPs), and the development of methods for efficient high-throughput genotyping. Currently, several large scale efforts are underway to develop high density SNP maps (12, 13). Although the available maps fall short of the density needed for full genome screening, higher density and more evenly spaced maps are soon anticipated (14, 15). In contrast, available microsatellite maps are more comprehensive and there is strong evidence that they may detect linkage disequilibrium over larger distances than SNPs and therefore may be better suited than SNPs for genome-wide association studies (16, 17). The advantages and disadvantages of each marker and estimated numbers required for use in an association genome screen are discussed below. An ideal study design, however, will include the combined use of both marker types.

Full genome association (or linkage disequilibrium) studies suggest laborious and costly individual genotyping of substantial sets of DNA samples. One approach that can significantly reduce time and expense of these process is DNA pooling, where equal amounts of DNA from many individuals sharing disease status are mixed together and genotyped. Pooling individual DNA samples renders the determination of allele frequencies much more efficient, as the same information obtained from the analysis of a large number of individuals can be extracted from pooled data using just a few co-amplifications. Here, affected individuals (patients or individuals with trait of interest) and ethnically matched controls can be grouped separately and then allele frequency estimates can be compared between the two pools. Nuclear or trio families in which patient, mother, and father DNA samples are collected can also be used in DNA pooling studies. In this case, parents are pooled separately from the affected offspring (patients) and 'control' or non-transmitted allele frequencies can be compared with those obtained from the patient pool (18–20). In general, a two to three stage approach is optimal whereby initial screens can be conducted using DNA pooling, and then only those sites yielding positive results are confirmed using individual genotyping.

This chapter includes detailed protocols for pooled DNA amplification and detection of microsatellite and SNP markers to facilitate efficient, cost-effective, high resolution genome screening for detection of disease loci by association (c.f. Chapter 6). Methods of analysis for pooled data and examples using both case-control and nuclear family-based samples are discussed. Correction methods for the two problems commonly associated with microsatellite typing—differential amplification and stutter artefact—are outlined. A discussion of experimental design, genetic mapping resources, and additional technical considerations is also included.

2 Quantification of DNA samples for pooled amplification

For the quantitation of individual DNA samples to be combined in pools, both spectrophotometric (OD_{260}) and fluorescent dye detection methods can be used with DNA extracted from whole blood and are available in high-throughput 96-well formats. However, a fluorescent detection method (described in *Protocol 1*) has the important advantage of greater sensitivity and specificity, although it can be less sensitive with degraded or single-stranded (denatured) DNA samples. This method of quantitation is highly recommended by authors and others (21). The use of UV absorbance as a method of DNA quantification for pooled amplifications is not recommended as the additional noise introduced may obscure true allele frequency differences between pools following PCR amplification and therefore lead to an increased error rate. Regardless of which method is used, all samples should be quantitated (minimally) in duplicate to ensure accuracy of each individual sample measurement. Duplicate samples showing greater than 5% difference should be quantitated again.

Protocol 1

DNA quantitation using fluorescence detection

Equipment and reagents

- 96-well spectrofluorometer, SPECTRAmax Gemini (Molecular Devices). Possible alternative machines: Fluoroscan *Ascent* (Life Sciences International, UK) fluorometer, DyNAQuant 200 (Hoefer/Pharmacia Biotech, not 96-well), or see Hitachi or Molecular-Dynamics for other options.

- Spectrophotometer (any)
- Nunc microplates (Applied Scientific)
- PicoGreen™ fluorescent dye (Molecular Probes, Inc.)
- Tris-EDTA (Molecular Probes, Inc.)
- DNA quantitation standards[a]

Method

1   Dilute samples to approximate concentrations of 50–100 ng/µl (based on spectrophotometric readings). If minimal amounts of DNA are available, samples can be diluted to a lower concentration for quantification. Control DNA standards can then be adjusted accordingly.

2   According to manufacturer's protocol, combine 1.0 µl each DNA sample with 100 µl of TE and 1 µl of PicoGreen™ quantitation reagent in 96-well Nunc microtitre plates.

3   Construct a standard curve from dilutions using a genomic DNA sample of known concentration and analyse samples according to manufacturer's protocol.

4   Dilute all DNA samples to the same concentration (between 10–25 ng/µl) for pooling. All samples should be routinely measured in duplicate or triplicate. If replicates are > 5% different, sample should be re-measured.

5   Construct DNA pools as appropriate for study: cases and controls, both parents vs. affected, unaffected sibs, parents separately, clinical subgroups, etc. (see discussion of study design in text). All pools should be constructed in *triplicate* for determination and comparison of microsatellite or SNP allele frequencies.

[a] Quantitation standards can either be made from DNA of known concentration or purchased. The same ones should be used for all quantitations made in a particular experiment to maintain consistency. A series of eight is recommended, for example: 0, 10, 25, 50, 75, 100, 150, 200 ng each, and run in duplicate.

3 Genetic analysis of microsatellite markers using pooled DNA samples

The amplification of microsatellite markers using pooled DNA samples will require first performing marker optimization using individual samples. Fluorescent labelled (5′ forward primer only, with HEX, TET, or FAM) primer-pairs should be selected for each marker of choice and independently optimized using individual DNA samples to determine Mg^{2+} concentration and thermo-cycling parameters for amplification efficiency. At this time, primer-pairs of interest can also be multiplexed for simultaneous amplification or just pooled for electrophoresis detection, provided they are selected and combined correctly by size and fluorescent label for detection on an automatic sequencer. Because three fluorescent dyes are available for primer labelling, the simultaneous detection of several groups of markers with overlapping sizes is possible. These initial steps will also allow you to determine whether stutter and/or differential amplification are present for a marker, which can be adjusted for in data analysis steps (discussed below), if desired. A general protocol for PCR amplification using an automatic sequencer for detection and analysis is presented below (*Protocol 2*). It is also possible to perform genotyping of individual and pooled DNA samples using capillary array electrophoresis (CAE) methodology; however, a full discussion and appropriate protocols are beyond the scope of this chapter (for more details, see ref. 21).

Most commercially available *Taq* polymerases carry out non-template addition of an adenosine base (dA) at the 3′ end of the polymerase chain reaction (PCR product). *Taq* polymerase adds an additional base, on average, 80% of the time. This can affect both individual genotyping and analysis of pooled amplifications, and can vary widely between markers and even between replicate PCR reactions. Two pools may therefore appear different due to differing plus-A artefacts rather than true actual allele frequency differences. Two strategies to overcome this process are included here (*Protocols 2 and 3*):

(a) Enzymatic removal of plus-dA by digestion of PCR products with Klenow fragment (22).

(b) An additional 72°C step of 50 min at the end of PCR to drive the plus-dA reaction to completion (23).

Depending on the individual marker characteristics, one or none of these strategies may be necessary. It is important to note that reaction parameters significantly influence the production of this plus-dA artefact. PCR conditions such as rapid cycling, short extension times, and lower Mg^{2+} concentration all minimize, whereas the opposite all increase production of artefact (24).

For electrophoresis detection and analysis of pooled DNA microsatellite amplifications (*Protocols 4 and 5*), sufficient product is necessary to place the highest allele peak in the upper half of the resolution range of the sequencer. Both over- and under-loading of PCR product can produce images that are unsuitable for accurate analyses. The dilution factors for each marker may vary

117

and must be examined to ensure accurate determination of allele frequencies. For clear resolution of pooled alleles, a concentration of 5–6% denaturing acrylamide should be used for all gel electrophoreses. Individual samples with known marker genotypes should be included on each gel to control for variation *between* gels that can often occur.

Protocol 2

PCR amplification of microsatellite markers

Equipment and reagents

- 96-well thermocycler (MJ Research or others e.g. Applied Biosystems)
- PCR 8- or 12-strip tubes and caps (Robbins Scientific)
- Pipettors (single and 12-tip multichannel—any manufacturer)
- PCR reagents: 10 × buffer II, 100 mM dNTPs, 25 mM MgCl$_2$, 5 U/μl *Taq* polymerase or Amplitaq Gold™ (Applied Biosystems)

- Fluorescent labelled primers (5′ forward primer only with HEX, TET, or FAM) (Research Genetics or Operon Technologies, Inc.)
- DNA (pooled and individual samples; n depends on experimental design)

Method

1 Prepare PCR reaction volumes[a] (10–15 μl) containing:

   (a) 5–20 ng total genomic DNA (pooled[b] or individual samples).

   (b) 1.5 mM MgCl$_2$, 10 mM Tris, 50 mM KCl, 200 μM of each dNTP (AmpliTaq™ buffer), 25 ng each primer.

   (c) 0.5 U of AmpliTaq™ polymerase (AmpliTaq Gold™ may be used).

2 Perform PCR using the following standard amplification parameters:[c]

   (a) 2 min at 94°C initial denaturation.

   (b) 28 cycles (1 min at 94°C, 1 min at 56°C, 45 sec at 72°C).

   (c) Final extension[d] of 50 min at 72°C.

[a] Reagents can be used to prepare as a mastermix and then aliquoted to each DNA sample tube for PCR.

[b] Pools should be amplified in duplicate (each replicate pool) to provide a control for variation in pool construction, PCR, and measurement.

[c] Each marker may need to be optimized independently and these conditions represent a good starting point. Annealing temperature may need to be raised and/or MgCl$_2$ and primer-pair concentrations adjusted. Optimization strategies for PCR conditions will not be discussed further in this chapter (see ref. 24).

[d] An additional 72°C step of 50 min is added at the end of PCR to drive the plus-dA reaction to completion.

Protocol 3

Elimination of A-overhang from PCR products

Equipment and reagents

- Thermocycler or 30 °C incubator
- Pipettors (single and 12-tip multichannel— any manufacturer)
- Klenow fragment (Amersham Pharmacia Biotech, Inc.)
- Klenow 10 × reaction buffer (Amersham Pharmacia Biotech, Inc.)

Method

1 Mix the following reagents:

(a) Klenow fragment (0.25 U).

(b) 12.5 μl of PCR product from pooled amplification[a] (Protocol 2).

(c) 1.5 μl of 10 × reaction buffer.

(d) 1.0 μl dd H_2O.

2 Incubate at 30 °C for 1.0–1.5 h.

[a] Reagents can be prepared as a mastermix and then added directly to PCR product in original tube following amplification.

Protocol 4

Preparation of denaturing polyacrylamide gel for electrophoresis

Equipment and reagents

- Sequencing gel cassette (Applied Biosystems)
- 36 cm 'well-to-read' sequencing plates (Applied Biosystems)
- 0.2 mm spacers and 34–96 well combs (Applied Biosystems)[a]
- SequaGel sequencing system: concentrate, diluent, and buffer (National Diagnostics)
- N,N,N′,N′-tetramethylethylenediamine (TEMED) (Sigma Chemical Company)
- 10% (w/v) ammonium persulfate (APS) (Sigma Chemical Company)[b]
- Alconox cleanser (Fisher Scientific)
- Ethanol (200 proof) (Fisher Scientific)
- Kimberly-Clark Kimwipes EX-L (Fisher Scientific)
- Applied Biosystems reference manuals for automated sequencer

Method

1 Clean glass plates using a light sprinkle of Alconox cleanser and gloved hand. Rinse the plates thoroughly and dry with large Kimwipes. Following this wash, rinse both plates with ethanol and wipe dry.

2 Assemble plates and spacers and place horizontally on blocks (or tip boxes, etc.) so that they are level for gel pouring. Alternatively, gel can be poured using gel cassette apparatus according to manufacturer's protocol (not discussed here).

3 Prepare denaturing gel mix according to manufacturer's protocol. Example for a 6% gel (50 ml total volume), gently mix the following reagents:
   - 12.0 ml gel concentrate
   - 33.0 ml gel diluent
   - 5.0 ml gel buffer
   - 40 μl TEMED
   - 500 μl of 10% (w/v) ammonium persulfate

4 Keep the glass plates horizontal and add the gel mix slowly to the upper end using large syringe. Allow the gel mix to evenly migrate between the plates by capillary action. Insert comb into end of plates and allow 1.5–2.0 h for complete polymerization.[c]

[a] Combs are available in 36-, 48-, 64-, and 96-well formats, depending on ABI sequencer model.

[b] Ammonium persulfate should be freshly prepared every few days and stored in the dark at 4 °C.

[c] Gel can be poured 24–36 h ahead of time of use. Cover top of gel with comb in place using Saran Wrap.

Protocol 5

Sample preparation and gel electrophoresis using automatic sequencer

Equipment and reagents

- Automated sequencing instrument ABI377 (Applied Biosystems)
- Thermocycler or 94 °C incubator
- GENESCAN (Ver. 2.0.1) software (Applied Biosystems)
- GENOTYPER (Ver.) software (Applied Biosystems)
- 96-well Falcon assay plates for sample preparation (Becton Dickinson)
- Internal lane sizing standard: Tamara-350 or Tamara-500 molecular weight marker (Applied Biosystems)

- Blue dextran sample loading buffer (Applied Biosystems)
- Formamide (Sigma Chemical Company)
- Pipettors (single and 12-tip multichannel— any manufacturer)
- Loading tips
- Denaturing acrylamide and buffer kit (National Diagnostics)
- 10 × TBE (Life Technologies, Inc.); working concentration is 1 × TBE
- Applied Biosystems reference manuals for automatic sequencer

Protocol 5 continued

Method

1 Remove comb and assemble gel cassette apparatus according to manufacturer's protocol. Place gel cassette apparatus onto the automatic sequencer and put top and bottom buffer chambers in place. Carefully fill top and bottom with $1 \times$ TBE and begin pre-run (30 min) of gel as described in manufacturer's protocol.

2 For each individual or pooled amplification, combine the following using a 96-well tray:[a]
   - 2.5 μl formamide
   - 0.5 μl internal lane size standard (Tamara-350)
   - 0.5 μl blue dextran loading buffer
   - 4.0 μl of PCR product[b]

3 Denature the samples for electrophoresis at 94 °C for 5 min.

4 Flush the gel wells with syringe to remove any urea.

5 Immediately load 0.5–2.0 μl of each sample onto gel[c] (obtained in Protocol 2).

6 Perform electrophoresis on automatic sequencer at 3600 V for 2.0–3.5 h.

7 Following electrophoresis, perform gel analysis using GENESCAN as described in the manufacturer's instruction manual:
   (a) Check gel lane tracking manually.
   (b) Define size standard peaks manually.
   (c) Use 2nd order least squares sizing method to calculate peak sizes to 0.01 of a base.

8 Import raw data for each amplification into Excel for analysis.

9 GENOTYPER can be used for allele image analysis (see discussion in Section 4.4).

[a] Reagents can be used to prepare as a mastermix and then aliquoted to wells in 96-well tray before adding PCR product.

[b] At this step, PCR products obtained for different markers can be pooled, depending on size and colour of fluorescent label. Sufficient product for each marker is needed to place the highest allele peak in the upper half of the resolution range of sequencer. Both over- and under-loading can produce images that are unsuitable for accurate analyses. Dilutions for each marker may vary and must be tested.

[c] The amount loaded onto each gel will depend on intensity of each marker (see footnote b) as well as number of wells used for each gel, e.g. if you are using a 64-well comb, only 0.5 μl of sample can be loaded as compared to 2.0 μl for 34-well comb.

4 Analysis of pooled microsatellite data

Several approaches can be used for the analysis of pooled microsatellite data depending on specific study objectives and required accuracy of allele frequency estimations. In the most general scenario, allele frequency estimates can be determined from pooled data and compared between two groups of interest (e.g. patients and controls, patient subgroups, or other groups), to identify significant associations. A typical electropherogram from a pooled DNA microsatellite amplification is shown in *Figure 1*. Peak heights obtained from electropherograms are used to estimate the approximate allele frequencies, assuming that peak height is directly proportional to the DNA amount for a particular allele. Allele frequencies are therefore estimated from the peak height for each allele (from N individuals) divided by the sum of the peak heights for all alleles (2N allele frequency counts) as shown in *Table 1*. Because each pool should be run in triplicate (three replicates were made for each pool in *Protocol 1*) the mean of the three values can then be used for further analysis.

4.1 Correction methods for stutter and differential amplification

The most challenging aspect of a pooling approach for microsatellite typing is the accurate interpretation of allele frequencies. Stutter bands are produced by the amplification of products one or two repeat units shorter than the correct sized PCR product (or allele) because of slippage of *Taq* polymerase on the repeated sequence (25). When pooled samples are used to determine allele frequencies for a particular marker, these stutter bands are included with the correct sized alleles one or two repeat units smaller. Stutter is more prevalent in dinucleotide repeats, the most common form of microsatellite markers, but also occurs to a much lesser extent in tri- and tetranucleotide repeats (26). Dif-

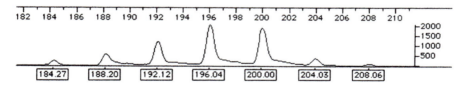

Figure 1 Electropherogram showing pooled amplification results for tetranucleotide microsatellite marker D4S1625 and a pool size of 60 individuals (using ABI377 automated sequencer). Allele sizes range from 184–208 base pairs.

Table 1 Allele frequencies determined from pooled amplification of D4S1625[a]

Allele (bp)	Peak height	Estimated allele frequencies	Estimated allele counts
184	253	0.042	5.0
188	506	0.084	10.1
192	1188	0.196	23.5
196	1952	0.322	38.7
200	1720	0.284	34.1
204	324	0.054	6.4
208	113	0.019	2.2

[a] Results based on pooled data from amplification of marker shown in Figure 1 (n = 60 individuals).

ferential amplification, another potential artefact, is observed in heterozygotes and is caused by the preferential amplification of the smaller allele. This is observed in all classes of microsatellites, to some extent, and is believed to result from the larger alleles reannealing at a faster rate (since they contain more repeat units) which reduces the efficiency of PCR amplification (27). Not all markers will demonstrate stutter artefact and/or differential amplification, and some of these difficulties, if present, may be overcome by modification of the PCR reaction parameters. However, both stutter artefact and differential amplification of microsatellite alleles can lead to a distortion in the estimated allele frequencies between two groups analysed with DNA pooling.

Several approaches to accurately estimate allele frequencies of microsatellite markers from pooled amplifications have been reported (28–30). More recently, Perlin *et al.* (31) described a more sophisticated method for the mathematical correction of stutter artefacts. The relative amount of product for the true allele and stutter bands is calculated individually for each allele of a microsatellite marker and then used to construct a matrix. This matrix is then used to adjust the results from a pool in which many alleles are represented (19). This method is more accurate than others that have been described because it takes into account the observation that each allele of a particular marker has its own unique stutter pattern.

While a full description of the theory underlying the matrix correction method is beyond the scope of this chapter, it is simply outlined here. Briefly, an observed vector distribution Y of band peak heights is characterized by:

$$Y = AX$$

where the vector X denotes the true distribution of allele proportions and the rectangular matrix A consists of known stutter profiles for the alleles derived from individual typings at a locus. Individual genotyping results are used to construct the allele-specific correction matrix. The pseudoinverse function in the program package Mathematica® (Wolfram Research—see Appendix) can be used to calculate the inverse of the rectangular matrix A, and is then used to determine X from the product of A^{-1} and Y.

An example of a matrix used for correction of data obtained from the pooled DNA microsatellite amplification is taken from Barcellos *et al.* (19) and is shown in *Table 2*. Here, significant stutter artefact peaks were observed for dinucleotide microsatellite marker D6S105, and an allele-specific matrix was designed using individual D6S105 genotyping profiles (data not shown) for correction of pooled data. In *Table 2*, the columns of matrix A represent the stutter profiles for each of the observed alleles derived from individual genotyping results. The distribution of fragments for allele 129 for example is 0.55, 0.27, and 0.18, for fragment sizes 129, 127, and 125, respectively. The pseudoinverse of this rectangular matrix was multiplied by a vector Y, the observed distribution of fragment sizes in the pooled samples to give the allele frequency estimates, vector X. The corrected frequencies were normalized in order to sum to a total of 100%. An example of the observed pooled DNA control frequency profile from a pool of 75 individuals,

Table 2 D6S105 stutter correction matrix, A, observed pooled fragment distribution of controls, Y, and resulting estimated allele frequencies X[a,b]

A											Y	X	Allele
133	131	129	127	125	123	121	119	117	115	113			
.68	0	0	0	0	0	0	0	0	0	0	2.19	3.22	133
.26	.68	0	0	0	0	0	0	0	0	0	4.22	4.97	131
.06	.26	.55	0	0	0	0	0	0	0	0	9.33	14.26	129
0	.06	.27	.73	0	0	0	0	0	0	0	16.89	17.45	127
0	0	.18	.27	.68	0	0	0	0	0	0	47.56	59.24	125
0	0	0	0	.26	.73	0	0	0	0	0	26.13	13.75	123
0	0	0	0	.06	.27	.73	0	0	0	0	28.03	29.38	121
0	0	0	0	0	0	.23	.73	0	0	0	8.73	2.70	119
0	0	0	0	0	0	.04	.27	.73	0	0	4.98	3.94	117
0	0	0	0	0	0	0	0	.23	.80	.83	1.94	1.33	115
0	0	0	0	0	0	0	0	.04	.20	.17	0.00	0.00	113

[a] Modified from ref. 31, and based on individual typing results for the D6S105 dinucleotide microsatellite.
[b] Reproduced with permission from *Am. J. Hum. Genet.* (ref. 19).

and the resulting allele frequency estimates following stutter correction are also presented in *Table 2*. Results determined using a pool of 75 control individuals are shown in *Figure 2* where the p-value for this comparison using goodness of fit chi-square testing, 0.91 (vs. $p < 10^{-5}$ uncorrected for stutter), demonstrates the closeness of corrected pooled allele counts to individual typing results.

Other methods have been recently described for correction of stutter effects and differential amplification (32). For stutter adjustment, individual genotype profiles are utilized as described above; however, instead of constructing a matrix, correction is performed progressively starting from the longest available allele for a particular marker using calculated ratios between height of stutter band and height of primary peak. It is not always possible to obtain values for rare alleles and these values can be obtained using the mean of the two adjacent alleles for a particular marker. No correction is made to the longest allele. The height of the next longest allele is reduced by the estimated size of the first stutter band of the longest allele. The height of the third longest allele is then reduced by the size of the second stutter band of the longest allele and the first stutter band of the (already corrected) second longest allele. The process is repeated down to the shortest allele, can incorporate any number of stutter bands, and can be performed using Microsoft Excel® software (32).

Correction for differential amplification involves recording the relative heights of alleles of several heterozygous individuals across the whole range of alleles for a particular marker. This allows the calculation of the average reduction in peak height per repeat unit (32). The shortest allele (already corrected for stutter) is left unchanged, and larger alleles are multiplied by this increasingly higher correction factor. As described above for matrix correction, allele frequencies are normalized following correction for stutter and differential amplification so that all allele frequencies sum to 100%.

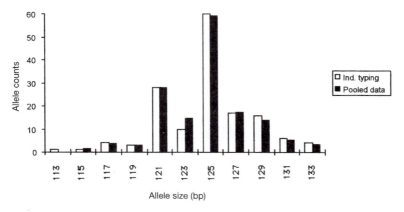

Figure 2 Pooled (pool size of 75) and individual typing results for D6S105 microsatellite. Pooled data adjusted for stutter artefact using matrix in Table 2 ($p = 0.91$ vs. 10^{-5} unadjusted). Reproduced with permission from *Am. J. Hum. Genet.* (ref. 19).

4.2 Example of a case-control study using pooled DNA amplification

PCR amplification of microsatellite markers and comparison of pools of patient and ethnically matched control DNA samples can be used to reveal disease associations (19). The locus responsible for haemochromatosis (HFE), for example, shows an association with allele 121 of the dinucleotide marker D6S105, located within a region 3.3 cM telomeric to HLA-A on chromosome 6p21 (33). A comparison of a pool of 51 haemochromatosis patients with a pool of 75 control individuals typed for D6S105 (shown in *Figure 3*) revealed a significant positive association of allele 121 in the patients, accompanied by a reduction in frequency of most other alleles ($\chi^2 = 47.6$, df = 7, p < 10^{-5}, corrected for stutter using matrix in *Table 2*), with values virtually identical to those obtained from individual typing ($\chi^2 = 47.9$, df = 7 , p < 10^{-5}). Significant differences were also detected between pooled patient and control data without mathematical correction for stutter artefact ($\chi^2 = 37.0$, df = 7, p < 10^{-5}), even though the determination of allele frequencies within each pooled sample was not as accurate. Multiple comparisons were made for D6S105 using independent amplifications of both patient and control pools to demonstrate reproducibility of these results (data not shown). This example shows that pooled DNA amplifications of a dinucleotide microsatellite marker can be used to clearly signal the presence of a disease locus in a case-control association study design.

Several statistical approaches can be used to determine the significance of comparisons using pooled case-control allele frequency data. CLUMP (34) assesses the significance of the result using a Monte Carlo approach, by performing repeated simulations to generate tables having the same marginal totals as the ones under consideration and counting the number of times that a chi-square value associated with the real table is achieved by the randomly simulated data.

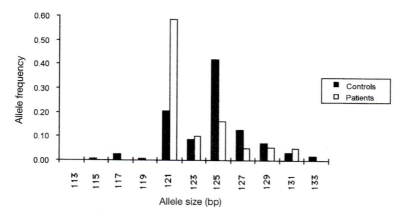

Figure 3 Haemochromatosis patients (n = 51) and control individuals (n = 75) typed using pooled samples for D6S105 microsatellite. Data adjusted for stutter artefact using matrix in Table 2 ($\chi^2 = 47.61$, df = 7, p < 10^{-5}). Reproduced with permission from *Am. J. Hum. Genet.* (ref. 19).

For each marker, 1000 simulations are run to estimate the nominal p-value. Overall chi-square contingency table testing can also be performed (19). For comparison of just one allele in patients vs. controls, the allele frequency differences can be tested under the null hypothesis that the frequencies within each group are equal, by use of a two sample test for binomial proportions with the unit normal distribution for assessing significance. As with Pearson χ^2 testing for specific alleles, a Bonferroni correction should be used to account for multiple testing. Other statistics for pooled data analyses have also been described (11). For case-control studies, comparisons can be performed using corrected or uncorrected allele frequency data, depending on the overall goals and design of a particular study.

4.3 DNA pooling using nuclear family-based samples

A DNA pooling strategy can also be used with nuclear (or trio) family-based sample collections to identify marker–disease associations. DNA samples obtained from mothers, fathers, and affected children (also, unaffected if available) are each pooled separately for PCR amplification of a particular marker. The subtraction method (18) can be applied to corrected pooled data to estimate a parental non-transmitted or affected family-based controls (AFBAC) 'control population' for comparison with patient allele frequencies. Several methods can be used to assess the significance of this comparison and have been described in Section 4.2. For comparison of just one allele, the allele frequency differences can be tested under the null hypothesis that the transmitted and non-transmitted frequencies are equal. If individual genotypes are used as follow-up using nuclear family-based samples, significance can be assessed by use of the transmission-disequilibrium test or (TDT) (35, 36). Examples of these approaches of analysis using pooled data are demonstrated in several recent studies (19, 20, 32, 37). Use of uncorrected DNA pool frequencies for family-based comparisons is not recommended.

4.4 Analysis of microsatellite allele image patterns from DNA pools

While more accurate estimation of allele frequencies from pooled DNA amplifications will be obtained following arithmetical corrections for stutter and differential amplification, this will require the individual genotyping of a number of individuals so that a unique matrix or adjustment factors based on these observations can be prepared to perform the correction. Because stutter and differential patterns will be unique to a given microsatellite marker, each must therefore be evaluated independently. The process can prove to be time-consuming, and another association marker screening process has been recently proposed which involves comparing microsatellite allele image patterns (AIPs) generated from PCR amplification of different DNA pools (38). Here, the difference in the areas of two AIPs produced using an automated sequencer is expressed as a fraction of the total area of the two AIPs or ΔAIP (see *Figure 4*). This

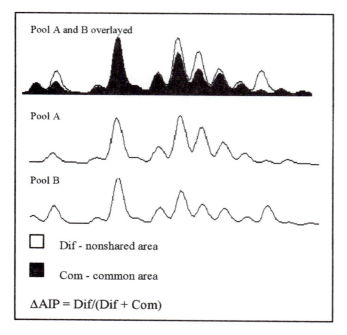

Figure 4 Overlaid allele image patterns (AIPs) of two different pools amplified with the marker D6S1666. Area 'Dif' and 'Com' are the non-shared and common areas, respectively, between the two AIPs. Reproduced with permission from *Am. J. Hum. Genet.* (ref. 38).

method can be quite useful in situations where the goal of a study is to identify significant differences between two groups, i.e. case-control or patient subtypes, etc. Assuming PCR amplification of two pools under the same conditions will result in similar stutter and differential amplification, any differences would then be due to different allele frequency distributions. This method may be appropriate for use as a screen for markers in two-stages that would then be confirmed using individual genotyping (37, 38).

Full details of this method are presented in Daniels *et al.* (38); however a brief description of the analysis method is presented here. Triplicate pools for each pool and duplicate PCR runs are recommended (as described above) for analysis using an ABI377 sequencer. The six resulting pooled images can be overlaid using GENOTYPER which scales all traces so that the height of the largest peak is equal in each. The baseline is determined automatically in GENOTYPER and images are not modified in any way, prior to analysis. The consensus image is taken to be representative of the allele frequencies in that pool. The consensus images for the two pools to be compared are overlaid in GENOTYPER and are sorted by use of the Apple Macintosh® screen capture facility. The pooled allele image is isolated as simple text (Macintosh) and then imported into the Debabelizer® graphics manipulation software for analysis (Equilibrium—see Appendix). Calculation of ΔAIP, the measure of the total area that is not shared by the two superimposed consensus allele image patterns is expressed as a fraction of the total shared and non-shared area. The area 'Com' is common to both allele image patterns. The non-shared area is denoted 'Dif'. Areas Com and Dif are measured in Debabelizer® by shading the shared and non-shared areas in different colours and calculating the pixel count for each. The ΔAIP test statistic is calculated from the expression Dif/(Dif + Com) (38).

Because the value of ΔAIP is influenced by factors such as number of marker alleles and the number of cases and controls in the sample, the largest AIP values will not necessarily correspond to the most statistically significant differences. Therefore, computer simulation is necessary to determine significance levels as described (38). Values of P for ΔAIP are obtained by simulating case and control samples from a population with allele frequencies estimated from the peak heights of the control sample—a software program for this purpose is available from co-author M. J. Owens (37, 38). Delta AIP should be used simply as an initial screening procedure prior to individual genotyping when precise significance levels are not usually required. Allele image patterns obtained for pools appear to be highly reproducible. Simulations have demonstrated that the power of ΔAIP to detect allele differences between pools is comparable with that of chi-square contingency table testing. For markers yielding significant ΔAIPs in an original sample, a replication sample can be used to test an allele-specific directional hypothesis (ASDH) derived from the allele showing the largest group difference in the original sample (39). The height of the allele's peak for each group is converted to a percentage of the total of all the peak heights for the group and tested for significance using Pearson χ^2 comparing that peak against all others.

While the ΔAIPs approach can serve as a valuable method for association screening, there are several disadvantages:

(a) Results from PCR reactions cannot be averaged, which would allow the reduction of error due to variation between replicate pools.

(b) The method does not allow the frequency of non-transmitted parental alleles to be estimated when nuclear or trio families are used, so family studies are not possible.

(c) It does not allow specific differences in individual alleles to be measured.

5 SNP allele frequency determination using kinetic PCR

SNPs have recently been recognized as attractive markers for association mapping of disease genes. Although SNPs are mostly biallelic, and therefore less informative than microsatellite markers, they occur much more frequently within the genome and are mutationally more stable (40–42). In addition, because SNPs have only two alleles, they are more amenable to automated methods of genotyping. Several robust and high-throughput methods exist for genotyping SNPs, including allele-specific PCR, high-density oligonucleotide hybridization arrays (12), multiplex PCR single base extension (SBE) methods

(43), denaturing high performance liquid chromatography (DHPLC) (44), and others. All of these methods require varying degrees of post-PCR processing, and currently it is unclear which method will be the most cost- and labour-efficient way to type the large numbers of both markers and individual samples that are necessary for full genome association screening.

A novel method for the determination of SNP allele frequencies using pooled DNA samples and kinetic PCR has recently been described (45). This typing method is extremely accurate and has a number of advantages over others that have been proposed. Genotyping of pools does not require expensive fluorescent labelled primers or probes; it does not involve any post-PCR processing, and it operates under uniform conditions without the need for marker-specific assay optimization. It promises to be inexpensive, time-saving, and precise enough to allow detection of the relatively weak but important genetic effects expected for complex traits using outbred populations.

As described in ref. 45, in order to measure a SNP allele frequency in a mixture of DNAs pooled from individual samples, two separate allele-specific PCR reactions are performed on equal aliquots of the pool. The specificity of the PCR amplifications is conferred by placing the 3′ end of one of the primers in each reaction directly over and matching one or the other of the variant nucleotides (46). This specificity can be enhanced particularly by using the Stoffel fragment of *Taq* DNA polymerase (47). Ideally, only completely matched primers are extended and only the matching allele is amplified. However, in practice the mismatched allele will frequently also be amplified, but much less efficiently so that many more amplification cycles are needed to generate detectable levels of PCR product. Using the conditions described below, mismatch amplification is frequently delayed by more than ten cycles when monitoring the amplification on a cycle-by-cycle basis (48) using fluorescent dsDNA binding dyes such as SYBR® Green I. A delay of around six cycles is adequate for the determination of allele frequencies of SNPs that have a minor allele frequency greater than a few per cent.

When the allele frequency in a pool is 50%, the two PCR amplifications are expected to require the same number of cycles to produce the same increase in fluorescent signal, assuming that both allele-specific primers amplify with equal efficiency. The number of cycles it takes for a reaction to cross a predetermined fluorescence threshold is called the C_t, and can be a fractional value. When one allele is more frequent in a pool, the PCR reaction specific to that allele will reach the threshold at an earlier cycle (i.e. have a smaller C_t value), than the PCR reaction amplifying the other allele. The difference in C_ts between the two PCR reactions, the ΔC_t, is a measure of the amplification bias and thus of the allele frequency. A one cycle delay means that the ratio of the amount of one allele to the other is ½; a two cycle delay, ¼; or in general, $1/2^{\Delta Ct}$. Converting a ratio to a frequency by adding the numerator to the denominator results in:

$$\text{frequency of allele}_1 = 1/(2^{\Delta Ct} + 1)$$

where $\Delta C_t = (C_t \text{ of allele}_1\text{-specific PCR}) - (C_t \text{ of allele}_2\text{-specific PCR})$.

Note that ΔC_t can be either positive or negative, depending on which specific PCR reaction exhibits the lowest C_t. The '2' in the denominator is properly '1 + the initial replication efficiency'. However, the initial replication efficiency is usually sufficiently close to 100% so that '2' is an adequate approximation (49).

The amplification efficiencies for the two allele-specific PCR amplifications may differ slightly. This can be measured and compensated for by performing the allele-specific PCR reactions on a DNA known to be heterozygous for the SNP of interest. The ΔC_t for this DNA should equal zero if the PCRs are equally efficient. Any deviation from zero indicates that they are not, and the deviation can be subtracted from the ΔC_t measurements to compensate for differential amplification efficiencies (*Table 3*). In practice, however, it should only be necessary to include heterozygote controls to correct for differential amplification efficiency when one is interested in determining the absolute allele frequency in a given pool. For an initial case-control screen of a large number of SNPs it would not be practical to include heterozygote controls for each SNP, and differential amplification efficiencies should not interfere with the ability to identify significant differences in allele frequency between pools of DNA. The subset of SNPs identified as potentially interesting in such a screen could then be re-amplified with the inclusion of heterozygote controls for differential amplification efficiency.

The conditions described here can be used in a screen of large number of SNP markers with little or no assay optimization. A number of assays will fail, but the failure rate can be estimated and controlled for in the subsequent analysis. Two forms of assay failure are possible:

(a) Failure to discriminate alleles adequately, leading to insensitivity to actual differences between DNA pools.

(b) Excessive assay variability leading to excess type I (false association) errors.

The frequency of the first type of failure can be estimated by 'spot-checking' a small subset of the total number of SNPs. Whether it has occurred in any given SNP cannot be known, but the effect of this type of error can be minimized by incorporating the failure rate into the subsequent analysis. A 20% failure rate, for instance, would mean that a study of 10 000 SNPs is actually only an 8000 SNP study. The occurrence of the second type of failure will be known for a particular SNP from the multiple measurements performed for each SNP as part of the screen. The SNP-specific variability can then be taken into account when assessing the significance of frequency differences at that particular SNP.

Figure 5 shows kinetic growth curves for two separate PCR reactions (four replicates of each) performed on a DNA sample that was prepared by adding 1 part of a DNA homozygous for one SNP allele to 19 parts of a DNA homozygous for the other allele. The amplified DNA thus contained a mixture of 5% allele$_1$ and 95% allele$_2$. Reactions amplified with the primer specific to allele$_1$ crossed the threshold at approximately cycle 26 (average 25.77), while reactions with the primer specific to allele$_2$ crossed the threshold at approximately cycle 30 (average 30.45). The ΔC_t, i.e. the difference between the two C_ts, was in this case

Protocol 6

SNP allele frequency determination on pooled DNA samples

Equipment and reagents

- Kinetic (real time, quantitative) thermocycler, GeneAmp® Sequence Detection System 5700 or 7700. Possible alternative machines: LightCycler™ (Idaho Technology, Inc.), iCycler™ (Bio-Rad Laboratories).

- Genomic DNA in 10 ng/µl concentration. To determine absolute values of an allele frequency at a given SNP, known heterozygous sample(s) (for the relevant SNP) can be used to control for differential amplification efficiency. Alternatively, differences in allele frequencies can be compared between two or more pools without the use of a heterozygous control.[a]

- Three oligonucleotide primers for each SNP: two allele-specific primers with alternate 3′ bases, and one common reverse primer. Design so that the calculated melting temperature is close to, but above 58 °C (ref. 50).

- Optical PCR tubes and caps (Perkin Elmer)

- Fluorescent dyes: SYBR® Green I fluorescent dye (Molecular Probes, Inc.), Rox dye (5-(and-6)-carboxy-X-rhodamine, Molecular Probes, Inc.)[b]

- Enzyme: *Taq* Stoffel Fragment 'Gold' polymerase (Roche Molecular Systems, available from the authors upon request) or *Taq* Stoffel Fragment (Applied Biosystems)

- 10 × Stoffel buffer: 10 mM Tris–HCl, 40 mM KCl pH 8.0

- PCR reagents: 25 mM $MgCl_2$; 2.5 mM each dATP, dCTP, dGTP, dTTP, and dUTP; 1 U/µl uracil-N-glycosylase (Perkin Elmer, AmpErase® UNG); 100% DMSO; and 80% (w/v) glycerol

A. PCR amplification

1 Design the PCR experiment. For allele frequency determinations on a pool of DNA samples (n is determined by experimental design), perform 4–12 replicate reactions with each set of allele-specific primers. Perform the same number of replicate reactions on individual sample(s) heterozygous for the SNP to use for adjustment in calculation of allele frequencies. If the accurate determination of allele frequencies within a pool of samples is not required, for example in a large case-control screening study where the primary goal is to detect significant frequency *differences* by comparison of the pools, then it may not be necessary to genotype known heterozygotes.

2 For each SNP allele frequency determination follow steps 2–6. Add the following components for a mastermix for 100.0 µl reactions, multiplied by the total number of reactions for a given SNP:

- 10 × Stoffel Gold buffer   10.0 µl
- 25 mM $MgCl_2$ 8.0 µl
- 2.5 mM dATP, dGTP, dCTP each   2.0 µl
- 2.5 mM dTTP   1.0 µl

- 2.5 mM dUTP   3.0 μl
- Stoffel Gold polymerase (12 U/μl)   1.0 μl
- UNG (1 U/μl)   2.0 μl
- ROX dye (200 μM)   1.0 μl
- SYBR Green (20 ×)   1.0 μl
- 100% DMSO[c]   4.0 μl
- 80% glycerol[d]   2.5 μl
- Sterile H_2O 58.5 μl

3   Add to this mastermix 2.0 μl (multiplied by the total number of reactions) from a 10 μM stock of the common primer.

4   Divide the mastermix into two aliquots (label primer mixes 'A' and 'B') of equal volumes. To each of the two primer mixes 'A' and 'B' add 2.0 μl (multiplied by half the total number of reactions) from a 10 μM stock of one or the other allele-specific primer. Note 'A' and 'B' each refer to one allele-specific primer.

5   Divide the two primer mixes each into two aliquots (mixes 'AP' and 'AH', 'BP' and 'BH') of equal volumes. Add to one of each of the two primer mixes, AP and BP, 2.0 μl (multiplied by 1/4 of the total number or reactions) from a 10 ng/μl stock of pooled DNA. Add to the other two primer mixes, AH and BH, 2 μl (multiplied by 1/4 of the total number of reactions) from a 10 ng/μl stock of heterozygous DNA.

6   Add 100.0 μl of each of the four mixes (AP, AH, BP, BH) into optical PCR tubes. Cover the optical tubes with optical caps.

7   Program the thermocycler with the following cycling conditions: An initial incubation step of 2 min at 50 °C;[e] an enzyme heat-activation step of 12 min at 95 °C; followed by 45 two-step amplification cycles of 20 sec at 95 °C and 20 sec at 58 °C; and a final 20 min product extension step at 72 °C.

8   Place the reactions in the thermocycler and start the PCR amplification.

B. Data analysis

1   Determine the C_t values for each amplification reaction.[f] Calculate the ΔC_t for each pair of allele frequency determinations, by subtracting the C_t value of the amplification with one allele-specific primer from the C_t value of the amplification with the other allele-specific primer.

2   In a similar manner determine the ΔC_t for the amplification of heterozygous DNA samples, and average the multiple values for replicate experiments. Subtract this average from all the replicate ΔC_t values obtained for the pooled DNA.

3   Calculate the allele frequency according to the following formula:

$$\text{frequency of allele}_1 = 1/(2^{\Delta Ct} + 1),$$

where $\Delta C_t = (C_t \text{ of allele}_1\text{-specific PCR}) - (C_t \text{ of allele}_2\text{-specific PCR})$.

Allele_2 frequency $= 1 - \text{allele}_1$ frequency.

4 Determine the standard deviation of the replicate allele frequency determinations. Accept only allele frequency determinations with variation below a certain predetermined threshold (e.g. 2 standard deviations).[g]

[a] It is possible to use a 1:1 mixture of samples homozygous for the relevant SNP instead of heterozygous sample(s). This mixture is used to correct for differences in amplification efficiency between the two allele-specific primers (see below). When comparing several pools to determine differences in allele frequencies, the accuracy of the absolute values obtained may not be relevant, and controlling for differential amplification efficiency may not be necessary.

[b] SYBR Green binds specifically to double-stranded DNA, and an increase in fluorescence is thus a measure of the amplification of DNA. Rox is added to reduce the relative contribution of light scatter to the baseline fluorescence measurement and minimize well-to-well variation in relative fluorescence increase.

[c] 1% DMSO added with SYBR Green, for a total of 5%.

[d] 0.2% glycerol added with Stoffel.

[e] This allows an UNG-mediated elimination of carryover PCR product contamination (51).

[f] The C_t values can either be read directly off the PE/ABI sequence detection software, or calculated by setting an arbitrary fluorescence threshold, and then determining at which cycle the fluorescence crosses that threshold.

[g] Too large variability (between allele frequency determinations) of any particular assay indicates that the allele-specific amplification is not functioning properly. The primers of that particular assay may have to be redesigned. Amplification growth curves (automatically generated with the PE/ABI 5700 or 7700) should also be consulted. Amplifications that cross the threshold or reach the exponential phase of amplification at a high cycle number (e.g. after cycle 35 for 20 ng initial template concentration under the conditions given here) may be the product of the amplification of non-specific template and will thus not provide reliable allele frequencies.

an average of 4.68 cycles (*Table 3*, B71 polymorphism). Using the equation given above, and correcting for differential amplification efficiency, this ΔC_t corresponded to an allele$_1$ frequency of 5% (45). Pooled case-control and family-based samples can both be used with this method to determine SNP allele frequencies in a pooled DNA association screen. For either study design, differences in pooled allele frequencies can be tested for significance as described in Section 4.2.

6 Experimental design considerations

Large scale association genome screening using pooled DNA samples will have several experimental advantages. In the case of complex diseases, both interaction effects and disease heterogeneity can be examined simultaneously by appropriately subdividing patient groups prior to pooling. Different loci in different individuals may be contributing to a single disease phenotype, and this

Table 3 SNP allele frequency measurements across a range of values[a,b]

Allele 1 frequency (by OD$_{260}$)	Expected ΔC_t	PON				B71			
		Average observed ΔC_t	Heterozygote corrected ΔC_t	Measured allele 1 frequency	Standard deviation ±	Average observed ΔC_t	Heterozygote corrected ΔC_t	Measured allele 1 frequency	Standard deviation ±
0.95	-4.25	-4.01	-4.05	0.94	0.016	-3.21	-3.77	0.93	0.012
0.90	-3.17	-2.99	-3.03	0.89	0.010	-2.23	-2.79	0.87	0.023
0.80	-2.00	-1.88	-1.92	0.79	0.014	-1.22	-1.78	0.77	0.040
0.67	-1.00	-1.02	-1.06	0.68	0.051	-0.21	-0.77	0.63	0.032
0.59	-0.50	-0.44	-0.48	0.58	0.030	0.24	-0.32	0.56	0.031
0.50	0.00	0.14	0.10	0.48	0.016	0.70	0.14	0.48	0.024
Het.	0.00	0.04	0.00	0.50	0.051	0.56	0.00	0.50	0.013
0.42	0.50	0.78	0.74	0.37	0.045	1.21	0.66	0.39	0.016
0.33	1.00	1.18	1.14	0.31	0.007	1.65	1.09	0.32	0.021
0.20	2.00	2.11	2.07	0.19	0.007	2.54	1.99	0.20	0.011
0.10	3.17	3.21	3.17	0.10	0.014	3.63	3.07	0.11	0.007
0.05	4.25	4.52	4.48	0.04	0.003	4.68	4.12	0.05	0.002

[a] C_t measurements are average of four replicates.

[b] Reproduced with permission from *Genome Research* (ref. 45).

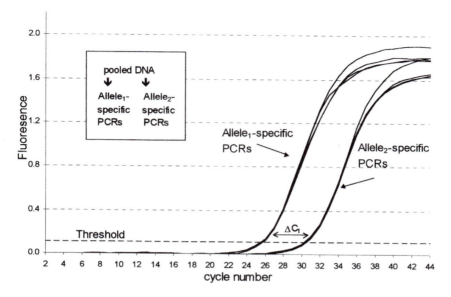

Figure 5 The basis of allele frequency measurement using kinetic PCR. Shown are amplification growth curves of PCR reactions performed for the ApoB71 polymorphism. A sample was constructed from two DNAs each homozygous for the different alleles of the ApoB71 SNP and contains 5% of allele 1. Equal aliquots of the pool (20 ng DNA each) were put into PCRs containing either of the two allele-specific primer sets. Four replicate reactions were performed with each primer set (eight PCRs total) The relative allele frequency is determined on the basis of the ΔC_t using equation (see text). Reproduced with permission from *Genome Research* (ref. 45).

possibility is particularly amenable to study in complex diseases where, for example, HLA associations have been determined and can be used to identify patient population pools (52, 53). In addition to predisposing genetic components within a subgroup of a particular disease, factors such as age of onset, sex, or other clinical phenotypes can also be used for classification, while at the same time maintaining use of large sample numbers for increased statistical power. The information and protocols presented here are relevant to all disease studies, but in particular to complex genetic diseases where the mode of inheritance is unknown, and multiple loci of modest effect, incomplete penetrance, heterogeneity, and interaction effects are likely to be involved.

An experimental design for association disease mapping must address two important issues: first, power, the probability of detecting a true disease association, and secondly, elimination of false associations which represent type I error. These form the basis of several important considerations in determining the best experimental design for association mapping given intrinsic properties of a particular disease such as population prevalence, age of onset, and laboratory resources to perform a genome screen. Power for association mapping is dependent on marker allele frequencies and a number of other unknown parameters such as mode of inheritance of the disease, disease allele frequencies, linkage disequilibrium between the marker and disease loci, and the recombination fraction between the marker and disease loci. However, using both case-control and family-based data and random mating assumptions, power will be determined only by the patient and control marker allele frequencies, in which the unknown parameters are subsumed (19). Power calculations serve only as a guide in designing an experimental protocol. The actual power in any real situation will depend on a large number of factors, including the number of marker alleles, analysis methods (54, 55), and the actual type of the association, i.e. positive or negative, one marker associated versus multiple markers, etc. Both the power and accuracy of microsatellite and SNP markers to detect disease genes in association (linkage disequilibrium) mapping depend on several other factors, such as the age of the disease mutation (or polymorphism), the strength of the genetic effect, the marker allele distribution in the population, mutation rates of the marker loci, the frequency of the disease allele, the recombination fraction, and also, the methods for mapping the disease genes. A study can be individually designed, taking account of power calculations, the availability of case-control and family samples, and the expected type I errors following the high resolution genome screen (see ref. 19; see Chapter 1 for further considerations of experimental design).

6.1 Selection of markers for full genome association screen

The central requirement for association mapping is that linkage disequilibrium be able to detect any locus within the map intervals available by marker densities. The extent of disequilibrium can vary widely across the human genome. In the HLA region, which is probably subject to strong balancing selection, disequilibrium extends over three megabases (56). In general, LD mapping using microsatellites has proven successful in heterogeneous populations over much smaller distances of 50–500 kb (57). Recent population studies have demonstrated LD between 400 kb and 2 cM (3, 58). Telomeric regions, however, have shown lower levels of disequilibrium than centromeric regions (59), and this must be accounted for in any study design. Although a 3000 (1 cM) microsatellite genomic screen could theoretically detect many disease genes, a much finer, e.g. at least 6000–12 000 (0.5–0.25 cM) screen, is the preferred goal. Even then some disease loci will be missed, due to lack of linkage disequilibrium in that particular region, or within the disease locus, e.g. BRCA1 in non-Ashkenazi Jewish populations, where each family carries a unique mutation.

Although denser maps are desirable, a 0.5–1 cM interval which means that a disease locus is within 0.25–0.5 cM of a marker appears to be a reasonable starting point for a genomic screen using microsatellite markers. Currently, it is estimated that 75% of the genome is covered with a map density of 1 cM or more (60) and this coverage is increasing at a rapid rate, particularly for SNPs; the goal of < 1 cM density across the genome will be a reality in the very near future. Although no single large integrated database for both SNPs and microsatellite markers is currently available, several comprehensive databases containing the location and in most cases laboratory typing protocols for both marker types are located on the WWW (see Table 4 and references). An ideal study design will include the combined use of both marker types. Although SNPs are likely to be more stable, they are less informative and much larger numbers will be needed for full genome screening—on the magnitude of 30–300000 (2, 66). Microsatellites should therefore be used for an initial association genome screen followed by screening with SNPs (and additional microsatellites markers) for candidate regions identified in initial screen. Once the human genome project is completed and the full DNA sequence is available, it will still be an extraordinary task to characterize each expressed gene product and variation within and between populations. Over the next five to seven years, microsatellite markers will gradually be replaced by full complements of SNPs within each candidate gene in the genome which can easily be facilitated by large scale pooled DNA association screens to identify disease predisposing variants.

6.2 Study guidelines

The combined use of case-control and nuclear (trio) family samples in a DNA pooling study design is optimal. With case-control pools, the rate of false negative results will drop because the differences in allele frequencies between patients and controls will be higher in the presence of the same genetic effect and sample size (11) at the expense of more false positive results. However, the use of pools derived from nuclear families can be used to replicate positive results and will help to identify false positive signals.

Application of the ΔAIP test statistic (38), or alternatively the uncorrected comparison of case and control pool frequencies for heterogeneity using the chi-square test may be the most effective approach to an initial screen for frequency

Table 4 Name and Web addresses for some SNP and microsatellite marker databases

Database name	Web address
The SNP Consortium (TSC) Database	http://snp.cshl.org/
National Center for Biotechnology Information (NCBI)	http://www.ncbi.nlm.nih.gov/SNP
Database for SNPs (dbSNP)	
Cooperative Human Linkage Center (CHLC)	http://lpg.nci.nih.gov/CHLC
Integrated maps, including SNP and microsatellite locations	
Human Genic Bi-Allelic Sequences (HGBASE)	http://hgbase.interactiva.de
European SNP database	
Marshfield Center for Medical Genetics	http://research.marshfieldclinic.org/genetics
Human genetic linkage maps	
University of Southampton	http://cedar.genetics.soton.ac.uk/
School of Medicine	public_html
Genetic Location Database (LDB)	

[a] See refs 61–65 for additional information.

differences. An issue to remain aware of in this case is the danger of false negative results, which could result in missing consequential genetic effects. This problem can be alleviated to some extent with the use of a very lenient significance level ($p < 0.05$ or even 0.10) for the first stage. False positives can be removed in a second stage using an independent case-control or nuclear family-based sample of equal or larger size. Markers that yield significant differences for DNA pools in both the original and replication samples should then be genotyped individually for all subjects in order to confirm the results of DNA pooling using traditional methods. This would also allow for much more informative haplotype assignment, which is an unfortunate drawback to using pooled data. Allele-specific hypothesis testing can be performed in second stage screen. Rather than accepting any significant pattern of allelic differences in the replication sample, the same allele must yield a significant difference in the replication sample, and any difference uncovered must be in the same direction (37). However, if very small differences (modest effects) are to be identified, then correction for stutter and differential amplification should be used (19, 32).

6.3 Technical considerations

Stutter artefacts and differential amplification of microsatellite alleles are marker-dependent and will vary. Ideally, each marker in a high resolution genomic screen should be independently optimized using individual samples before initiating pooled DNA amplifications. Preliminary experiments could be performed on a large number of microsatellite polymorphisms using the root mean square error approach (RMSE) (20), correlation comparisons, or goodness-of-fit X^2 tests (19) to identify reliable markers for DNA pooling experiments. The specific study and levels of desired significance would determine the maximum values that could be tolerated. Optimization runs could include the same 20 randomly selected control individuals (40 chromosomes) which would also serve to measure specific allelic stutter or differential amplification for mathematical correction of pooled data, if desired. A sample of this size will yield useful information on population frequencies and marker heterozygosity (if unknown), and could also signal strong disequilibrium with adjacent markers.

In some laboratories, however, it may be impossible to completely validate each microsatellite and SNP assay before utilizing it in a genome screen. Instead, standard conditions could be established under which most primer sets will work adequately without optimization, and then only spot checking of a small subset of assays be done to ensure quality control. For microsatellites, artefacts produced by stutter or differential amplification will act without bias on both patient and control samples. Assuming PCR amplification of two pools under the same conditions will result in similar stutter and differential amplification, any differences would then be due to different allele frequency distributions. If a marker association is strong enough, significant differences will be observed between pooled patient and control allele frequencies even without adjustment for stutter or differential amplification artefact. However, if the disequilibrium of a marker, or the association strength of a disease locus to a disease were moderate or low, then the signal from such a marker could be buried in the noise of stutter artefact and differential amplification.

The practical laboratory definition of several thousand microsatellite markers for use in pooled genomic screens is an enormous task, but must only be completed once to make the method generally available for association mapping of human disease and trait loci. An automated sequencer or scanner for detection of fluorescently labelled PCR products is the ideal instrument for initial association screening with pooled DNA samples using microsatellites, because it allows a large amount of information to be obtained from each gel. To reduce labour and cost, the most efficient scheme for completing a pooled screen, including the preliminary marker optimization phase for both micro-satellites and SNPs, would be a large collaborative study of several diseases with independent laboratories typing all diseases, and a division of microsatellite (and eventually SNP) markers among laboratories.

The advantage of using pooled DNA samples for microsatellite and SNP screening is especially clear in terms of cost and labour when compared to individual typing. Calculations reveal that since there are approximately 1200 copies of the human genome in 1 ng of DNA, then using 25 ng of DNA in a PCR would still give an average of 30 complete copies of each person's DNA in a pool of 1000 individuals (21). For an initial screen of 1000 cases and 1000 controls, for example, the number of gels necessary to investigate 6000–12000 microsatellite markers would be reduced 300–600 fold from approximately 16500 for indi-vidual typing (6000 markers), to 50–100 for the pooled screen (based on 12 markers per lane, three replicate pools for each marker, and 64 lanes on an ABI377). For a screen of 10000 SNPs in 1000 cases and 1000 controls the number of assays is reduced from 20 million to 160000, if four replicate reactions are done for each SNP (45). Although careful quantitation of DNA samples and construction of pools are both necessary when using pooled amplifications, this is performed just once for an entire screen and constitutes a small fraction of the actual typing effort.

7 DNA pooling in the era of the human genome sequence

At the time of this writing, a first draft of the human genomic sequence has been reported (67, 68), and is publicly available. The potential utility of this remark-able record for disease gene discovery will be realized only after three derivative databases are completed: locus annotation, protein expression, and locus-specific polymorphism. A first generation annotation of the human genome, the identification and functional and phylogenetic classification of each locus, should be forthcoming with the entire sequence itself. Gene array methods are currently being employed to define the proteome, or expression profile for each locus, according to characteristics of health and development for each tissue and cell type. Past efforts to compile genome-wide marker systems, including SNPs and microsatellites, will need to be redirected to the issues of thoroughness and completeness of coverage for each locus-containing region of the genome. Because it will be impossible to accrue information on all polymorphic sites potentially responsible for disease gene effects, inferences based on linkage disequilibrium will continue to be important in the identification of disease genes. Nonetheless, examination of markers near specific candidate loci for a disease will remain indispensable for disease gene identification. In general, haplotypes identified from two or more polymorphic sites will continue to be an invaluable adjunct for defining nearby consequential genetic variation.

This brief sketch of the future terrain of genetic epidemiology must also include DNA pooling in candidate gene screening utilizing the background information outlined above. Although future methodological improvements can be anticipated for DNA pooling, the basic steps of DNA quantification, marker selection, and recommendations for study design and analysis as described in this review will remain pertinent. Familiar issues surrounding a candidate locus screen with DNA pooling will remain. The absence of a signal for disease gene association cannot be taken as absence of effect, as such, because the markers available for a disease locus may not include or be in linkage disequilibrium with the actual disease-causing variant. The number of examined sites will remain large, even after refining a search to include only loci physiologically pertinent, appropriately expressed, and covered by suitable polymorphism. This means that the twin concerns of statistical power and false positives must still be dealt with by sample size and study replication. It should be remembered, however, that one great advantage will be present: positive signals for a disease gene association can be examined by immediately focusing experiments on the one or few loci identified by the positive signal.

Acknowledgements

Many thanks to Jorge R. Oksenberg for helpful comments on this manuscript and to Jill Hollenbach and Stacy Caillier for valuable assistance with figures. L. F. Barcellos is a post-doctoral fellow of the National Multiple Sclerosis Society (NMSS).

References

1. Huttley, G. A., Smith, M. W., Carrington, M., and O'Brien, S. J. (1999). *Genetics*, **152**, 1711.
2. Krugylak, L. (1999). *Nature Genet.*, **22**, 139.
3. Kendler, K. S., MacLean, C. J., Ma, Y., O'Neill, F. A., Walsh, D., *et al.* (1999). *Am. J. Med. Genet.*, **88**, 29.
4. Jorde, L. B., Watkins, W. S., Viskochil, D., O'Connell, P., Ward, K., *et al.* (1993). *Am. J. Hum. Genet.*, **53**, 1038.
5. Pugliese, A. (1999). *Diabetes Rev.*, **7**, 39.
6. Mein, C. A., *et al.* (1998). *Nature Genet.*, **19**, 297.

7. Concannon, P., *et al.* (1998). *Nature Genet.*, **19**, 292.

8. Risch, N. and Merikangas, K. (1996). *Science*, **273**, 1516.

9. Morton, N. E. and Collins, A. (1998). *Proc. Natl. Acad. Sci. USA*, **95**, 11389.

10. Camp, N. J. (1997). *Am. J. Hum. Genet.*, **61**, 1424.

11. Risch, N. and Teng, J. (1998). *Genome Res.*, **8**, 1273.

12. Wang, D. G., Fan, J. B., Siao, C. J., Berno, A., Young, P., *et al.* (1998). *Science*, **280**, 1077.

13. Cargill, M., Altshuler, D., Ireland, J., Sklar, P., Ardlie, K., *et al.* (1999). *Nature Genet.*, **22**, 231.

14. Collins, F. S., Brooks, L. D., and Chakravarti, A. (1998). *Genome Res.*, **8**, 1229.

15. Marshall, E. (1999). *Science*, **284**, 406.

16. Xiong, M. and Jin, L. (1999). *Am. J. Hum. Genet.*, **64**, 629.

17. Martin, E. R., Gilbert, J. R., Lai, E. H., Riley, J., Rogala, A. R., *et al.* (2000). *Genomics*, **63**, 7.

18. Thomson, G. (1995). *Am. J. Hum. Genet.*, **57**, 487.

19. Barcellos, L. F., Klitz, W., Field, L. L., Tobias, R., Bowcock, A. M., *et al.* (1997). *Am. J. Hum. Genet.*, **61**, 734.

20. Shaw, S. H., Carrasquillo, M. M., Kashuk, C., Puffenberger, E. G., and Chakravarti, A. (1998). *Genome Res.*, **8**, 111.

21. Breen, G., Sham, P., Li, T., Shaw, D., Collier, D. A., and St. Clair, D. (1999). *Mol. Cell. Probes*, **13**, 359.

22. Ginot, F., Bordelais, I., Nguyen, S., and Gyapay, G. (1996). *Nucleic Acids Res.*, **24**, 40.

23. Smith, J. R., Carpten, J. D., Brownstein, M. J., Ghosh, S., Magnuson, V. L., *et al.* (1995). *Genome Res.*, **5**, 312.

24. Innis, M. A. and Gelfand, D. H. (1999). *PCR applications: protocols for functional genomics* (ed. M. A. Innis, D. H. Gelfand, and J. J. Sninsky), pp. 3–22. Academic Press, San Diego, CA.

25. Litt, M. and Luty, J. A. (1989). *Am. J. Hum. Genet.*, **44**, 397.

26. Sheffield, V. C., Nishimura, D. Y., and Stone, E. M. (1995). *Curr. Opin. Genet. Dev.*, **5**, 335.

27. Demers, D. B., Curry, E. T., Egholm, M., and Sozer, A. C. (1995). *Nucleic Acids Res.*, **23**, 3050.

28. Khatib, H., Darvasi, A., Plotski, Y., and Soller, M. (1994). *PCR Methods Appl.*, **4**, 13.

29. Pacek, P., Sajantila, A., and Syvanen, A. C. (1993). *PCR Methods Appl.*, **2**, 313.

30. LeDuc, C., Miller, P., Lichter, J., and Parry, P. (1995). *PCR Methods Appl.*, **4**, 331.

31. Perlin, M. W., Lancia, G., and Ng, S. K. (1995). *Am. J. Hum. Genet.*, **57**, 1199.

32. Kirov, G., Williams, N., Sham, P., Craddock, N., and Owen, M. J. (2000). *Genome Res.*, **10**, 105.

33. Feder, J. N., Gnirke, A., Thomas, W., Tsuchihashi, Z., Ruddy, D. A., *et al.* (1996). *Nature Genet.*, **13**, 399.

34. Sham, P. C. and Curtis, D. (1995). *Ann. Hum. Genet.*, **59**, 97.

35. Spielman, R. S., McGinnis, R. E., and Ewens, W. J. (1993). *Am. J. Hum. Genet.*, **52**, 506.

36. Spielman, R. S. and Ewens, W. J. (1996). *Am. J. Hum. Genet.*, **59**, 983.

37. Fisher, P. J., Turic, D., Williams, N. M., McGuffin, P., Asherson, P., *et al.* (1999). *Hum. Mol. Genet.*, **8**, 915.

38. Daniels, J., Holmans, P., Williams, N., Turic, D., McGuffin, P., Plomin, R., *et al.* (1998). *Am. J. Hum. Genet.*, **62**, 1189.

39. Hill, L., Craig, I. W., Asherson, P., Ball, D., Eley, T., *et al.* (1999). *Neuroreport*, **10**, 843.

40. Collins, F. S., Euyer, M. S., and Chakravarti, A. (1997). *Science*, **278**, 1580.

41. Landegren, U., Nilsson, M., and Kwok, P.-Y. (1998). *Genome Res.*, **8**, 769.

42. Brookes, A. J. (1999). *Gene*, **234**, 177.

43. Lindblad-Toh, K., Winchester, E., Daly, M. J., Wang, D. G., Hirschhorn, J. N., *et al.* (2000). *Nature Genet.*, **24**, 381.

44. Hoogendoorn, B., Norton, N., Williams, N., Hamshere, M. L., Spurlock, G., *et al.* (2000). *Hum. Genet.*, **107**, 488.
45. Germer, S., Holland, M. J., and Higuchi, R. (2000). *Genome Res.*, **10**, 258.
46. Newton, C. R., Graham, A., Heptinstall, L. E., Powell, S. J., Summers, C., *et al.* (1989). *Nucleic Acids Res.*, **17**, 2503.
47. Germer, S. and Higuchi, R. (1999). *Genome Res.*, **9**, 72.
48. Higuchi, R., Rockler, C., Dollinger, G., and Watson, R. (1993). *Bio/Technology*, **11**, 1026.
49. Higuchi, R. and Watson, R. M. (1999). *PCR applications: protocols for functional genomics* (ed. M. A. Innis, D. H. Gelfand, and J. J. Sninsky), pp. 263–84. Academic Press, San Diego, CA.
50. Wetmur, J. G. (1991). *Crit. Rev. Biochem. Mol. Biol.*, **26**, 227.
51. Longo, M. C., Berninger, M. S., and Hartley, J. L. (1990). *Gene*, **93**, 135.
52. Klitz, W., Aldrich, C. L., Fildes, N., Horning, S. J., and Begovich, A. B. (1994). *Am. J. Hum. Genet.*, **54**, 497.
53. Haines, J. L., Terwedow, H. A., Burgess, K., Pericak-Vance, M. A., Rimmler, J. B., *et al.* (1998). *Hum. Mol. Genet.*, **7**, 1229.
54. Terwilliger, J. D. (1995). *Am. J. Hum. Genet.*, **56**, 777.
55. Schaid, D. J. (1996). *Genet. Epidemiol.*, **13**, 423.
56. Klitz, W., Thomson, G., Borot, N., and Cambon-Thomsen, A. (1992). *Evol. Biol.*, **26**, 35.
57. Jorde, L. B., Watkins, W. S., Carlson, M., Groden, J., Albertsen, H., *et al.* (1994). *Am. J. Hum. Genet.*, **54**, 884.
58. Cox, A., Camp, N. J., Nicklin, M. J., *et al.* (1998). *Am. J. Hum. Genet.*, **62**, 1180.
59. Watkins, W. S., Zenger, R., O'Brien, E., Nyman, D., Eriksson, A. W., *et al.* (1994). *Am. J. Hum. Genet.*, **55**, 348.
60. Bowcock, A. M., Chipperfield, M. A., Ceverha, P., Yetman, E., and Phung, A. (1996). In *Human gene mapping 1995: a compendium* (ed. A. J. Cuticchia, M. A. Chipperfield, and P. A. Foster), pp. 1454–68. Johns Hopkins University Press, Baltimore.
61. Smigielski, E. M., Sirotkin, K., Ward, M., and Sherry, S. T. (2000). *Nucleic Acids Res.*, **28**, 352.
62. Sherry, S. T., Ward, M., and Sirotkin, K. (2000). *Hum. Mutat.*, **15**, 68.
63. Brooks, A. J., Lehvaslaiho, H., Siegfried, M., Boehm, J. G., Yuan, Y. P., *et al.* (2000). *Nucleic Acids Res.*, **28**, 356.
64. Porter, C. J., Talbot, C. C., and Cuticchia, A. J. (2000). *Hum. Mutat.*, **15**, 36.
65. Marth, G., Yeh, R., Minton, M., Donaldson, R., Li, Q., *et al.* (2001). *Nat. Genet.*, **27**, 371.
66. Roberts, L. (2000). *Science*, **287**, 1898.
67. MacIlwain, C. (2000). *Nature*, **405**, 983.
68. Butler, D. and Smaglik, P. (2000). *Nature*, **405**, 984.

Chapter 6

Single-sperm typing: a rapid alternative to family-based linkage analysis

Michael Cullen

Basic Research Program, SAIC, National Cancer Institute-Frederick, Frederick, MD, USA

Graduate Genetics Program, GWIBS, The George Washington University, Washington DC, USA

Mary Carrington

Basic Research Program, SAIC, National Cancer Institute-Frederick, Frederick, MD, USA

1 Introduction

Single-sperm typing provides an efficient means of measuring recombination frequencies relative to the traditional methods of genetic cross and pedigree analysis. Using this method, it is possible to rapidly determine the haplotype of each meiotic product directly using PCR to identify alleles at multiple polymorphic markers along the chromosome. Traditional pedigree analysis, on the other hand, requires genotypes collected from children of parents informative (heterozygous) for markers of interest. For example, mapping resolutions of 1–2 cM were reported for the Genethon human linkage map based on 5264 microsatellites genotyped for eight CEPH (Centre d'Etudes du Polymorphisme Humaine) families, totalling 134 individuals (186 meioses) (1). However, markers used to construct a family-based linkage map must have high joint polymorphic information content (PIC), i.e. a high proportion and number of informative meioses per marker pair (2). In regions of low marker density this is problematic since the total number of markers with high PIC values is decreased. This issue becomes less relevant with the use of single-sperm typing because donors who are heterozygous at the appropriate markers can be selected regardless of the PIC value of those markers. Furthermore, unlimited numbers of meiotic events provide a means of analysing tightly linked markers at resolutions of 0.1–0.2 cM, presently not possible by pedigree analysis (3–5). Thus, single-cell typing is quite useful for ordering loci along a chromosome and it is applicable to any species with haploid gametes from which semen samples can be obtained. Sperm typing has been used to determine phase when parental information is not available (6) and order tightly linked polymorphic markers (4, 7–10), some less than 1 cM apart (11, 12). It has also proven useful in the characterisation of recombination hotspots (13, 14), individual variation in recombination rates (9, 10, 14–18), chiasma interference (19), segregation distortion (20–23), germline frequency of mutations (24–31), and gene conversion events (27, 32).

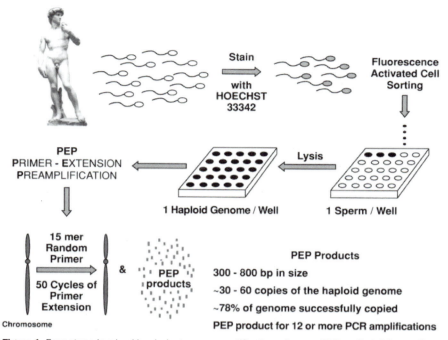

Figure 1 Four steps involved in whole genome amplification of sperm DNA: cell staining, cell sorting, cell lysis, and primer extension pre-amplification (PEP). Viable sperm are washed and stained with Hoechst 33342 (*Protocol 1*). Stained sperm are sorted, one per well, into 96-well microtitre plates containing alkaline lysis buffer, by fluorescence activated cell sorting (*Protocol 2*). Haploid DNA is released upon heat/alkaline lysis (*Protocol 2*). 50 cycles of primer extension using 15-mer random oligonucleotide primers generates millions of fragments that collectively represent the equivalent of 30–60 copies of the haploid genome and sufficient template for numerous PCR amplifications (*Protocol 3*).

Single-sperm typing involves the procurement of haploid DNA from semen, whole genome amplification of individual sperm (optional step), and PCR amplification of sperm DNA with oligonucleotide primers flanking the desired marker(s). Sperm are stained and sorted, one cell per well of a microtitre plate, by fluorescence activated cell sorting (FACS). Upon cell lysis every well contains one haploid genome. *Taq* polymerase-dependent primer extension utilising 15-mer random primers replicates roughly 78% of the genome 30–60 times as a series of 300–800 bp amplification products (*Figure 1*) (33). Whole genome amplification of single-sperm DNA is carried out when multiple PCR amplifications need be performed from one haploid sample. Upon completion, a small aliquot of this reaction serves as template for single or multiplex PCR amplification of short tandem repeats (STRs) and single nucleotide polymorphisms (SNPs). The following chapter provides an introduction to single-sperm typing, including protocols and discussion on:

(a) Single-sperm isolation.

(b) Whole genome amplification of haploid DNA.

(c) PCR amplification of STRs and SNPs using PEP product as a source of DNA.

(d) Nested and multiplex PCR amplification.

(e) Allele determination by gel electrophoresis.

(f) Interpretation of sperm typing data.

(g) General approaches for analysing recombination data.

2 Isolation of single sperm

The isolation of haploid DNA from individual sperm cells for genetic analysis can be divided into three steps: cell staining (*Protocol 1*), cell sorting (*Protocol 2*), and cell lysis (*Protocol 2*). Cell staining is carried out with Hoechst 33342, a non-intercalating fluorophore that preferentially binds AT-rich regions in the minor groove of DNA and fluoresces blue upon UV excitation (34). Hoechst 33342, as well as other bis-benzimidazoles, readily cross the plasma membrane, preserving cell viability and eliminating the need to fix or permeabilize cells. After staining, sperm cells are sorted and deposited, one per well, into a 96-well microtitre plate by fluorescence activated cell sorting. The cell sorter discriminates among stained sperm, diploid cells, and debris by excluding objects that fall outside a given range of fluorescence (a function of DNA content) and signal scatter (a function of cell size, shape, and texture). Critical to the sort is the ability of the cell deposition unit to capture a target cell in a small volume of cell lysis solution at the centre of each microtitre well. Proper alignment of the cell deposition unit ensures one sperm per well, and therefore, one haploid genome per well after sperm lysis (*Figure 2*). Following heat and alkaline lysis, the pH of each sample is neutralised and ready for direct PCR amplification or whole genome amplification.

Critical parameters to consider when sorting sperm include setting the FACS sort window, selecting an appropriate microtitre plate for sorting, and the pH of DNA after sperm lysis. Stained cells flowing through the FACS machine are recorded as events on a plot of fluorescence versus signal scatter. Cells highlighted within a sort window will be deflected into trays based on the extent of fluorescence and scatter. Setting a sort window too wide will allow unwanted material to be collected with your sample, and setting too tight will cause exclusion of single-sperm based on differential staining (*Figure 3*). After setting the window, a few cells should be sorted into an empty microtitre plate to confirm the presence of one sperm per well under a fluorescence microscope. Sorting into round-bottom microtitre plates will improve the odds of a sperm hitting the denaturing solution at the centre of the well, not the side. The plates must be thin-walled for proper heat transfer during the PEP amplification step discussed in Section 3. Difficulty amplifying DNA from a lysed and neutralised sample may reflect a sample pH outside the optimum for *Taq* polymerase (pH 8.3). Prior to adding the neutralisation buffer (*Protocol 2*) confirm that a 1:1 mixture of cell lysis and neutralisation buffer is pH 8.25–8.35. A more thorough discussion of cell sorting can be found in *Current protocols in cytometry* (34) and *Flow cytometry: a practical approach* (35).

Studies involving small numbers of individually isolated sperm are possible

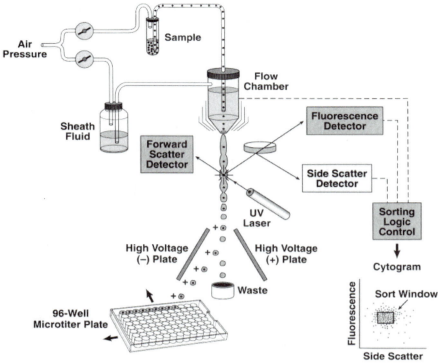

Figure 2 Fluorescence activated cell sorter. A stream of droplets containing one cell each is generated when cells are forced, under pressure, through a vibrating fluid filled flow chamber. Individual cells passing through the beam of a UV laser scatter light, and fluoresce when stained. The amount of light scatter and fluorescence is measured with detectors and sent to the FACS sorting logic control where it is displayed as a cytogram. Cells fluorescing and scattering light within a range determined by the sort window meet the selection criteria and are positively charged. Uncharged cells flow into the waste while selected cells are deflected into the wells of a 96-well tray, as they pass through an electric field. A cell deposition unit positions the 96-well tray so each well receives the specified number of cells.

without the assistance of a flow cytometer. Laboratories equipped with an inverted phase-contrast microscope and tabletop centrifuge can isolate individual sperm by one of two methods involving micromanipulation. Li *et al.* purified sperm from semen by sucrose step gradient centrifugation followed by isolation of individual cells by micromanipulation under a microscope (5, 36). Lien *et al.* isolated individual sperm embedded in small dried pieces of low-melting point agarose (6, 10, 18).

Sources of viable sperm for sorting are limited to cryobanks and volunteer donor programs. Sperm from a cryobank is viably frozen and shipped overnight. Donor information accompanying the frozen sample may include ethnic background, health, and infectious disease status. Sperm from a donor program is often unprocessed and potential disease status of the donor is usually unknown. Appropriate safety precautions should be taken when sorting cells of unknown background.

Protocol 1

Wash and stain sperm

Equipment and reagents

- 120 ml sterile polypropylene specimen container (Fisher Scientific)
- Falcon 50 ml polypropylene conical tubes (Becton Dickinson)
- Beckman TJ6 tabletop centrifuge
- Haemocytometer
- Inverted microscope
- Semen from donor[a,b]
- 1 × PBS pH 7.4, without $CaCl_2$ and $MgCl_2$ (Gibco BRL)
- 10 mg/ml Hoechst 33342 (Sigma Chemical Company)
- QIAamp® DNA extraction kit (Qiagen)

Method

1 Dilute the entire semen sample to 80 ml with 1 × PBS pre-heated to 37°C. Mix well by inversion and split equally into eight 50 ml conical tubes.

2 Rinse the specimen container with 80 ml of fresh PBS and divide among the same eight tubes. Repeat this step until each tube has a final volume of 40 ml.

3 Pellet the sperm by centrifuging 20 min at 200 g, room temperature. Discard the supernatant.

4 Gently resuspend each pellet in 12.5 ml of 37°C PBS, pool the eight aliquots, and divide into two new 50 ml conical tubes.

5 Pellet the sperm by centrifuging 20 min at 200 g, room temperature. Discard the supernatant.

6 Resuspend both pellets in 4 ml of 37°C PBS, then remove an aliquot for counting on a haemocytometer.

7 Dilute 25 × 10^6 sperm to 5 ml with 37°C PBS and add 100 µl of Hoechst 33342 (50 µg/ml).[c,d]

8 Pellet the sperm by centrifuging 10 min at 200 g, room temperature. Discard the supernatant.

9 Resuspend the pellet in 2 ml of PBS and incubate 1–3 h at 37°C.[e]

[a] The semen specimen should be collected on the morning of the sort to assure processing is begun within 4 h of collection. Sperm staining and sorting must be done with living cells, so protect the specimen from light damage and temperature extremes by storing in the dark at room temperature.

[b] Treat semen as biohazardous and perform all work in a laminar flow safety cabinet.

[c] Unused cells can be pelleted by centrifugation and stored at –70°C or genomic DNA extracted as described for the QIAamp® DNA extraction kit (Qiagen).

[d] Dilute 5 µl of Hoechst 33342 (10 mg/ml) 200-fold with water prior to use.

[e] Sperm stained and incubated for at least an hour can be stored overnight at 4°C and sorted the following day.

Protocol 2

Isolate individual sperm by fluorescence activated cell sorting

Equipment and reagents

- Fluorescence activated cell sorter (FACStar Plus, Becton Dickinson; 753 or Elite, Coulter)[a]
- Fluorescence microscope
- Beads coated with a UV excitable molecule (Flow Cytometry Standards Corporation)
- 65°C incubator
- Flexible, thin-walled, 96-well U-bottom microtitre plate (Becton Dickinson)

- Electronic 8- or 12-channel pipettor (Fisher Scientific)
- Aluminium foil adhesive covers (Beckman Instruments)
- Sperm stained with Hoechst 33342 (Protocol 1)
- Cell lysis buffer:[b] 200 mM KOH, 50 mM DTT (Sigma Chemical Company)
- Neutralisation buffer:[c] 950 mM Tris–HCl pH 8.3, 300 mM KCl

Method

1 Power up the UV laser and align the FACS optics and fluidics to optimize the fluorescence and scatter signal, stream, and drop delay using UV excitable beads.

2 Verify alignment of the machine by sorting beads onto a microscope slide and checking for one bead per drop by fluorescence microscopy. Once aligned, set the machine for a two or three drop sort.

3 Align the automated cell deposition unit to deliver one sorted bead centred directly into each well of a Falcon flexible 96-well U-bottom microtitre plate per second.

4 Flush beads from the system with buffer, apply the sperm sample (Protocol 1), and set the sort window using fluorescence on the vertical axis and side or forward scatter on the horizontal axis (Figure 3).

5 A dot plot of all events detected will appear as either one or two distinct populations of cells, the latter of which is due to differences in stain uptake. Align the sort window to include only the desired population of cells (Figure 3).

6 As the FACS operator aligns the machine, aliquot 5 μl of cell lysis buffer[b] per well of a 96-well U-bottom microtitre plate, in a room free of cell or PCR contaminants. Store microtitre plates at 4°C immediately prior to sort.[d]

7 Sort one cell per well of the 96-well plate with the exception of wells B5, D5, F5, and H5 used as negative controls and reference wells for matching the genotyping data with the appropriate well.

8 Seal each plate with an adhesive aluminium foil cover and heat 10 min at 65°C.[e]

9 Carefully remove foil from each tray and aliquot 5 μl of neutralisation buffer per

Protocol 2 continued

well (final volume = 10 μl/well). Seal each plate with a new foil cover and store at −20 °C. The DNA is stable for at least a year.

[a] The FACS machine must be capable of sorting by UV band excitation and include an automated cell deposition unit.

[b] Prepare cell lysis buffer with concentrated KOH and 0.5 M dithiothreitol[c] (DTT) immediately prior to use.

[c] Sterile filter prior to storage at −20 °C.

[d] To avoid loss by evaporation do not store microtitre plates prepared with cell lysis buffer in the laminar flow hood.

[e] Take precautions not to crush the round-bottom wells. Apply and remove adhesive cover with the 96-well plate secured to the heating block of the thermal cycler used in *Protocol 3*.

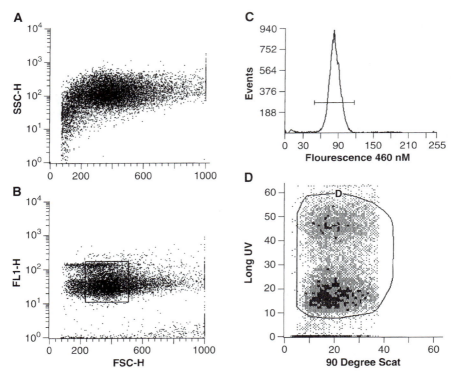

Figure 3 Stained sperm passing through a fluorescence activated cell sorter are recorded as events on a cytogram. The FACS operator highlights the desired cell population within a sort window by setting the range of fluorescence and signal scatter. Cells that fluoresce and scatter light outside this range are excluded. Four cytograms illustrate the parameters used to define the target sperm population. (A) Dot plot of side scatter vs. forward scatter. (B) Dot plot of fluorescence vs. forward scatter. (C) Histogram of events vs. fluorescence. (D) Dot plot of fluorescence vs. side scatter. Sort windows are displayed on cytograms (B) and (D). Differential uptake of stain accounts for the two populations of sperm highlighted in the sort window of cytogram (D).

3 Whole genome amplification of haploid DNA

DNA from haploid cells remains an indispensable tool for studies of recombination. Traditionally, the amount of information available from a single sperm was limited to the number of markers simultaneously amplified in a reaction. Large multilocus (multiplex) PCR amplifications using picogram amounts of target DNA were difficult to carry out, and lacked the benefit of data verification by repetition. The capacity to amplify greater numbers of markers per haploid genome was crucial to the improved efficacy of sperm typing over family-based linkage studies. Responding to this need, Zhang *et al.*, in 1992, developed the method of whole genome amplification (also known as primer extension pre-amplification) that circumvents many of the problems associated with single-sperm typing (33). Haploid DNA from a sperm cell is amplified non-exponentially, creating sufficient template for 12 or more PCR reactions (see *Protocol 3*). The whole genome amplification method differs from conventional PCR with regard to target yield and coverage. In PCR, multiple cycles of primer annealing and extension bring about an exponential increase in the copies of a unique target sequence. In contrast, the PEP reaction employs 10^9 random primer sequences to maximise genome coverage at the expense of target yield. It was reported experimentally (33) and by mathematical modelling (37) that from one haploid genome, 50 cycles of primer extension using a 15-mer random oligonucleotide primer would replicate 78% of the genome as a series of 300–800 bp DNA fragments. The average yield for target sequences measured was 60 copies per haploid cell, or 1 copy/μl of completed PEP reaction, as described in *Protocol 3*. Some markers will amplify more efficiently than others when using PEP products as a source of DNA for PCR.

Critical parameters to consider when performing whole genome amplification on single-sperm include 15-mer random primer quality, the PEP amplification buffer, type of *Taq* polymerase, and retro-fitting a thermal cycler with a modified heating block. Maximum coverage of the genome is subject to the availability of 10^9 different 15-mer primers. Therefore, it is critical that random primer synthesis is monitored for consistent quality and frozen stocks are handled appropriately to avoid primer degradation. Difficulties with the PEP reaction are often traced to poor primer quality or incorrect sample pH. DNA released from sperm upon alkaline lysis followed by pH neutralisation with concentrated buffer (*Protocol 2*) contains sufficient potassium, eliminating the need for it in the PEP reaction buffer. Therefore, never substitute *Taq* DNA polymerase reaction buffer for the PEP amplification buffer described in *Protocol 3*. Whole genome amplification involves random priming at millions of sites along the genome followed by polymerase-dependent primer extension. Attempts to increase PCR specificity with 'Hot Start' thermal cycling conditions or high specificity *Taq* DNA polymerase (e.g. Perkin Elmer TaqGold® DNA polymerase) are unnecessary and may negatively affect the outcome. The thermal cycler used for the PEP reaction must be able to accommodate the same thin-walled 96-well U-bottom microtitre plate used in the sperm sort.

Protocol 3

Primer extension pre-amplification (PEP)

Equipment and reagents

- 96-well tray of sorted, denatured, and neutralised sperm (*Protocol 2*)
- Aluminium foil adhesive covers (Beckman)
- Electronic 8- or 12-channel pipettor (Fisher Scientific)
- Thermal cycler fitted with a 96-well heating block that accommodates U-bottom microtitre plates (MJ Research)

- 10 × potassium-free amplification buffer:[a] 100 mM Tris–HCl pH 8.3, 25 mM $MgCl_2$
- dNTPs at 2 mM each (Gibco BRL)
- 400 μM random 15-mer oligonucleotide primer (Gibco BRL)[b]
- 5 U/μl AmpliTaq® DNA polymerase (Perkin Elmer)
- Mineral oil (paraffin oil, heavy) (Fisher Scientific)

Method

1 Prepare PEP reaction cocktail (100 reactions):
   - 3400 μl distilled water
   - 600 μl of 10 × potassium-free amplification buffer
   - 600 μl random 15-mer oligonucleotide primer (40 μM final concentration)
   - 300 μl of 2 mM each dNTPs (200 μM final concentration each)
   - 100 μl *Taq* DNA polymerase (5 U/μl)

2 Remove a tray of sorted, denatured, and neutralised sperm (*Protocol 2*) from the freezer to thaw.

3 Aliquot 50 μl of PEP reaction cocktail per well using a multichannel pipettor. Mix thoroughly by pipetting (final volume = 60 μl/well).

4 Layer mineral oil over each well and seal the tray with an aluminium foil adhesive cover.[c]

5 Perform the PEP reaction under the following conditions:

(a) Initial denaturation:	5 min	95 °C
(b) 50 cycles:	1 min	92 °C
	2 min	37 °C
	(3 min ramp time from 37 °C to 55 °C)	
	4 min	55 °C
(c) Final extension:	10 min	72 °C
(d) Hold:		4–15 °C

6 Upon completion store the microtitre plate at –20 °C.[d,e] PEP products are good for at least three years.

[a] The absence of K^+ in the PEP 10 × amplification buffer compensates for the KOH and KCl present in the sperm lysis and neutralisation buffers. A final reaction concentration of 42 mM K^+ is attained when the reaction cocktail is added to the sample.

[b] No additional purification is necessary when synthesising random 15-mer oligonucleotide primers. Resuspend the primer in $1 \times$ potassium-free amplification buffer and store in 600 μl aliquots (enough for 100 reactions) at –20 °C.

[c] PEP reactions carried out in a thermal cycler with a heated cover should still use mineral oil overlays to prevent loss of PEP product by evaporation during storage.

[d] Allow 9–11 h for completion of the PEP amplification reaction.

[e] Microtitre plates stored frozen are less likely to be contaminated by inter-well leakage.

4 PCR amplification using PEP reaction products as a source of DNA

Successful amplification of short tandem repeats (STRs) and single nucleotide polymorphisms (SNPs) from PEP reaction products can be achieved with only minor modifications to the standard PCR protocol. Ideally, a 60 μl PEP reaction contains on average 60 copies of a given target sequence or one copy per μl of completed reaction (33). PCR conditions capable of amplifying one copy of target DNA should work with PEP amplified sperm DNA. Although this is often the case for SNPs (Section 4.2), modifications are necessary to achieve robust results when amplifying STRs (Section 4.1). Nested PCR effectively amplifies STRs when single round PCR fails. The method entails one round of normal PCR by means of forward and reverse primers, for 25 cycles. Upon completion an aliquot of the reaction products is transferred into a second PCR reaction (nested) utilising one internal and one original primer (hemi-nested), or two internal primers (fully nested), for 30 cycles (*Figure 4*). Nested PCR is necessary when amplifying more than one locus at a time (multiplex PCR). Primers designed for single or nested PCR should not amplify a region larger than 280 bp since PEP products range in size from 300–800 bp. Primers 20 bp in size with a G·C content of $\approx$ 50% are chosen to closely flank the polymorphic nucleotide (SNPs) or nucleotide repeat (STRs). Nested PCR requires an internal primer(s) that does not overlap either the forward or reverse primer. When selecting a marker (SNP or STR) for single-sperm typing, issues of experimental design, including single versus multiplex (multilocus) PCR, method of allele detection, and contamination should be considered. For instance, simultaneous amplification of multiple markers in one reaction entails nested PCR, thus doubling the number of amplification steps and opportunity for contamination. Additionally, allele discrimination of SNPs in a multiplex reaction is difficult given the complex DNA migration patterns produced upon electrophoresis through a single-strand conformational poly-morphism (SSCP) gel. Such limitations are compelling reasons to use techniques such as allele discrimination by primer length (ADPL), amplification created restriction sites (ACRS), or allele-specific oligonucleotide hybridisation (ASO), discussed in Section 4.2 (see Chapter 7 for a description of DNA-based typing techniques). Given a choice between SNPs and STRs, select a class of markers based on density across the region of interest and the method of detection that

A. Hemi-nested PCR

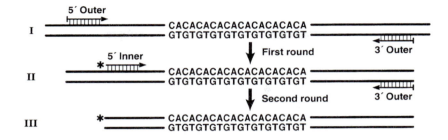

B. Fully Nested PCR

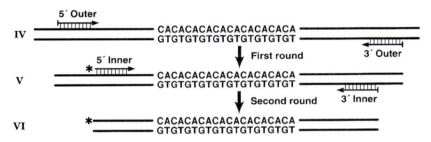

Figure 4 Nested PCR amplification is carried out in a hemi-nested or fully nested format. (A) Hemi-nested PCR. (I) One round of normal PCR amplification using forward and reverse primers flanking a dinucleotide repeat. (II) A small aliquot of the first reaction is re-amplified using a primer from the first round (3′ Outer) and a fluorescent or radiolabelled (*) internal primer (5′ Inner). (III) Upon completion, second round product is labelled and distinguishable from first round product. (B) Fully nested PCR is similar to hemi-nested PCR except step (V) requires two internal primers (5′ Inner and 3′ Inner).

suits your time and resources. Descriptions of techniques for amplifying haploid DNA and the appropriate method of allele detection follows. All PCR protocols discussed emphasise a 96-well format.

4.1 Amplification of polymorphic short tandem repeats (STRs)

STRs or microsatellites are tandemly repeated sequence motifs of 2–6 base pairs present in the genome of all organisms studied to date (38). STRs occur throughout the genome at a frequency greater than expected given their base composition (38). They can be very polymorphic (39, 40) and are distributed evenly across the genome (1, 41). The high mutation rate of STRs (estimated at 10^{-3} events per locus per generation) makes them appropriate for evolutionary studies over short periods of time (42, 43). The high degree of polymorphism and density of STRs make them ideal genetic markers for disease gene mapping and population genetics studies that employ linkage disequilibrium analysis. Recent efforts toward constructing high resolution linkage maps were carried out using STR data generated from large pedigrees. Abundant DNA from family members provided ample resources for genotyping large numbers of markers. Recently, STRs have been used in sperm typing for the purpose of determining the order of and genetic distance separating tightly linked markers (10–19, 44–46). Unlike DNA from family studies, the number of markers amplified per individual sperm is limited. Primer extension pre-amplification of DNA from a single sperm provides template for at least 12 amplifications. Multiplex PCR increases the number of markers amplified per reaction furthering the amount of information that can be generated from a single sperm.

An advantage to performing multiplex PCR is the ability to amplify multiple markers in one PCR reaction and resolve all the alleles on one lane of an electrophoresis gel. Multiplex PCR amplification from PEP reaction products can greatly extend the number of markers screened per sperm sample. The design and execution of multiplex PCR is easily accomplished for STRs by nested PCR amplification. By staggering the size of PCR products it is possible to discriminate alleles for multiple markers. As many as 11 STRs have been amplified simultaneously from a single lysed sperm (16). Multiple primer-pairs can be pooled into a single reaction to amplify PEP product or single-sperm DNA. An aliquot of the completed multiplex PCR reaction is re-amplified either separately in multiple reactions containing a pair of primers where one or both of the pair are nested (*Figure 5A*) or pooled into one reaction (*Figure 5B*). Upon completion, reaction products are resolved by polyacrylamide gel electrophoresis. Alleles are visualised by incorporation of radiolabelled primers into the reaction product (see *Protocols 4–6*), silver staining (*Protocol 12*), ethidium bromide staining (*Protocol 13* and *Table 1*), or fluorescence on a DNA sequencer (*Table 1*).

Visualising amplification products requires selecting a method of allele detection that best suits the resources of the laboratory and the goal of the analysis (*Table 1*). The method selected will influence the PCR amplification conditions as well as the reporter molecule used. The choices include:

(a) Labelling product during the reaction by incorporating fluorescent or radio-labelled oligonucleotide primers.

(b) Directly visualising the product by ethidium bromide or silver nitrate staining.

In protocols described herein, radiolabelled alleles are distinguished by differences in the number of repeats as reflected in the size of products upon gel electrophoresis. It is essential that primers used in multiplex reactions be designed to avoid overlap in product size. Differences in product size for a given marker may vary significantly among individuals and should be determined in advance. Therefore, optimize all multiplex reactions using a plentiful source of (e.g. PBL) DNA from individuals involved in the study and/or control DNA representing the scope of alleles present in a population. Detection by fluorescence eliminates the need to avoid overlap if each marker is labelled with a different fluorescent dye. A multiplex reaction will often contain one or more markers that amplify at levels difficult to visualise by ethidium bromide or silver nitrate staining, so the more sensitive isotopic or fluorescent-labelled primers are preferable in the amplification reaction.

Nested PCR amplification of STRs from single sperm involves three separate amplification steps, providing multiple opportunities for PCR contamination. Given that single-sperm typing requires only picogram amounts of DNA, it is not unlikely for a contaminant to be preferentially amplified. Care must be taken to avoid cross-contamination from adjacent wells of a microtitre plate or exogenous PCR products. A conservative approach involves division of the workspace into four separate work areas:

(a) A PCR clean room for preparing all PEP and PCR reaction cocktails, adding sperm DNA to the PEP reaction, and adding PEP product to the first amplification reaction.

(b) A second room dedicated to transferring an aliquot of PCR product from the first to the second amplification reaction.

(c) A separate room for post-PCR analysis.

(d) A radiation area free of PCR product (if necessary). Always maintain a separate set of pipettors and aerosol barrier tips for each work area, and clean all equipment and surfaces with dilute bleach before use.

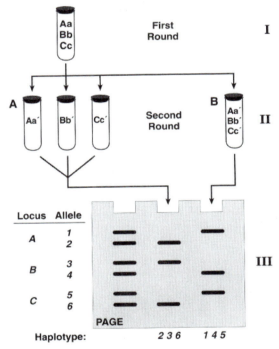

Figure 5 Multiplex PCR options. (I) Markers A, B, and C are co-amplified in the first round using forward and reverse primers Aa, Bb, and Cc respectively. (II) A small aliquot of the completed reaction is re-amplified using one primer from the first round (A, B, and C) and one nested primer (a′, b′, and c′) separately (A) or pooled (B). (III) PCR products (A) are pooled prior to electrophoresis (lane 2), whereas products from the second round multiplex PCR (B) are loaded directly (lane 3). Both alleles for markers A, B, and C are shown in lane 1. The three marker haplotypes for haploid DNA genotyped in wells 2 and 3 are A*2 B*3 C*6 and A*1 B*4 C*5 respectively.

Table 1 Method of allele detection

Method	Multiplex PCR	Nested PCR	Label PCR product with	Polyacrylamide gel	Visualize alleles	Protocols	Reference
STRs							
Size	Yes	Recommended	32P-labelled primer	Denaturing	Autoradiograph	4,5,6,9,10	–[a]
Size	Yes	Recommended	[32P]dCTP	Denaturing	Autoradiograph	–	11,14,17,28
Size	Yes	Recommended	Fluorescent primer	Denaturing	ABI sequencer	–	10,16,23,25, 28,29,45,46
Size	Yes	Recommended	Nothing	Non-denaturing[b]	EtBr staining[c]	4,5,9, 11,13	13,15,18,19, 21,24,25, 33,44
Size	Yes	Recommended	Nothing	Denaturing	Silver staining	4,5,9,10,12	–
Size	Yes	Recommended	Nothing	Non-denaturing	Silver staining	–	12,66
SNPs							
SSCP[d]	No	Optional	[32P]dCTP	Non-denaturing	Autoradiograph	7,8,9,10	57,59
SSCP	No	Optional	Nothing	Non-denaturing	EtBr staining	–	58
SSCP	No	Optional	Nothing	Non-denaturing	Silver staining	7,8,9,10,12	–
ASO[e]	Yes	Recommended	32P-labelled probe	No gel	Autoradiograph	–	3,5,19,36,60
ADPL[f]	Yes	Required	Nothing	Non-denaturing	EtBr staining	–	5,7,54,55
ACRS[g]	Yes	Required	Nothing	Non-denaturing	EtBr staining	–	6,45,56

[a] Author's unpublished data.
[b] Substitute agarose for polyacrylamide gel.
[c] Ethidium bromide.
[d] Single-strand conformational polymorphism.
[e] Allele-specific oligonucleotide hybridization.
[f] Allele discrimination by primer length.
[g] Amplification created restriction sites.

Protocols 4, 5, and *6* detail the steps involved in amplifying a single STR using PEP product as a source of DNA. Adding additional markers (multiplex PCR) requires modifying the reaction by adjusting the relative amounts of each primer in the first round of amplification only (*Protocol 4*). If multiple sets of primers will be used, select the best outcome when primers for marker *A* at 0.2 μM are amplified with primers for marker *B* at increasing concentrations of 0.2, 0.4, 0.8, and 1.6 μM. Next, repeat the same series of amplifications with primers for marker *A* at 0.4 μM, 0.8 μM, and so on. The second round of multiplex amplification remains unchanged from *Protocol 5* with the exception of substituting into the reaction the appropriate internal primer for each marker in the reaction, whether pooled or individually amplified. Multiplex reactions of three or more markers amplify more efficiently when their primers are pooled in the first round of amplification and re-amplified separately in multiple individual second round reactions as illustrated in *Figure 5A*. Direct amplification of sperm DNA, without prior PEP amplification, is carried out as described in *Protocols 4* and *5*, with two exceptions:

(a) Substitute the 10 $\times$ potassium-free amplification buffer used in PEP reactions (Protocol 3) for the 10 $\times$ PCR buffer routinely used in the first round of amplification.

(b) Reduce the 15 μl reaction cocktail used in the first round of amplification to 10 μl when amplifying a 10 μl aliquot of sperm DNA per microtitre well.

PCR product generated as described in *Protocols 4, 5,* and *6* is radiolabelled and alleles are resolved by size on a denaturing polyacrylamide gel (*Protocols 9* and *10*). Water is substituted for [γ-^{32}P]dATP labelled internal primer when the analysis is performed non-radioactively and PCR product is visualised by silver nitrate staining (*Protocols 9, 10,* and *12*) or ethidium bromide staining (*Protocols 9, 11,* and *13*). For a more thorough discussion of multiplex PCR amplification of sperm DNA using fluorescent labelled primers, refer to the citation provided in *Table 1*.

Protocol 4

First round of PCR amplification (STRs only)

Equipment and reagents

- 96-well, thin-wall PCR tray (Pegasus Scientific)
- 96-well full plate rubber cover (Perkin Elmer)
- Clear acetate foil adhesive covers (Sarstedt)
- Electronic 8- or 12-channel pipettor (Fisher Scientific)
- Thermal cycler that accommodates a 96-well PCR plate and has a heated cover (9700, Perkin Elmer; PTC-100, MJ Research)

- 96-well tray of PEP amplified sperm DNA (*Protocol 3*)
- 10 $\times$ PCR buffer: 100 mM Tris–HCl pH 8.3, 500 mM KCl (Perkin Elmer)[a]
- 25 mM MgCl$_2$ (Perkin Elmer)[b]
- dNTPs at 2 mM each (Gibco BRL)
- 10 μM forward and reverse oligonucleotide primers (Gibco BRL)[b]
- 5 U/μl AmpliTaq® DNA polymerase (Perkin Elmer)

Protocol 4 continued

Method

1   Prepare 1st PCR reaction cocktail (100 reactions):
    - 200 μl of 10 × PCR buffer
    - 200 μl of 25 mM MgCl$_2$ (2.5 mM final concentration)
    - 200 μl of 2 mM each dNTPs (200 μM final concentration each)
    - 40–320 μl of 10 μM forward primer (0.2–1.6 μM final concentration)
    - 40–320 μl of 10 μM reverse primer (0.2–1.6 μM final concentration)
    - 25 μl *Taq* DNA polymerase (5 U/μl)
    - q.s. to 1500 μl with distilled water

2   Aliquot 15 μl of PCR reaction cocktail per well using a multichannel pipettor.

3   Thaw a tray of PEP amplified sperm DNA (*Protocol 3*) and using a multichannel pipettor transfer 5 μl of product from the PEP tray to a well containing reaction cocktail.[c,d]

4   Cover the PCR tray with a 96-well rubber cover[e] and perform the PCR reaction under the following conditions:

(a) Initial denaturation:	9 min	94 °C
(b) 10 cycles:	1 min	94 °C
	4 min	60 °C
(c) 15 cycles:	1 min	94 °C
	3 min	60 °C
(d) Final extension:	10 min	72 °C
(e) Hold:		4 °C

5   Label internal primer used in the second round of nested PCR (*Protocol 5*) with [γ-^{32}P]dATP as described in *Protocol 6*.

6   Upon completion, transfer 2 μl of PCR product from the first round of amplification to a second 96-well PCR tray.[f] Seal the second tray with a clear adhesive cover and store at 4 °C no longer than 24 h.

[a] Use MgCl$_2$-free 10 × PCR buffer.

[b] The final concentration needs to be determined empirically for each set of primers.

[c] The amount of PEP product transferred for the first PCR amplification needs to be determined empirically and ranges from 1–5 μl.

[d] PEP reaction products are considered safe to handle in clean rooms designated for the initial PCR set up.

[e] 96-well rubber covers are preferred over strip caps for reducing contamination between wells, during step 6.

[f] Carry out the transfer in a dedicated area of the laboratory not used for the initial PCR set up or the post-PCR analysis. Keep a separate multichannel pipettor for this purpose.

Protocol 5

Second round (nested) PCR amplification (STRs only)

Equipment and reagents

- PCR micro-caps for 96-well PCR tray (Pegasus Scientific)
- Electronic 8- or 12-channel pipettor (Fisher Scientific)
- Thermal cycler that accommodates a 96-well PCR tray and has a heated cover (9700, Perkin Elmer; PTC-100, MJ Research)
- 96-well tray containing PCR product transferred from the first amplification reaction (*Protocol 4*)
- 10 × PCR buffer: 100 mM Tris–HCl pH 8.3, 500 mM KCl (Perkin Elmer)[a]

- 25 mM MgCl$_2$ (Perkin Elmer)[b]
- dNTPs at 2 mM each (Gibco BRL)
- 10 μM forward or reverse oligonucleotide primers used in *Protocol 4* (Gibco BRL)[b,c]
- 10 μM internal oligonucleotide primer (Gibco BRL)[b]
- 5 U/μl AmpliTaq® DNA polymerase (Perkin Elmer)
- [γ-^{32}P]dATP labelled internal primer (*Protocol 6*)

Method

1 Prepare 2nd PCR reaction cocktail (100 reactions):
   - 785 μl distilled water
   - 200 μl of 10 × PCR buffer
   - 200 μl of 25 mM MgCl$_2$ (2.5 mM final concentration)
   - 200 μl of 2 mM each dNTPs (200 μM final concentration each)
   - 200 μl of 10 μM forward or reverse primer (1 μM final concentration)
   - 180 μl of 10 μM internal primer (0.9 μM final concentration)
   - 25 μl *Taq* DNA polymerase (5 U/μl)
   - 10 μl [γ-^{32}P]dATP labelled internal primer (*Protocol 6*) (0.016 μM final concentration)[d]

2 Aliquot 18 μl of PCR reaction cocktail into a well containing 2 μl of PCR product from the first amplification reaction (*Protocol 4*), using a multichannel pipettor. Mix thoroughly by pipetting.

3 Seal the PCR tray with strip caps and perform the PCR reaction under the following conditions:

(a) Initial denaturation:	9 min	94 °C
(b) 5 cycles:	1 min	94 °C
	1 min	60 °C
(c) 25 cycles:	30 sec	94 °C
	1 min	60 °C
(d) Final extension:	60 min	72 °C
(e) Hold:		4 °C

4 Upon completion store the PCR tray at 4 °C.

Protocol 5 continued

[a] Use MgCl$_2$-free 10 × PCR buffer.

[b] The final concentration needs to be determined empirically for each set of primers.

[c] The orientation of the internal primer has a bearing on whether the forward or reverse primer is used.

[d] The amount of labelled internal primer can vary from 7–15 μl per 100 reactions.

Protocol 6

Radiolabelling oligonucleotide primers with [γ-^{32}P]dATP

Equipment and reagents

- 37 °C incubator
- 10 μM internal oligonucleotide primer (Gibco BRL)
- 10 × T4 polynucleotide kinase buffer: 700 mM Tris–HCl pH 7.6, 100 mM MgCl$_2$, 50 mM DTT (New England Biolabs)
- 10 U/μl T4 polynucleotide kinase (New England Biolabs)
- [γ-^{32}P]dATP (6000 Ci/mmol) (New England Nuclear)

Method

1 Prepare the kinase reaction cocktail (300 reactions):[a]
- 5 μl distilled water
- 10 μl of 10 μM internal oligonucleotide primer
- 3 μl of 10 × polynucleotide kinase buffer
- 2 μl T4 polynucleotide kinase (10 U/μl)
- 10 μl of [γ-^{32}P]dATP (6000 Ci/mmol)

2 Incubate the reaction for 30 min at 37 °C.

3 Store the labelled primer at –20 °C.[b]

[a] Provides enough labelled primer for the amplification of three PCR trays or 300 samples.

[b] No further processing of the labelled primer is necessary.

4.2 Amplification of single nucleotide polymorphisms (SNPs)

SNPs are the most common variant identified within the human genome, accounting for approximately 90% of all human DNA polymorphisms (47). SNPs are single base substitutions existing as bi-allelic polymorphisms, where a given allele is present at a frequency greater than 1% (48). Large scale mapping of the human genome suggests that one base substitution exists every 1000 bases (47, 49, 50). Recent advances in high-throughput sequencing, PCR, and chip-based technologies account for thousands of candidate SNPs identified from expressed sequence tag (EST) and sequence-tagged site (STS) sequence data (50, 51). Presently, a SNP map of the human genome exists that could be useful in family-based linkage studies with over 2000 markers at an average density of one marker every 2 cM (50). However, the use of SNPs in linkage studies is hampered because they are not very informative, with average heterozygosity values as low as 34% (50). Family-based linkage studies require polymorphic markers with a high degree of polymorphic information content (PIC) to achieve sufficiently large numbers of informative meioses. In contrast a single-sperm based linkage study with multiple donors heterozygous at the appropriate markers provides sufficient numbers of sperm (meiotic events) for a thorough analysis (52). Single-sperm linkage studies have employed SNPs as a source of polymorphic markers (3, 6, 9, 19, 33, 45, 53), and demonstrated the feasibility of SNPs in multiplex PCR amplification (7, 8, 20, 36, 54, 55).

Multiplex PCR amplification of SNPs requires additional effort tailoring allele-specific primers to a set of markers. Allele detection of multiple SNPs in one lane necessitates allele-specific primer design or restriction digestion to convey differences in base composition as differences in PCR product size. Despite this drawback, quick, non-radioactive, sperm typing of multiple SNPs is possible. Two available methods, ADPL (allele discrimination by primer length) (5, 7, 54, 55) and ACRS (amplification created restriction sites) (6, 45, 56) are amenable to multiplexing, see *Table 1*. Both distinguish between alleles of a locus based on product size, making it possible to amplify and electrophorese multiple markers together. Unlike STRs, alleles of a SNP vary in base composition and not size. Therefore, allele-specific primers must be designed to create differences in PCR product length between alleles (ADPL), or create a restriction site in one allele and not the other (ACRS). Multiplex amplification and discrimination of alleles by either method is accomplished non-radioactively by nested PCR. SSCP (single-strand conformational polymorphism) (described in *Protocols 7–10* and *12*) (57–59) and ASO (allele-specific oligonucleotide hybridisation) (3, 5, 19, 36, 60) can also be used to genotype SNPs. SSCP analysis distinguishes single base substitutions between alleles by differential migration of folded single-strand DNA through a polyacrylamide gel (see Chapter 4). Allelic differences are identified by changes in the pattern, not size, of PCR products on a gel. Therefore alleles of multiple SNPs run in a single lane of an SSCP gel will not give easily interpretable results. However, SSCP analysis of multiple SNPs co-amplified in a single PCR reaction is possible as described in *Figure 5A* with one exception, products of the separate second round reactions are not pooled prior to electrophoresis. Nested PCR amplification of PEP DNA involves numerous steps and increases the odds of PCR contamination. Therefore SNP amplification should be carried out under similar contamination safeguards as described for STRs in Section 4.1.

Protocol 7 details the steps involved in single round PCR amplification of a SNP using PEP product as a source of DNA. Unlike the amplification of STRs described in *Protocol 4*, individual SNPs require a single round of amplification incorporating radiolabelled dCTP in the final product. *Protocol 8*, recommended for SNPs difficult to amplify, details the steps involved in a second round of PCR amplification using internal primers and an aliquot of the first round reaction product. Similar to *Protocols 4* and *5*, [α-³²P]dCTP is substituted for [γ-³²P]dATP labelled internal primer during the second round of amplification. Direct amplification of sperm DNA, without prior PEP amplification, is carried out as described in *Protocols 7* and *8*, with two exceptions:

(a) Substitute the 10 × potassium-free amplification buffer used in PEP reactions (*Protocol 3*) for the 10 × PCR buffer routinely used in *Protocol 7*.

(b) Reduce the 15 μl reaction cocktail used in the first round of amplification to 10 μl when amplifying a 10 μl aliquot of sperm DNA.

PCR product generated as described in *Protocols 7* and *8*, is radiolabelled during amplification and alleles are resolved by SSCP analysis (*Protocols 9* and *10*). Water is substituted for [α-³²P]dCTP when SSCP analysis is performed non-radioactively and PCR product is visualised by silver nitrate staining (*Protocols 9, 10,* and *12*). For a more thorough discussion of the non-radioactive techniques ADPL and ACRS, refer to the citations provided in *Table 1*.

Protocol 7

Single round PCR amplification from PEP product (SNPs only)

Equipment and reagents

- 96-well, thin-wall PCR tray (Pegasus Scientific)
- Clear acetate foil adhesive covers (Sarstedt)
- PCR micro-caps for 96-well PCR tray (Pegasus Scientific)
- Electronic 8- or 12-channel pipettor (Fisher Scientific)
- Thermal cycler that accommodates a 96-well PCR tray and has a heated cover (9700, Perkin Elmer; PTC-100, MJ Research)
- 96-well tray of PEP amplified sperm DNA (*Protocol 3*)

- 10 × PCR buffer: 100 mM Tris–HCl pH 8.3, 500 mM KCl (Perkin Elmer)[a]
- 25 mM MgCl₂ (Perkin Elmer)[b]
- dNTPs at 2 mM each with the exception of dCTP at 1 mM (Gibco BRL)
- 10 μM forward and reverse oligonucleotide primers (Gibco BRL)[b]
- 5 U/μl AmpliTaq® DNA polymerase (Perkin Elmer)
- [α-³²P]dCTP (3000 Ci/mmol) (New England Nuclear)

Method

1 Prepare PCR reaction cocktail (100 reactions):
   - 200 μl of 10 × PCR buffer
   - 200 μl of 25 mM MgCl₂ (2.5 mM final concentration)
   - 200 μl of 2 mM dNTPs (1 mM dCTP)
   - 40–320 μl of 10 μM forward primer (0.2–1.6 μM final concentration)
   - 40–320 μl of 10 μM reverse primer (0.2–1.6 μM final concentration)
   - 25 μl *Taq* DNA polymerase (5 U/μl)

- q.s. to 1500 μl with distilled water
- 8 μl of [α-^{32}P]dCTP

2 Thaw a tray of PEP amplified sperm DNA (*Protocol 3*) and transfer 5 μl of product from the PEP tray to a second 96-well PCR tray using a multichannel pipettor. Seal the second tray with a clear adhesive cover and transfer to an area dedicated to radioisotope use.[c]

3 Aliquot 15 μl of PCR reaction cocktail per well using a multichannel pipettor.

4 Seal the PCR tray with strip caps and perform the PCR reaction under the following conditions:[d]

(a) Initial denaturation:	9 min	94°C
(b) 30 cycles:	30 sec	94°C
	1 min	55°C
	90 sec	72°C
(c) Final extension:	10 min	72°C
(d) Hold:		4°C

5 Upon completion store the PCR tray at 4°C.

[a] Use MgCl$_2$-free 10 × PCR buffer.

[b] The final concentration needs to be determined empirically for each set of primers.

[c] The amount of PEP product transferred for the first PCR amplification needs to be determined empirically and ranges from 1–5 μl.

[d] Modifications to the thermal cycler program may be required to successfully amplify a SNP without nested PCR. Avoid thermal cycler programs exceeding 35 cycles.

Protocol 8

Optional second round (nested) PCR amplification (SNPs only)

Equipment and reagents

- 96-well, thin-wall PCR tray (Pegasus Scientific)
- 96-well full plate rubber cover (Perkin Elmer)
- PCR micro-caps for 96-well PCR tray (Pegasus Scientific)
- Electronic 8- or 12-channel pipettor (Fisher Scientific)
- Thermal cycler that accommodates a 96-well PCR tray and has a heated cover (9700, Perkin Elmer; PTC-100, MJ Research)
- 96-well tray containing PCR product transferred from the first amplification reaction (*Protocol 7*)
- 10 × PCR buffer: 100 mM Tris–HCl pH 8.3, 500 mM KCl (Perkin Elmer)[a]
- 25 mM MgCl$_2$ (Perkin Elmer)[b]
- dNTPs at 2 mM each with the exception of dCTP at 1 mM (Gibco BRL)
- 10 μM forward or reverse oligonucleotide primers (Gibco BRL)[c]
- 10 μM internal primer (Gibco BRL)
- 5 U/μl AmpliTaq® DNA polymerase (Perkin Elmer)
- [α-^{32}P]dCTP (3000 Ci/mmol) (New England Nuclear)

Method

1 The first round of amplification is carried out as described in *Protocol 7* with the following exceptions:

    (a) Distilled water is substituted for [α-^{32}P]dCTP in the reaction cocktail.

    (b) A 96-well full plate rubber cover is substituted for strip caps.

    (c) The thermal cycler conditions described in *Protocol 7* are replaced with those described in *Protocol 4*.

2 Upon completion transfer 2 μl of PCR product from the first round of amplification to a second 96-well PCR tray.[d] Seal the second tray with clear acetate cover and store at 4°C no longer than 24 h.

3 Prepare 2nd PCR reaction cocktail (100 reactions):

    • 767 μl distilled water

    • 200 μl of 10 × PCR buffer

    • 200 μl of 25 mM MgCl$_2$ (2.5 mM final concentration)

    • 200 μl of 2 mM dNTPs (1 mM dCTP)

    • 200 μl of 10 μM forward or reverse primer (1 μM final concentration)

    • 200 μl of 10 μM internal primer (1 μM final concentration)

    • 25 μl *Taq* DNA polymerase (5 U/μl)

    • 8 μl of [α-^{32}P]dCTP

4 Aliquot 18 μl of PCR reaction cocktail into a well containing 2 μl of PCR product from the first amplification reaction using a multichannel pipettor. Mix thoroughly by pipetting.

5 Seal the PCR tray with strip caps and perform the PCR reaction under the following conditions:

(a) Initial denaturation:	9 min	94°C
(b) 5 cycles:	1 min	94°C
	1 min	60°C
(c) 25 cycles:	30 sec	94°C
	1 min	60°C
(d) Final extension:	60 min	72°C
(e) Hold:		4°C

6 Upon completion store the PCR tray at 4°C.

[a] Use MgCl$_2$-free 10 × PCR buffer.

[b] The final concentration needs to be determined empirically for each set of primers.

[c] The orientation of the internal primer has a bearing on whether the forward or reverse primer is used.

[d] Carry out the transfer in a dedicated area of the laboratory not used for the initial PCR set up or the post-PCR analysis. Keep a separate multichannel pipettor for this purpose.

5 Discriminating alleles by gel electrophoresis

Having selected the class of marker for sperm analysis and the method of allele detection, it is necessary to resolve the amplification products by gel electrophoresis and discriminate which allele is present for a given sperm. The methods discussed in this chapter are largely radioisotope based, but non-radioactive methods are briefly discussed and highlighted in *Table 1*. Discriminating between alleles of a short tandem repeat simply involves determining size differences of di-, tri-, or tetranucleotide repeat units present within a short stretch of amplified DNA. Differences in repeat length are reflected in the relative mobility of the DNA fragment during electrophoresis through a denaturing polyacrylamide gel. DNA fragments containing few repeats (smaller alleles) migrate farther than fragments containing many repeats (larger alleles). Electrophoresis of amplified STRs is performed on a 72-well denaturing polyacrylamide gel (37.5 × 45 cm). Radiolabelled samples are electrophoresed, transferred to blotting paper, dried, and the PCR products visualised on autoradiography film as exposed bands (*Protocols 9* and *10*). Non-radiolabelled samples are electrophoresed, and the PCR products visualised directly by silver staining (*Protocols 9*, *10*, and *12*). In addition, small numbers of samples can be electrophoresed on a miniature non-denaturing polyacrylamide gel (18 × 16 cm) and the PCR product visualised by ethidium bromide staining (*Protocols 9*, *11*, and *13*).

Discriminating between alleles of a single nucleotide polymorphism by SSCP involves identifying single base substitutions present within a short stretch of amplified DNA. Differences in sequence are reflected in the number and relative mobility of folded single-strand DNA fragments during electrophoresis through a non-denaturing polyacrylamide gel. Electrophoresis by SSCP is performed on a 72-well non-denaturing polyacrylamide gel (37.5 × 45 cm). Radiolabelled samples are electrophoresed, transferred to blotting paper, dried, and the PCR products visualised on autoradiography film as exposed bands (*Protocols 9* and *10*). Non-radiolabelled samples are electrophoresed, and the PCR products visualised directly by silver staining (*Protocols 9*, *10*, and *12*).

A major concern when genotyping a large number of sperm is whether an allele identified on an autoradiograph corresponds with the correct sperm sorted into the well of a tray. DNA from a sample that undergoes PEP and nested PCR amplification followed by gel electrophoresis is transferred from one plate to the next as many as four times. Transfer errors can be reduced using a 12-channel pipettor to move DNA between plates and a 12-channel syringe for loading 72-well gels. Assigning the proper sample number to an allele identified in the lane of a gel can be difficult when multiple samples at the beginning or end of the gel fail to amplify. To prevent this, four wells (B5, D5, F5, and H5) are routinely left empty when sorting sperm. Functioning as both a reference point and negative control, they dictate the order of samples on the autoradiograph (see *Figure 6*). Maintaining this order is essential when a sample bearing a recombination event between two markers needs to be located and the results confirmed by re-amplification.

Multiplex PCR (*D6S439* and *MOGCA*)

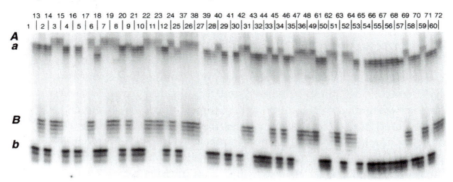

Figure 6 A two-marker analysis of sperm DNA co-amplified with *D6S439* and *MOGCA*. PCR product was radioactively labelled and resolved by polyacrylamide gel electrophoresis. Allele *a* of *D6S439* segregates with allele *b* of *MOGCA* in 32 sperm. Allele *A* of *D6S439* segregates with allele *B* of *MOGCA* in 26 sperm. Lanes 2, 7, and 60 are recombinants. Lanes 17, 41, and 65 are blanks corresponding with wells B5, D5, and F5 of the original PEP amplified sperm DNA tray (*Protocol 3*). The three blanks are used to align the autoradiograph data with the samples.

Protocol 9

Preparing polyacrylamide gels

Equipment and reagents

- 37.5 × 43/45 cm glass sequencing plates and clamps (IBI)
- 0.4 mm spacers and 72-well shark-tooth comb (IBI)
- STS-45 vertical electrophoresis apparatus (IBI)
- 18 × 16 cm glass electrophoresis plates and clamps (Pharmacia)
- 1.5 mm spacers and 28-well comb (Pharmacia)
- Hoefer SE 400 vertical electrophoresis apparatus (Pharmacia)

- Denaturing gel mix: 6% (v/v) acrylamide/bis-acrylamide (37.5:1), 50% (w/v) urea, 0.6 × TBE buffer
- 30% (w/v) acrylamide/bis-acrylamide (37.5:1) (Boehringer Mannheim)
- 10 × TBE: 1.3 M Tris–HCl, 450 mM boric acid, 25 mM EDTA (Bio-Rad)
- 10% (w/v) ammonium persulfate (Gibco BRL)[a]
- *N,N,N',N'*,-tetramethylethylenediamine (TEMED) (Boehringer Mannheim)

A. Denaturing gel

1 Clean and assemble a set of glass plates (37.5 × 43/45cm) using 0.4 mm spacers and clamps.

2 Mix by gentle inversion the following reagents:
- 75 ml of denaturing gel mix
- 450 μl of 10% (w/v) ammonium persulfate
- 45 μl of TEMED

3 Keep the glass plates horizontal and add the gel mix to the upper end of the set.

Allow the mix to slowly and evenly migrate between the plates by capillary action. Do not use tape to seal the bottom and sides of the sequencing plates. Insert the shark-tooth comb inverted into the unpolymerized gel and allow 45–60 min for complete polymerization.

4 Remove comb and rinse trough with 1 × TBE.

5 Assemble electrophoresis apparatus and denaturing gel at room temperature. Fill unit with 0.6 × TBE, insert 72-well comb into trough, and check for leaks.

B. SSCP gel (non-denaturing)

1 Clean and assemble a set of glass plates (37.5 × 43/45cm) using 0.4 mm spacers and clamps.

2 Mix the following reagents by gentle inversion:
   - 52 ml distilled water
   - 15 ml of 30% (w/v) acrylamide/bis-acrylamide
   - 7.5 ml of 10 × TBE
   - 450 μl of 10% (w/v) ammonium persulfate
   - 45 μl of TEMED

3 Keep the glass plates horizontal and add the gel mix to the upper end of the set. Allow the mix to slowly and evenly migrate between the plates by capillary action. Do not use tape to seal the bottom and sides of the sequencing plates. Insert the shark-tooth comb inverted into the unpolymerized gel and allow 45–60 min for complete polymerization.

4 Remove comb and rinse trough with 1 × TBE.

5 Assemble electrophoresis apparatus and SSCP gel in a 4°C cold room. Fill unit with 1 × TBE, insert 72-well comb into trough, and check for leaks.

C. Non-denaturing gel (small)

1 Clean and assemble a set of glass plates (18 × 16 cm) using 1.5 mm spacers and clamps.

2 Mix by gentle inversion the following reagents:
   - 28 ml distilled water
   - 8 ml of 30% (w/v) acrylamide/bis-acrylamide
   - 4 ml of 10 × TBE
   - 280 μl of 10% (w/v) ammonium persulfate
   - 28 μl of TEMED

3 Add the gel mix to the vertical gel assembly, insert comb, and allow 45–60 min for complete polymerization.

4 Remove comb and rinse wells with 1 × TBE.

5 Assemble electrophoresis apparatus and non-denaturing gel at room temperature, fill unit with 1 × TBE, and check for leaks.

[a] Ammonium persulfate should be freshly made every few days and stored away from light.

Protocol 10

Sample preparation and polyacrylamide gel electrophoresis

Equipment and reagents

- Clear acetate foil adhesive covers (Sarstedt)
- Electronic 8- or 12-channel pipettor (Fisher Scientific)
- Hamilton 12-channel syringe gel loader (Fisher Scientific)
- 3000 volt power supply (Pharmacia Biotech)
- Whatman 3MM filter paper (Fisher Scientific)
- 35 × 43 cm autoradiography film (Kodak)
- Gel dryer

- 95 °C incubator
- 4 °C cold room
- 96-well tray containing PCR amplified PEP product from *Protocol 5, 7, or 8*
- 96-well round-bottom microtitre plate (Sarstedt)
- Gel loading dye: 95% formamide, 10 mM NaOH, 0.25% bromphenol blue, 0.25% xylene cyanol

A. Denaturing gel electrophoresis

1 Transfer 5 µl of PCR amplified PEP product (*Protocol 5*) to a 96-well microtitre plate containing 10 µl of gel loading dye, using a multichannel pipettor. Seal the plate with a clear acetate cover.

2 Heat the samples for 2 min at 95 °C, and then quickly chill them on ice.

3 Load 2–3 µl of samples onto a 72-well denaturing gel (*Protocol 9*) by means of a Hamilton 12-channel syringe loader.

4 Electrophoresis proceeds for 2–3 h at 1600 volts constant, maximum amps and watts.[a]

5 Gels containing radioactive products proceed to step 6, but for silver staining follow *Protocol 12*.

6 Carefully separate the glass plates, transfer the gel to Whatman 3MM filter paper, cover the gel side with plastic wrap, and vacuum dry with heat.

7 Expose to autoradiography film 4–24 h before developing.

B. SSCP gel electrophoresis

1 Carried out as described for denaturing gel electrophoresis with the following exceptions:

   (a) Step 1, transfer 5 µl of PCR amplified PEP product (*Protocol 7 or 8*)...

   (b) Step 3, load samples onto a non-denaturing SSCP gel (*Protocol 9*)...

   (c) Step 4, electrophoresis proceeds at 4 °C for 3–4 h at 50 watts constant, maximum amps and volts...[a]

[a] Electrophoresis time varies with the size of the product and the gel composition.

Protocol 11

Sample preparation and non-denaturing gel electrophoresis

Equipment and reagents

- Clear acetate foil adhesive covers (Sarstedt)
- Electronic 8- or 12-channel pipettor (Fisher Scientific)
- 3000 volt power supply (Pharmacia Biotech)
- PCR amplified PEP product from *Protocol 5*[a]

- 96-well round-bottom microtitre plate (Sarstedt)
- 10 × gel loading dye: 50% (v/v) glycerol, 0.2 M EDTA, 0.42% (w/v) bromphenol blue, 0.42% (w/v) xylene cyanol

Method

1 Using a multichannel pipettor transfer 2 μl of 10 × gel loading dye to the 96-well thin-wall PCR tray containing PCR amplified PEP product from *Protocol 5*. Mix by pipetting and seal the plate with a clear acetate cover.

2 Load 10–15 μl of sample onto a 28-well non-denaturing polyacrylamide gel (*Protocol 9*).

3 Electrophoresis proceeds for 1–1.5 h at 200 volts constant, maximum amps and watts.[b]

4 When completed carefully separate the upper glass plate from the gel and notch the corner of the gel corresponding to the first well loaded.

5 Proceed to *Protocol 13* (ethidium bromide staining).

[a] Nested PCR amplification in the absence of [γ-^{32}P]dATP labelled internal primer.

[b] Electrophoresis time varies with the size of the product and the gel composition.

Protocol 12

Silver staining of DNA in polyacrylamide gels

Equipment and reagents

- Shallow stainless steel tray large enough to accommodate a polyacrylamide gel
- Whatman 3MM filter paper (Fisher Scientific)
- Gel dryer
- 1 × fixing solution: 0.6% (w/v) benzene sulfonic acid, 19% (v/v) ethanol (Pharmacia Biotech)
- 1 × staining solution: 0.2% (w/v) silver nitrate, 0.07% (w/v) benzene sulfonic acid (Pharmacia Biotech)

- 1 × developing solution: 2.5% (w/v) sodium carbonate, 0.037% (w/v) formaldehyde, 0.002% (w/v) sodium thiosulfate (Pharmacia Biotech)
- 1 × stopping and preserving solution: 1% (v/v) acetic acid, 5% (w/v) sodium acetate, 10% (v/v) glycerol (Pharmacia Biotech)

Protocol 12 continued

Method

1. Carefully separate the upper glass plate from the gel. When possible cut a line across the gel above and below the point containing the PCR product and lift away excess gel with 3MM filter paper.

2. Soak the gel, still attached to a glass plate, in $1 \times$ fixing solution for at least 30 min.[a]

3. Rinse the gel with distilled water before soaking in $1 \times$ staining solution for 30 min.

4. Rinse the gel with distilled water for 1 min before soaking in $1 \times$ developing solution for 6 min[b].

5. Soak the gel in $1 \times$ stopping and preserving solution for at least 30 min.

6. Transfer the gel to 3MM filter paper, cover the gel side with plastic wrap, and vacuum dry with heat. The dried gel can be photographed or serve as a permanent record.

[a] All solutions should be used at room temperature (20–27 °C).

[b] The developing solution should be prepared immediately before use.

Protocol 13

Ethidium bromide staining of DNA in polyacrylamide gels

Equipment and reagents

- UV transilluminator with video or Polaroid camera
- Gel staining solution: 1/1000 dilution of ethidium bromide (0.5 μg/ml)

Method

1. Carefully separate the upper glass plate from the gel and notch the corner of the gel corresponding to the first well loaded.

2. Slide the gel into enough gel staining solution to cover it and gently rock for 10 min.[a]

3. Rinse gel in distilled water briefly.

4. Place the gel on a UV transilluminator and photograph.[b]

[a] Caution: ethidium bromide is a known mutagen and carcinogen. Take necessary precautions when handling staining solution and gel.

[b] Avoid prolonged exposure to UV light and always wear a face shield when illuminating stained gels.

6 Interpretation of sperm typing data

Single-sperm typing of polymorphic markers provides a rapid means of establishing phase of alleles on a chromosome (haplotype), ordering markers on a chromosome, measuring germline mutation rates, measuring segregation patterns, mapping recombination hotspots, and assessing heterogeneity in recombination rates among individuals. Estimates of the recombination fraction between polymorphic markers are easily attained by dividing the number of recombinant haplotypes identified by the total number of haplotypes observed. The probability that a recombination event will occur between two markers is in proportion to the physical distance separating the markers. Therefore the frequency of recombination within an interval defines the genetic distance of the interval. Estimates of recombination fractions between multiple markers can be used to infer their order on a chromosome when multi-point mapping techniques are applied. Careful interpretation of sperm typing data is critical when undertaking an analysis of linkage. The following discussion is limited to the collection of single-sperm haplotype data and considerations when mapping recombination breakpoints, estimating the recombination fraction between markers, and ordering markers on a chromosome.

6.1 Single-sperm haplotype scoring

Accurate scoring of single-sperm haplotypes is critical to estimating the recombination fraction between two polymorphic markers. Under ideal conditions, estimates would simply involve dividing the number of two marker haplotypes observed (parental + recombinant) into the number of recombinant haplotypes identified. In reality, sperm typing conditions are far from ideal. Despite the presence of a single haploid genome per well of a 96-well tray, an allele at one or more markers may occasionally fail to amplify. Similarly, a small fraction of sperm samples may amplify both alleles of a marker if there are two or more sperm per well. Because single-cell sorting and amplification is less than 100% efficient, genotyping errors resulting from lack of amplification, contamination, or presence of zero or two sperm per well are not uncommon. Data generated from a two-marker analysis consists of 16 potential outcomes: two parental haplotypes, two recombinant haplotypes, and 12 erroneous genotypes resulting from experimental error. *Figure 7A* illustrates the 16 potential outcomes identified in a two-marker multiplex amplification of the short tandem repeats *D6S291* and *MOGCA*. Considering the sizeable number of sperm screened per donor, care must be taken when scoring alleles identified per sperm. The ability to discriminate between two alleles of a marker that differ by a single dinucleotide repeat must be resolved before amplifying a particular marker or donor. Situations where the donor is irreplaceable and alleles of a marker are difficult to resolve require designing the primers to closely flank the repeat. This will reduce the size of the amplification product enough to possibly discriminate a two nucleotide difference. Prior to scoring an autoradiograph, align the sample numbers with the proper wells of the PEP amplified sperm DNA tray using the four negative control wells B5, D5, F5, and H5 as reference points (*Figure 6*). The transfer of genotyping data should be done using simple and arbitrary allele designations to reduce data transfer errors, e.g. locus *D6S439*: alleles *A* and *a*, locus *MOGCA*: alleles *B* and *b* (*Figure 6*). Always score autoradiographs one marker at a time so previous knowledge of the first allele does not influence the interpretation of the second allele. Having scored all single-sperm genotypes for a given donor, determine the frequency of each genotype as seen in *Figure 7B* and then proceed to the analysis.

Direct estimates of the recombination fraction (θ) between two markers makes use of frequency estimates for both parental and both recombinant haplotypes while excluding data from the 12 erroneous genotypings. Estimates of θ calculated without consideration for the errors inherent in single-sperm typing can be misleading and may result in erroneous estimations of θ. Direct estimates of the recombination fraction are limited to tightly linked markers of known chromosomal order and carried out for the sake of comparing recombination rates between different genomic intervals, as well as fine mapping recombinational hotspots (61). A direct comparison of recombination rates between markers located in different regions of the genome does not require a statistical program to generate maximum likelihood estimates of the recombination fraction and associated standard errors. Instead, a sperm identified with a crossover event between markers of interest is independently confirmed by amplifying the sample again for the original markers as well as an additional pair of tightly linked flanking markers. The number of confirmed recombinants identified in a genomic interval are compared to the number of confirmed recombinants in a second interval. Similarly, recombination breakpoints can be fine mapped by genotyping the recombinant sample with informative markers flanked by the markers used to identify the crossover. In contrast an analysis of recombination data can be carried out using the complete data set (erroneous genotypes included) in a statistical approach to constructing linkage maps. This approach calculates maximum likelihood estimates of a recombination fraction, taking into consideration errors inherent in the sperm typing technique (discussed in Section 6.2). Deciding whether to perform a direct analysis or a statistical analysis requires first defining the questions to be addressed by single-sperm typing then selecting the appropriate analytical tool.

6.2 General approaches for analysing recombination data

High-throughput single-sperm typing provides a means of generating high resolution genetic maps in the 0.1–0.2 cM range with a high degree of precision (small SE of 0.016) (3–5). The key to mapping at this resolution is large sample size, increased amplification efficiency, reduced contamination, and efficient sorting of one sperm per well. Consider the following scenario, described by Leeflang *et al.*, wherein two markers 0.5 cM apart are selected to screen 1000 sperm for recombinants. A distance of 0.5 cM is equivalent to a recombination fraction of 0.005. Therefore five recombinants should be identified for every 1000 sperm genotyped. In contrast, if we assume that each recombination is an independent event, then based on the Poisson distribution there is only a 56% chance of identifying at least five recombinants and an 88% chance of identifying at least three recombinants (61). A larger sample size would provide a more accurate estimate of the recombination fraction, unless the raw data contained a significant number of erroneous genotypes. Therefore, the greater the frequency

A. Potential Outcome When Genotyping Two Markers

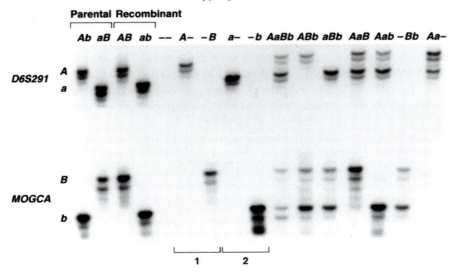

B. Genotype Frequencies

Genotype	Number of Sperm	
1 (–aB–)	1422	} Parental
2 (A––b)	1489	
3 (A–B–)	29	} Recombinant
4 (–a–b)	48	
5 (––––)	164	
6 (A–––)	74	
7 (––B–)	113	
8 (–a––)	101	
9 (–––b)	93	
10 (AaBb)	26	
11 (A–Bb)	5	
12 (–aBb)	24	
13 (AaB–)	1	
14 (Aa–b)	17	
15 (––Bb)	0	
16 (Aa––)	1	

Total genotyped (1-16)	3607	
Successfully genotyped (1-4)	2988 (83%)	
Parental haplotypes (1&2)	2911	
Recombinant haplotypes (3&4)	77	
Recombination fraction	0.0257 (77/2988)	

Figure 7 A two-marker analysis of sperm DNA co-amplified with *D6S291* and *MOGCA*.
(A) Amplification yields two *D6S291* alleles (*A* and *a*) and two *MOGCA* alleles (*B* and *b*). 16
potential genotyping outcomes exist: two parental haplotypes (*Ab* and *aB*), two recombinant
haplotypes (*AB* and *ab*), and 12 erroneous genotypes (lanes 5–16). Two sperm incompletely
amplified in lanes 6 and 7 are easily mistaken for a recombinant when sorted together in one
well. The same applies for wells 8 and 9. (B) A two-marker analysis of 3607 sperm is summed
up in a table of 16 frequencies (authors unpublished data).

175

of errors, the larger the sample size needed to achieve accurate statistical estimates.

Responding to the significant impact of experimental error on estimates, software was developed that generates maximum log likelihood estimates of the recombination fraction for testing different locus orders. The multi-point mapping strategies of the program SPERM and its predecessors TWOLOC, THREELOC, and MENDEL use multilocus haplotype frequencies, as seen in *Figure 7B*, to generate a maximum likelihood estimate and standard error for the recombination fraction in addition to parameters including amplification efficiency, contamination rate, and number of wells containing 0, 1, or 2 sperm. Estimates will vary for every locus order tested and the resulting maximum log likelihoods are compared to determine the best locus order. The SPERM program performs the analysis under a number of different assumptions regarding the above mentioned parameters. The different assumptions or models dictate whether amplification and contamination rates are allele-specific, locus-specific, or non-specific. In practice it is wise to perform an initial analysis of data under the most stringent of conditions using the general model where alleles of a locus have variable amplification and contamination rates. Next, re-analyse the data with several of the less complex submodels in which amplification and contamination rates are locus-specific or non-specific. The ideal submodel from which locus order and recombination fraction estimates are established should be the most parsimonious model featuring amplification and contamination parameters that are non-specific. Nevertheless, a submodel should be abandoned if a likelihood ratio test demonstrates a departure in the log likelihood estimate from that calculated under the general model, or it lacks the goodness-of-fit between the data and the model. The general model is sufficient when estimating the recombination fraction between markers of known order on a chromosome (61). It is not uncommon for direct estimates of the recombination fraction, discussed in Section 6.1, to agree with estimates generated statistically (3, 7). Nonetheless, conclusions drawn from sperm data processed through a statistical program are less likely to be biased, more likely to be accurate and provide the investigator with valuable information regarding potential sources of experimental error (62).

The frequency of false recombinants generated by experimental error has a bearing on the limit of resolution when mapping by single-sperm typing. Sperm analysis programs estimate amplification and contamination frequencies from the data to account for potential recombinants missed or falsely identified when generating log likelihoods estimates. High resolution mapping by single-sperm typing requires the lowest possible rate of genotyping errors achievable in order to maximise the number of successful meiotic events and increase the precision of estimates (low SE). In the event that genotyping errors cannot be reduced it is possible to assess the magnitude of their impact on results by estimating the frequency of false recombinants empirically. A sample genotyped as a recombinant could occur when a microtitre well receives two sperm during the cell sort and only one marker amplifies per sperm genome. Illustrated in *Figure 7A*, single-sperm DNA genotyped and loaded onto lanes 6–9 (see brackets 1 and 2 below gel) were unsuccessfully amplified at either *MOGCA* (lanes 6 and 8) or *D6S291* (lanes 7 and 9). A well containing DNA from two sperm independently genotyped as an *A*- and -*B* (lanes 6 and 7) would be perceived as the recombinant *AB* (lane 3). Likewise, a well containing DNA from two sperm independently genotyped as an *a*- and -*b* (lanes 8 and 9) would be perceived as the recombinant *ab* (lane 4). The probability of either scenario would be small, but testable empirically by sorting two sperm per well and genotyping each for the same markers used in the single cell analysis. Genotype an equivalent number of wells containing two sperm as done for the single-sperm analysis. The probability of two recombinant sperm sorting into the same well, e.g. two *AB* recombinants/well or two *ab* recombinants/well, or one recombinant sperm sorting into the well is small enough that any well identified as a recombinant is likely to reflect a false recombinant. If recombinants are identified in this fashion care should be taken to validate any recombination data generated from a single-sperm analysis performed under similar conditions.

A very thorough discussion of sperm data analysis and programs can be found in Lange *et al.* (63), Cui *et al.* (3), Goradia *et al.* (4), Leeflang *et al.* (61), Lazzeroni *et al.* (62), Farrall *et al.* (64), and McPeek *et al.* (65). The programs MENDEL and SPERM are available from Kenneth Lange at http://www.biomath.medsch.ucla.edu/faculty/klange/software.html (63). The program TWOLOC is available from Martin Farrall at http://www.well.ox.ac.uk/pub/genetics/twoloc (64). The program SPERMSEG, useful in the study of segregation distortion in single-sperm data, is available from Mary Sara McPeek at http://galton.uchicago.edu/~mcpeek/software/spermseg (65).

References

1. Dib, C., Faure, S., Fizames, C., Samson, D., Drouot, N., Vignal, A., *et al.* (1996). *Nature*, **380**, 152.
2. Chakravarti, A. (1991). *Hum. Genet.*, **87**, 721.
3. Cui, X., Li, H., Goradia, T. M., Lange, K., Kazazian, H. H., Galas, D., *et al.* (1989). *Proc. Natl. Acad. Sci. USA*, **86**, 9389.
4. Goradia, T. M. and Lange, K. (1990). *Ann. Hum. Genet.*, **54**, 49.
5. Li, H., Cui, X., and Arnheim, N. (1991). *Methods: a companion to methods in enzymology*, **2**, 49.
6. Lien, S., Kaminski, S., Alestrom, P., and Rogne, S. (1993). *Genomics*, **16**, 41.
7. Goradia, T. M., Stanton, V. P., Cui, X., Aburatani, H., Li, H., Lange, K., *et al.* (1991). *Genomics*, **10**, 748.
8. van Eijk, M. J. T., Russ, I., and Lewin, H. A. (1993). *Mamm. Genome*, **4**, 113.
9. Park, C., Russ, I., Da, Y., and Lewin, H. A. (1995). *Genomics*, **27**, 113.
10. Lien, S., Cockett, N. E., Klungland, H., Arnheim, N., Georges, M., and Gomez-Raya, L. (1999). *Anim. Genet.*, **30**, 42.
11. Furlong, R. A., Goudie, D. R., Carter, N. P., Lyall, J. E. W., Affara, N. A., and Ferguson-Smith, M. A. (1993). *Am. J. Hum. Genet.*, **52**, 1191.
12. Zhao, S., Li, K., Yu, M., and Peng, Z. (2000). *Anim. Biotechnol.*, **11**, 45.
13. Hubert, R., MacDonald, M., Gusella, J., and Arnheim, N. (1994). *Nature Genet.*, **7**, 420.

14. Park, C., Frank, M. T., and Lewin, H. A. (1999). *Genomics*, **59**, 143.

15. Yu, J., Lazzeroni, L., Qin, J., Huang, M., Navidi, W., and Erlich, H. (1996). *Am. J. Hum. Genet.*, **59**, 1186.

16. Simianer, H., Szyda, J., Ramon, G., and Lien, S. (1997). *Mamm. Genome*, **8**, 830.

17. Brown, G. M., Leversha, M., Hulten, M., and Ferguson-Smith, M. A. (1998). *Am. J. Hum. Genet.*, **62**, 1484.

18. Lien, S., Szyda, J., Schechinger, B., Rappold, G., and Arnheim, N. (2000). *Am. J. Hum. Genet.*, **66**, 557.

19. Schmitt, K., Lazzeroni, L. C., Foote, S., Vollrath, D., Fisher, E. M. C., Goradia, T. M., *et al.* (1994). *Am. J. Hum. Genet.*, **55**, 423.

20. Williams, C., Davies, D., and Williamson, R. (1993). *Hum. Mol. Genet.*, **2**, 445.

21. Leeflang, E. P., McPeek, M. S., and Arnheim, N. (1996). *Am. J. Hum. Genet.*, **59**, 896.

22. Grewal, R. P., Cancel, G., Leeflang, E. P., Durr, A., McPeek, M. S., Draghinas, D., *et al.* (1999). *Hum. Mol. Genet.*, **8**, 1779.

23. Girardet, A., McPeek, M. S., Leeflang, E. P., Munier, F., Arnheim, N., Claustres, M., *et al.* (2000). *Am. J. Hum. Genet.*, **66**, 167.

24. Zhang, L., Leeflang, E. P., Yu, J., and Arnheim, N. (1994). *Nature Genet.*, **7**, 531.

25. Leeflang, E. P., Zhang, L., Tavare, S., Hubert, R., Srinidhi, J., MacDonald, M. E., *et al.* (1995). *Hum. Mol. Genet.*, **4**, 1519.

26. Zhang, L., Fischbeck, K. H., and Arnheim, N. (1995). *Hum. Mol. Genet.*, **4**, 303.

27. Huang, M. M., Erlich, H. A., Goodman, M. F., and Arnheim, N. (1995). *Hum. Mutat.*, **6**, 303.

28. Kunst, C. B., Leeflang, E. P., Iber, J. C., Arnheim, N., and Warren, S. T. (1997). *J. Med. Genet.*, **34**, 627.

29. Grewal, R. P., Leeflang, E. P., Zhang, L., and Arnheim, N. (1998). *Neurogenetics*, **1**, 249.

30. Takiyama, Y., Sakoe, K., Amaike, M., Soutome, M., Ogawa, T., Nakano, I., *et al.* (1999). *Hum. Mol. Genet.*, **8**, 453.

31. Leeflang, E. P., Tavare, S., Marjoram, P., Neal, C. O., Srinidhi, J., MacFarlane, H., *et al.* (1999). *Hum. Mol. Genet.*, **8**, 173.

32. Zangenberg, G., Huang, M. M., Arnheim, N., and Erlich, H. (1995). *Nature Genet.*, **10**, 407.

33. Zhang, L., Cui, X., Schmitt, K., Hubert, R., Navidi, W., and Arnheim, N. (1992). *Proc. Natl. Acad. Sci. USA*, **89**, 5847.

34. Dean, P. N. (1997). In *Current protocols in cytometry* (ed. J. P. Robinson, *et al.*), Vol. 1, p. 1-0-1. John Wiley & Sons, Inc.

35. Ormerod, M. G. (1994). In *Flow cytometry: a practical approach* (ed. M. G. Ormerod), p. 27. IRL Press, Oxford.

36. Li, H., Gyllensten, U. B., Cui, X., Saiki, R. K., Erlich, H. A., and Arnheim, N. (1988). *Nature*, **335**, 414.

37. Sun, F., Arnheim, N., and Waterman, M. S. (1995). *Nucleic Acids Res.*, **23**, 3034.

38. Hancock, J. M. (1999). In *Microsatellites: evolution and applications* (ed. D. B. Goldstein and C. Schlotterer), p. 1. Oxford University Press, Oxford.

39. Litt, M. and Luty, J. A. (1989). *Am. J. Hum. Genet.*, **44**, 397.

40. Weber, J. L. and May, P. E. (1989). *Am. J. Hum. Genet.*, **44**, 388.

41. Dietrich, W. F., Miller, J., Steen, R., Merchant, M. A., Damron-Boles, D., Husain, Z., *et al.* (1996). *Nature*, **380**, 149.

42. Weissenbach, J., Gyapay, G., Dib, C., Vignal, A., Morissette, J., Millasseau, P., *et al.* (1992). *Nature*, **359**, 794.

43. Weber, J. L. and Wong, C. (1993). *Hum. Mol. Genet.*, **2**, 1123.

44. Hubert, R., Weber, J. L., Schmitt, K., Zhang, L., and Arnheim, N. (1992). *Am. J. Hum. Genet.*, **51**, 985.

45. Klungland, H., Gomez-Raya, L., Howard, C. J., Collins, R. A., Rogne, S., and Lien, S. (1997). *Mamm. Genome*, **8**, 573.
46. Girardet, A., Lien, S., Leeflang, E. P., Beaufrere, L., Tuffery, S., Munier, F., *et al.* (1999). *Eur. J. Hum. Genet.*, **7**, 239.
47. Collins, F. S., Brooks, L. D., and Chakravarti, A. (1998). *Genome Res.*, **8**, 1229.
48. Brookes, A. J. (1999). *Gene*, **234**, 177.
49. Li, W. and Sadler, L. A. (1991). *Genetics*, **129**, 513.
50. Wang, D. G., Fan, J., Siao, C., Berno, A., Young, P., Sapolsky, R., *et al.* (1998). *Science*, **280**, 1077.
51. Buetow, K. H., Edmonson, M. N., and Cassidy, A. B. (1999). *Nature Genet.*, **21**, 323.
52. Arnheim, N., Li, H., and Cui, X. (1990). *Genomics*, **8**, 415.
53. Lewin, H. A., Schmitt, K., Hubert, R., van Eijk, M. J., and Arnheim, N. (1992). *Genomics*, **13**, 44.
54. Li, H., Cui, X., and Arnheim, N. (1990). *Proc. Natl. Acad. Sci. USA*, **87**, 4580.
55. Hubert, R., Stanton, V. P. Jr., Aburatani, H., Warren, J., Li, H., Housman, D. E., *et al.* (1992). *Genomics*, **12**, 683.
56. Eiken, H. G., Odland, E., Boman, H., Skjelkvale, L., Engebretsen, L. F., and Apold, J. (1991). *Nucleic Acids Res.*, **19**, 1427.
57. Carrington, M., Miller, T., White, M., Gerrard, B., Stewart, C., Dean, M., *et al.* (1992). *Hum. Immunol.*, **33**, 208.
58. Glavac, D. and Dean, M. (1995). *Methods Neurosci.*, **26**, 194.
59. Dean, M. and Milligan, B. G. (1998). In *Molecular genetic analysis of populations: a practical approach* (ed. A. R. Hoelzel), p. 263. IRL Press, Oxford.
60. Saiki, R. K., Bugawan, T. L., Horn, G. T., Mullis, K. B., and Erlich, H. A. (1986). *Nature*, **324**, 163.
61. Leeflang, E. P., Schmitt, K., Hubert, R., Zhang, L., and Arnheim, N. (1994). In *Current protocols in human genetics* (ed. A. L. Boyle), Vol. 1, p. 1-6-1. John Wiley & Sons, Inc.
62. Lazzeroni, L. C., Arnheim, N., Schmitt, K., and Lange, K. (1994). *Am. J. Hum. Genet.*, **55**, 431.
63. Lange, K., Weeks, D., and Boehnke, M. (1988). *Genet. Epidemiol.*, **5**, 471.
64. Farrall, M. (1997). *Genet. Epidemiol.*, **14**, 103.
65. McPeek, M. S. (1999). *Am. J. Hum. Genet.*, **65**, 1195.
66. Neilan, B. A., Leigh, D. A., Rapley, E., and McDonald, B. L. (1994). *Biotechniques*, **17**, 708.

Chapter 7
PCR-based methods of HLA typing

Henry A. Erlich
Roche Molecular Systems, 1145 Atlantic Ave., Alameda CA 94501, USA
Children's Hospital Oakland Research Institute, 5700 Martin Luther King Jr. Way, Oakland, CA 94609, USA

Elizabeth A. Trachtenberg
Children's Hospital Oakland Research Institute, 5700 Martin Luther King Jr. Way, Oakland, CA 94609, USA

1 Introduction

Over the last two decades, molecular genetic techniques have been used to isolate the genes encoding the HLA class I and class II molecules and to characterize their genomic organization as well as their sequence diversity. The allelic sequence polymorphism at the HLA class I and II loci, revealed by extensive sequencing studies on a variety of human populations, is far greater than the antigenic variation detected by conventional serological typing (1). For example, there are about 280 DRB1 alleles defined by the second exon sequence but only about 15 different DR serological specificities or serotypes. Similarly, for the HLA-B locus, more than 450 alleles have been reported, compared to about 48 serological specificities. For the DPA1 and DPB1 loci, which encode the DP molecule, no serological typing system has been available and, consequently, most functional investigations of DP polymorphism, such as disease association studies or the analysis of DP mismatching in transplantation, have been possible only since the development of DNA-based HLA typing methods (2). The HLA class I and class II loci are the most polymorphic coding sequences in the human genome. The study of their allelic sequence diversity as well as the development of simple and rapid DNA-based typing methods has been greatly facilitated by the development of PCR amplification in the mid 1980s (3–6).

In general, PCR-based analysis of HLA polymorphism allows a much more accurate (fewer errors) and precise (more discriminating) method of typing than serology. Moreover, the primers, probes, and thermostable DNA polymerase that are used in PCR-based HLA typing can be produced as standardized reagents; this represents a critical advantage over serological and cellular typing methods. In addition, DNA methods permit the typing of a much wider variety of samples because, unlike serological methods, the viability of the cells or the expression of the relevant antigen on the cell surface is not required. PCR amplification makes possible the typing of minute samples, such as single cells or individual sperm (5, 7). Thus, HLA typing can, with PCR-based methods, be carried out on buccal swabs, hairs, dried blood spots, as well as archival material, such as paraffin-embedded tissue biopsy sections. This capability has made possible valuable retrospective epidemiological (8) and population genetics studies (9, 10) as well as forensics applications (11). The ability to type individual sperm for multiple loci has enabled studies of recombination rates of closely linked loci and the possibility of comparing such rates among different individuals (12) (see Chapter 6).

In addition, PCR-based typing data from which the nucleotide sequence of the sample can be inferred can reveal **how** and **where** alleles differ, allowing the analysis of the role of specific polymorphic amino acid residues in peptide binding and presentation as well as in disease association and in clinical transplantation. For example, the DR4 specificity can be encoded by any one of the more than 30 DRB1*04 alleles; some DR4 associated diseases (e.g. type 1 diabetes, rheumatoid arthritis, pemphigus vulgaris) are positively associated with specific DR4 alleles, and negatively associated with others (13–15). The negatively and positively associated alleles can differ by as little as a single codon. These critical polymorphic sequence motifs can now be readily distinguished by PCR-based HLA typing methods. In this chapter, we review briefly some of the PCR methods that have been developed since the first reported amplification of an HLA gene in 1986 to carry out DNA-based HLA typing (16, 17) and provide protocols for the probe-based typing methods used in our lab.

2 The HLA loci

The HLA loci on the short arm of human chromosome 6 encode two distinct classes of highly polymorphic cell surface molecules that bind and present processed antigens in the form of peptides to T lymphocytes. Recognition by the T cell of the HLA–peptide complex, along with co-stimulatory signals, results in T cell activation. The class I molecules, HLA-A, -B, and -C, are found on most nucleated cells. They are cell surface glycoproteins that bind and present peptides derived primarily from endogenously synthesized proteins (e.g. viral and tumour peptides) to $CD8^+$ T cells. These heterodimers consist of a polymorphic HLA-encoded α chain associated with the non-MHC encoded monomorphic polypeptide, β_2-microglobulin. The other HLA class I loci are significantly less polymorphic and HLA class I typing is generally restricted to the polymorphism at the HLA-A, -B, and -C loci.

The class II molecules consist of MHC-encoded α and β glycoprotein chains associated as heterodimers on the cell surface of antigen-presenting cells such as B cells and macrophages. Class II molecules serve as receptors for processed peptides; however, these peptides are derived predominantly from membrane and extracellular proteins (e.g. bacterial peptides) and are presented to $CD4^+$ T cells. The HLA-D region contains several class II genes and has three subregions: HLA-DR, -DQ, and -DP. Both the HLA-DQ and -DP regions contain one functional gene for each of the α and β chains. The HLA-DR subregion contains one functional gene (DRA) for the α chain; the number of functional genes for the β

chain varies from one to two per chromosome. All haplotypes express a DRB1-encoded polymorphic polypeptide that is found on the cell surface in association with the DRA-encoded polypeptide. The other functional class II DRB genes, DRB3, DRB4, and DRB5 encode polypeptides which are also found on the cell surface in association with the DRA-encoded polypeptide but at a lower level and only in certain class II haplotypes. In general, the DRB3 locus is found on haplotypes where the DRB1 allele is in the *03, *11, *12, *13, or *14 groups; the DRB3 gene product types serologically as DRW52. The DRB4 locus is found on haplotypes where DRB1 is in the *04, *07, or *09 groups, and the DRB4 gene product types serologically as DRW53. The DRB5 locus is found on haplotypes where DRB1 is *02 (either *15 or *16), and DRB5 types serologically as DRW51. There are, however, rare exceptions to this pattern.

With the exception of the DRA and the DPA1 loci, the genes encoding the functional class II molecules are highly polymorphic. The HLA-A, -B, and -C loci also exhibit extensive allelic diversity. Analyses of the HLA class I and II structures have shown that these polymorphic amino acid residues line the peptide binding cleft and interact directly with the peptide and/or the T cell receptor (18–20). The extensive polymorphism at both the class I and II loci and its localization to the peptide binding groove, as well as the analyses of sequence substitution patterns (non-synonymous vs. synonymous changes), have led to the notion that the extensive allelic sequence diversity observed at virtually all HLA loci is maintained by selective forces, such as balancing selection and overdominance (heterozygote advantage) or frequency-dependent selection (21–23).

3 HLA allelic sequence diversity

The allelic sequence diversity of the HLA class I and class II loci is the highest among mammalian coding sequence polymorphisms. The functional significance of this extensive polymorphism as well as the genetic mechanisms and the evolutionary forces that have generated and maintained this sequence diversity continue to be the subject of many immunological, genetic, and evolutionary investigations (24–26). For the HLA class II genes, the loci encoding the α and β chains of the DR, the DQ, and the DP antigens, virtually all of the polymorphism is localized to the second exon. This exon encodes the α-helical 'walls' and the β-pleated sheet 'floor' of the peptide binding groove formed by the α–β heterodimer. Among the class II α chain loci, only the DQA1 locus, with over 15 alleles, shows extensive polymorphism. The β chain loci, however, are highly polymorphic. Population surveys in a variety of human populations, have identified over 85 alleles at the DPB1 locus and over 221 at the DRB1 locus as of 1999 (27). A small number of these alleles are identical in amino acid sequence and differ only at the nucleotide level through silent substitutions. The other DRB loci (i.e. DRB3) show a relatively modest number of alleles although some of the alleles at DRB3 differ at many different sites.

In contrast, the HLA class I HLA-A, -B, and -C antigens contain polymorphic α1 and α2 protein domains that comprise the peptide binding groove encoded within a single heavy chain locus. The α1 and α2 domains are encoded in the second and third exons respectively. Like the class II loci, the class I loci are highly polymorphic: as of 1999, population studies had revealed 124 alleles at the HLA-A locus, 259 alleles at the HLA-B locus, and 70 alleles at the HLA-C locus (27). In general, a given population contains only a subset of the class I or class II alleles that have been identified world-wide and different populations often have significantly different allele frequency distributions. Different populations can also have varying patterns of linkage disequilibrium, that is, the non-random association of alleles at the linked HLA loci.

In general, the pattern of allelic sequence diversity at all the polymorphic HLA loci is a patchwork of discrete sequence motifs. This patchwork pattern of polymorphism is thought to reflect the operation of gene conversion-like events that have generated the extensive sequence diversity observed in human populations by recombining these short sequence motifs (24). One consequence of this pattern is that, in PCR-based HLA typing, a large number of different alleles can be distinguished by using a relatively modest number of oligonucleotide primers or probes (see below) that recognize these sequence motifs. On the other hand, sometimes a given pattern of sequence motifs, detected either with probes or primers or by sequencing, may be consistent with more than a single genotype because the observed sequence motifs can be combined into more than a unique pair of alleles. This issue of 'ambiguity' in DNA-based typing is discussed below.

4 Nomenclature

In the World Health Organization (WHO) nomenclature for HLA alleles, the locus designation (e.g. DRB1) is followed by an asterisk (*) and by two digits that identify the allele group (e.g. DRB1*04 which, in this case, corresponds to the serological DR4 type), and two more digits that identify the allele or DR4 subtype (e.g. DRB1*0401, DRB1*0402, etc.). An additional digit is used to designate silent or synonymous variants, that is, different nucleotide sequences that encode the same amino acid sequence (e.g. DRB1*08041 and *08042). Recently, rare sequence variants that prevent the expression of a given gene have been identified; these so-called 'null' alleles can be promoter mutations, nonsense mutations, or mutations that affect mRNA splicing (28). For example, the nomenclature for this category of variants for an HLA-A*2402 allele that is not expressed is HLA-A*2402N. Most of the HLA 'null' alleles reported thus far are for subtypes of HLA-A2, -A3, -A4, and -A24 and are very rare. In general, the allele groups, designated by the first two digits (i.e. DRB1*04 or *08), correspond to serological specificities (i.e. DR4 or DR8). There are, however, exceptions. For the HLA-B locus, all the alleles within a single allele group designation (e.g. HLA-B*15) do not necessarily encode the same serological type. For example, several different serological specificities are associated with different B15 alleles (e.g. B*1522 with B35 and B*1501, B*1504, B*1505–1508, B*1515, B*1520, B*1524 with B62). A recent report on the serological equivalents of HLA alleles serves as a 'dictionary', relating alleles and serological specificities for HLA-A, -B, -C, DRB1/3/4/5, and DQB1 (29).

5 HLA typing: a brief history

5.1 Serological and cellular methods

Historically, HLA typing has been performed by using a combination of the serological microcytotoxicity test (30) and, in some cases, a cellular assay, the mixed lymphocyte reaction (MLR) (31) for the class II antigens. In the micro-cytotoxicity assay, which can be used to type both class I and II antigens, an antiserum (or monoclonal antibody) is mixed with live lymphocytes and allowed to bind to the cell surface molecules. Specific binding is then detected with the addition of complement which lyses the cells and allows the uptake of a dye. The microcytotoxicity assay requires viable cells and uses antisera obtained primarily from individuals who have been sensitized to HLA differences such as multiparous women (women who have had multiple pregnancies) or individuals who have received multiple transfusions. Consequently, these reagents are limiting in quantity and difficult to standardize. Although, as noted above, over 200 DRB1 alleles (different amino acid sequences) have been identified, serological reagents can distinguish only 15 different groups of DR molecules encoded by these alleles.

5.2 DNA-based techniques

The initial approach to HLA typing at the DNA level involved the restriction fragment length polymorphism (RFLP) method using labelled cDNA clones or genomic fragments as hybridization probes (32, 33). Different HLA serotypes exhibited different banding patterns. In some cases, the probes cross-hybridized to related genomic sequences, yielding a complex pattern of bands (restriction fragments). The use of short locus-specific probes, often derived from the 3'UT region, typically simplified the banding patterns and facilitated typing. RFLP typing required neither cell surface expression nor cell viability and, provided that several restriction enzymes were used, could often subdivide HLA class II serotypes. Although an informative approach, RFLP typing required a large amount of high molecular weight genomic DNA and the Southern blotting procedure was somewhat cumbersome. This approach, consequently, was not well-suited to routine clinical typing. In addition, since the majority of the polymorphic restriction sites used for RFLP typing were not in exon 2 or exon 3, this method relied heavily on linkage disequilibrium of the polymorphic restriction sites with the sequence polymorphisms in these exons. Most importantly, RFLP typing failed to distinguish much of the HLA class II sequence polymorphism.

The development of the PCR greatly facilitated the analysis of sequence polymorphism at both the class I and II loci and, in turn, the HLA region was a primary model system for developing PCR genetic typing methods. The second region, after beta-globin, to be amplified from genomic DNA using this newly developed amplification method was the HLA-DQA1 second exon (16, 17). By generating billions of copies of the specific target sequence from a complex template like genomic DNA, this technique enabled the use of simple, non-radioactive methods to analyse sequence information. Based on the available database of class I and class II allelic sequence diversity, a variety of relatively simple and rapid PCR-based methods has been developed to carry out HLA typing at the DNA level.

Most typing methods involve the design of primer pairs that are capable of amplifying all alleles at the target locus with the polymorphic sequence motifs localized between the primer sites (for more information regarding primer design of highly polymorphic loci, see Chapter 3). The sequences between the primers are subsequently characterized by a variety of approaches, including hybridization probes, restriction enzymes, chain-termination sequencing reactions, or inferred from the conformation-based mobility of the PCR products using gel electrophoresis. The other main approach to HLA typing uses the PCR itself as a method of distinguishing polymorphisms by exploiting the specificity of oligonucleotide primer extension and places the 3′ end of the primer at the polymorphic site.

5.2.1 SSO

The first PCR-based approaches to HLA typing utilized labelled sequence-specific oligonucleotide (SSO) probes to hybridize to PCR products amplified from the sample and immobilized on a nylon or nitrocellulose filter, the 'dot blot' method (17). SSO probes had been previously applied to restriction enzyme digested genomic DNA in gels (34) but the probes often cross-hybridized to non-target genomic fragments and the procedure was very complex and cumbersome. PCR amplification of specific sequences from genomic DNA created millions of copies of the specific target sequence greatly simplifying the use of SSO probes. In SSO dot blot typing with immobilized PCR products, under appropriate hybridization and wash conditions, the labelled SSO probes would bind only to the complementary sequence in the amplified DNA and were able to distinguish single nucleotide differences. Using a panel of probes specific for informative sequence motifs, the HLA alleles in the sample could be inferred from the pattern of probe reactivity. The initial methods utilized ^{32}P-labelled probes for typing of the HLA-DQA1 locus but shortly thereafter, non-radioactively labelled probes were introduced (4) and are now commonly used. The probes can be labelled either directly with an enzyme (e.g. HRP) or with biotin. The biotin labelled probes can be detected with streptavidin conjugated to HRP (or AP) and can be used with chromogenic or chemoluminescent substrates for sensitive, simple, and robust detection. More recently, digoxigenin labelled probes and antibody to digoxigenin detection methods have been introduced (35, 36).

Currently, computer programs are routinely used to infer the genotype from the probe reactivity pattern. The genotype interpretation programs have to be updated periodically to incorporate newly identified alleles. In some cases, these new alleles will require the addition of probes to the typing system. In most cases, however, the new allele represents a new combination of known poly-morphic sequence motifs and thus, does not create the need for additional probes. In this case, however, the incorporation of the new allele into the typing system and software may create additional ambiguities. Such ambiguities arise when a given probe reactivity pattern is consistent with more than one genotype. Given enough primers and probes, the PCR/SSO method is, in princi-ple, capable of distinguishing all of the alleles at a given HLA locus. To achieve allele level typing, however, it is usually necessary to amplify separately the alleles of a heterozygote (see below) and analyse the probe reactivity pattern for each individual allele.

In the SSO probe typing approach, the sequence of the primers and the amplification reaction conditions (thermal profile, Mg^{2+} concentration, primer concentrations, etc.) are designed so that all alleles at the target locus are amplified and, whenever possible, the amplification is locus-specific. In some cases, such as generic DRB1 typing, the same primer pairs amplify the DRB1, DRB3, DRB4, and DRB5 second exons. This approach allows the typing of all these loci from a single PCR. On the other hand, amplification of more than one locus can complicate the interpretation of probe reactivity if the complementary sequence motif is found in more than one locus. In the case of DRB1, it is difficult to find a single primer pair that is locus-specific and that also amplifies all alleles of DRB1.

In the design of SSO probes, the position of the mismatched base pair is generally placed toward the middle of the probe to minimize the stability of the mismatched probe–target duplex. Not all base pair mismatches are equally destabilizing; the G-T mismatch is the least destabilizing and, if possible, should be avoided to minimize cross-hybridization to the non-target allele. To simplify the hybridization conditions for multiple probes, buffer systems, such as those including tetramethylammonium chloride (TMAC), have been developed to minimize the effect of GC% differences between probes. However, due to its cost, many labs have designed probes and conditions to simplify hybridization analy-sis without addition of TMAC.

Following the initial SSO probe typing system for DQA1, PCR/SSO dot blot typing systems for DRB1, DQB1, DPB1, and DPA1 have been developed (37–41), as well as, more recently for the HLA-A, -B, and -C loci (42, 43). Reverse hybridiza-tion approaches using immobilized SSO probe arrays, developed to simplify SSO typing, are described below.

Detailed protocols for the dot blot method and the reverse line blot method are described below. *Table 1* describes the locus-specific primers used for ampli-fying the DRB1 (DRB3, DRB4, and DRB5), DQB1, and DPB1 loci. *Tables 2* and *3* describe the group-specific primers for the class II loci for amplifying separately the two alleles of a heterozygote sample. *Figure 1* shows the pattern of DQB1 probe reactivity for homozygous samples.

Table 1 Class II DRB1, DQB1, and DPB1 locus-specific primers utilized in dot blot typing formats

Locus	5' Primer[a] (5' → 3')	3' Primer[a] (5' → 3')	PCR profile[b]	Reference[c]
DRB1, 3, 4, 5	GH46: CCGGATCCTTCGTGTCCCCACAGCACG	AB60: CCGAATTCCGCTGCACTGTGAAGCTCTC	95°C 1 min → 60°C 1 min → 72°C 30 sec × 35 cycles	GH46: Ref. 1 AB60: Ref. 2
DQB1	DB130: AGGGATCCCGCAGAGAGGATTTCGTGTAC	GH29: GAGCTGCAGGTAGTTGTGTCTGCACAC	95°C 1 min → 55°C 1 min → 72°C 15 sec × 35 cycles	DB130: Ref. 2 GH29: Ref. 2
DPB1	UG19: GCTGCAGGAGAGTGGCGCCTCCGCTCAT	UG21: CGGATCCGGCCCAAAGCCCTCACTC	95°C 1 min → 65°C 1 min → 72°C 30 sec × 35 cycles	UG19: Ref. 3 UG21: Ref. 3

[a] PCR mastermixes for the primers in this table include 15% glycerol, 50 pmoles each primer, and 1.5 mM $MgCl_2$.

[b] PCR profiles for the primers in this table begin with a 95°C for 5 min step, continue as described above, then end with a 72°C extension for 10 min, and a hold at 15°C.

[c] Ref. 1: Scharf, et al. (1991). *Hum. Immunol.*, **30**, 190.
Ref. 2: Erlich, et al. (1991). *Eur. J. Immunogenet.*, **18**, 33.
Ref. 3: Bugawan, et al. (1991). *Immunogenetics*, **34**, 413.

Table 2 Class II DRB1 group-specific primers utilized in dot blot typing formats

Group-specific region/alleles	5' Primer sequence[a]	3' Primer sequence[a]	PCR profile[b]	Reference[c]
DRB1 WLF	RAP90: GGGGATCCTGGAGTACTCTACGGGTG	AB60: CCGAATTCCGCTGCACTGTGAAGCTCTC	95°C 1 min → 65°C 1 min → 72°C 30 sec × 35 cycles	RAP90: Unpublished AB60: Ref. 1
DRB1 WPR	AB83: GGGGATCCTGTGGCAGCCTAAGAGG	AB60: CCGAATTCCGCTGCACTGTGAAGCTCTC	95°C 1 min → 65°C 1 min → 72°C 1 min × 35 cycles	AB83: Ref. 2 AB60: Ref. 1
DRB1 VH	AB54: GGGGATCTTGGAGCAGGTTAAACA	CA05: CGCTGCACTGTGAAGCTCTC	95°C 1 min → 65°C 1 min → 72°C 30 sec × 35 cycles	AB54: Ref. 2 CA05: Unpublished

	Primer 1	Primer 2	Profile[b]	Reference[c]
DRB1 YSTG	RAP59: GGGGATCCTGGAGTACTCACGGGTG	AB60: CCGAATTCCGCTGCACTGTGAAGCTCTC	95°C 1 min → 65°C 1 min → 72°C 30 sec × 35 cycles	RAP59: Ref. 3 / AB60: Ref. 1
DRB1 YSTS	AB82: GGGGATCCTGGAGTACTCTACGTC	AB60: CCGAATTCCGCTGCACTGTGAAGCTCTC	95°C 1 min → 65°C 1 min → 72°C 30 sec × 35 cycles	AB82: Ref. 2 / AB60: Ref. 1
DRB1 YSTS- 3'V @ 86	AB82: GGGGATCCTGGAGTACTCTACGTC	AB131: CGCTGCACTGTGAAGCTCTCCA	95°C 1 min → 67°C 2 min → 72°C 1 min × 35 cycles	AB82: Ref. 2 / AB131B: Unpublished
DRB1 YSTS- 3'G @ 86	AB82: GGGGATCCTGGAGTACTCTACGTC	AB132: CGCTGCACTGTGAAGCTCTCAC	95°C 1 min → 67°C 2 min → 72°C 1 min × 35 cycles	AB82: Ref. 2 / AB132B: Unpublished
DRB1 GYK	CHO-120: CGTTTCCTGTGGCAGGGTAAGTATA	AB60: CCGAATTCCGCTGCACTGTGAAGCTCTC	95°C 1 min → 65°C 1 min → 72°C 30 sec × 35 cycles	CHO-120: Unpublished / AB60: Ref. 1
DRB1 3'R @71	GH46: CCGGATCCTTCGTGTCCCCACAGCAC	CHO-32: TGTCCACCGCGGCCGCCT	95°C 1 min → 65°C 1 min → 72°C 30 sec × 35 cycles	GH46: Ref. 4 / CHO-32: Unpublished
DRB1 3'E @71	GH46: CCGGATCCTTCGTGTCCCCACAGCACG	CHO-33: TGTCCACCGCGGCCCGCTC	95°C 1 min → 65°C 1 min → 72°C 30 sec × 35 cycles	GH46: Ref. 4 / CHO-33: Unpublished

[a] PCR mastermixes for the primers in this table include 15% glycerol, 50 pmoles each primer, and 1.5 mM $MgCl_2$.

[b] PCR profiles for the primers in this table begin with a 95°C for 5 min step, continue as described above, then end with a 72°C extension for 10 min, and a hold at 15°C.

[c] Ref. 1: Erlich, et al. (1991). Eur. J. Immunogenet., **18**, 33.

Ref. 2: Begovich, et al. (1992). J. Immunol., **148**, 249.

Ref. 3: Apple, et al. (1992). Tissue Antigens, **40**, 69.

Ref. 4: Scharf, et al. (1991). Hum. Immunol., **30**, 190.

Table 3 Class II DQB1 and DPB1 group-specific primers utilized in dot blot typing formats

Group-specific region/alleles	5′ Primer sequence[a]	3′ Primer sequence[a]	PCR profile[b]	Reference[c]
DQB1 Asp @ 57 (0301/0303 ambiguity)	DB130: AGGGATCCCCGCAGAGAGGATTTCGTGTAC	CHO-04: CTGGCTGTTCCAGTACTCGGCGT	95°C 1 min → 70°C 20 sec → 72°C 15 sec × 35 cycles	DB130: Ref. 1 CHO-04: Unpublished
DQB1 Ala @ 57 (0302/0304 ambiguity)	DB130: AGGGATCCCCGCAGAGAGGATTTCGTGTAC	CHO-03: CTGGCTGTTCCAGTACTCGGCGG	95°C 1 min → 65°C 30 sec → 72°C 15 sec × 35 cycles	DB130: Ref. 1 CHO-03: Unpublished
DPB1 DEE(F)	CHO-5′DEE: GAGCTGGGGCGGCCTGATGA	UG21: CGGATCCGGCCCAAAGCCCTCACTC	95°C 1 min → 70°C 1 min → 72°C 15 sec × 35 cycles	CHO-5′DEE: Unpublished UG21: Ref. 2
DPB1 DEE(R)	UG19: GCTGCAGGAGAGTGGCGCCTCCGCTCAT	CHO-3′DEE: GTCCTTCTGGCTGTTCCAGTACTCCTCAT	95°C 1 min → 70°C 1 min → 72°C 15 sec × 35 cycles	UG19: Ref. 2 CHO-3′DEE: Unpublished
DPB1 V(R)	UG19: GCTGCAGGAGAGTGGCGCCTCCGCTCAT	CHO-3′V: CTCGTAGTTGTGTCTGCATAC	95°C 1 min → 65°C 1 min → 72°C 15 sec × 35 cycles	UG19: Ref. 2 CHO-3′V: Unpublished
DPB1 AAE(R)	UG19: GCTGCAGGAGAGTGGCGCCTCCGCTCAT	CHO-3′AAE: GTCCTTCTGGCTGTTCCAGTACTCCGCAG	95°C 1 min → 70°C 1 min → 72°C 15 sec × 35 cycles	UG19: Ref. 2 CHO-3′AAE: Unpublished
DPB1 VYQL	CHO-01 VYQL: CCAGAGAATTACGTGTACCAGTT	UG21: CGGATCCGGCCCAAAGCCCTCACTC	95°C 1 min → 65°C 30 sec → 72°C 15 sec × 35 cycles	CHO-01 VYQL Unpublished UG21: Ref. 2

[a] PCR mastermixes for the primers in this table include 15% glycerol, 50 pmoles each primer, and 1.5 mM MgCl$_2$.

[b] PCR profiles for the primers in this table begin with a 95°C for 5 min step, continue as described above, then end with a 72°C extension for 10 min, and a hold at 15°C.

[c] Ref. 1: Erlich, et al. (1991). Eur. J. Immunogenet., **18**, 33.

Ref. 2: Bugawan, et al. (1991). Immunogenetics, **34**, 413.

ERRATUM

Carrington and Hoelzel *Molecular Epidemiology*

This is the correct version of Figure 1 in Chapter Seven, p.191.

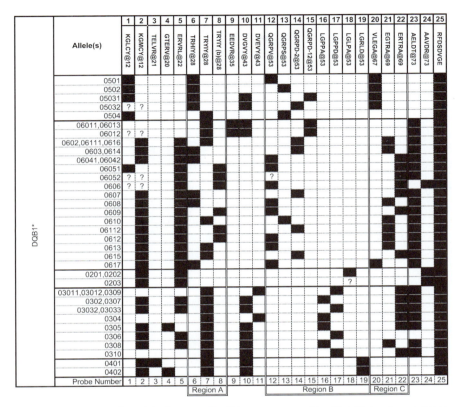

Figure 1 DQB1 Probe Reactivity Patterns. Peptide sequence motifs with initial codon positions are shown underneath each probe number (1–25), listed at top and bottom of figure. Positive probe hits are designated by black boxes for each allele, listed in left column. The presence of more than 2 positive probes within a defined region (A, B, C) indicates a mixed sample or contamination.

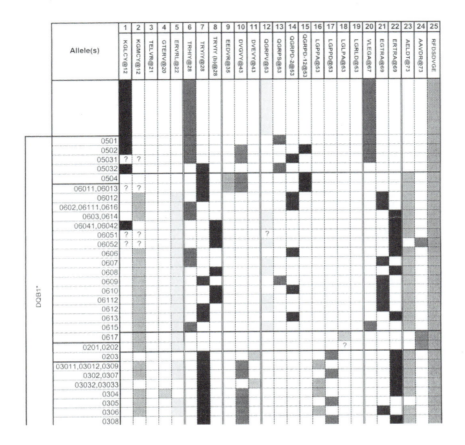

Figure 1 DQB1 Probe Reactivity Patterns. Peptide sequence motifs with initial codon positions are shown underneath each probe number (1–25), listed at top and bottom of figure. Positive probe hits are designated by black boxes for each allele, listed in left column. The presence of more than 2 positive probes within a defined region (A, B, C) indicates a mixed sample or contamination.

Protocol 1

High-throughput PCR amplification for HLA typing

Equipment and reagents

- Thermal cycler(s)
- Micropipetters (e.g. Pipetmen) and tips
- Repeat pipettor (e.g. Easy Step Pipettor and Combitips)
- PCR workstation with UV light
- Vortex

- Microcentrifuge and other centrifuge tubes (1.5–15 ml) for amplification cocktail preparation and mixing
- PCR tubes (0.2 ml; e.g. Perkin Elmer (PE) TC9600) and racks
- Thin-walled tubes (0.5 ml; e.g. PE TC480) and racks

191

- PCR tube caps (0.2 ml tube caps—strips of 8 or 12 caps)
- Cap roller tool
- 6 mM or 8 mM MgCl$_2$, stored in small aliquots at 4 °C

- Primers: 50 μM stock, stored in 200 μl aliquots in freezer (–20 °C)
- 10 × PCR mastermix (recipe follows)
- Sterile distilled and deionized water (ddH$_2$O), in small aliquots stored at 4 °C

Note: all reagents used for amplification are dispensed in single or limited use volumes.

A. In clean room

Note: a separate 10 × PCR mastermix with primers for each locus amplified can be set up and frozen in single or daily use aliquots. This 10 × PCR mastermix should include the following:

Stock concentration	Final concentration
• 50 μM 5′ and 3′ primers	50 pmoles per locus-specific amplification or
	25 pmoles per epitope- or group-specific amplification
• *Taq* polymerase	5 U/100 μl reaction
• 100 mM each dNTP	0.1875 mM (each dNTP: dATP, dGTP, dCTP, dTTP)
• 80% glycerol	10–15%
• 1 M Tris–HCl	10 mM
• 3 M KCl	50 mM

It is advisable to set up Amplification Log worksheets for each locus amplified. Include on the worksheets specific primers, MgCl$_2$, dNTP, *Taq*, and glycerol concentrations, as well as cycling profile and instrument information. A 96-well grid with sample identifiers for ease of set up and tracking purposes is also useful on this worksheet.

All amplification set up should be performed in an enclosed PCR workstation with UV light. This unit will limit exposure to the open laboratory environment, protecting against cross-contamination or airborne contamination during experiments. The UV radiation of working area prior to use blocks the replication of contaminating DNA sequences. All materials used in this area should be marked clearly 'NO PCR' so as not to be contaminated with PCR product. Gloves should be changed frequently, whenever they may be contaminated with DNA.

1 Clean set up area with 10% bleach and/or expose to UV light for ~ 20 min.

2 Put down a fresh assay mat or bench matting.

3 Thaw samples and 10 × PCR mastermix (with specific primers for locus to be amplified) on ice.

4 Select appropriate controls from working aliquots stored at 4 °C. Controls are chosen based on locus or region to be analysed.

5 Fill out appropriate Amplification Log(s) and identify all samples and controls (both positive and negative) to be amplified.

    (a) A negative control (no nucleic acid template) should be set up in the last and every ~ 20th tube.

    (b) Positive controls are best situated in the last lane to allow for easier probe analysis.

6 Label tubes.

7 Fill 96-well thermocycling plates with 0.2 ml PCR tubes and snap the tube stabilizing plate into place. Cover tubes/plates with fresh Saran (or similar) Wrap, to keep clean.

8 Calculate amount of each reagent needed for amplification cocktail (including PCR mastermix with primers, sterile ddH$_2$O, and MgCl$_2$) based on number of samples to be amplified and volume of amplification reaction (usually 100 μl), and enter that information onto the amplification worksheet. Include an extra ~ 5–10% for pipetting 'error'. The sample volume must be considered in setting up the amplification cocktail. For calculating the sample volume, consider the following:

    (a) Use between 50–500 ng DNA per PCR reaction. In general, if using QIAamp extracted DNA, allow 10 μl DNA per 100 μl reaction. If using other extracted material, use between 1–20 μl DNA, depending on viscosity and/or known concentration and adjust amplification cocktail accordingly.

    (b) For positive controls, use 25–500 ng DNA per 100 μl reaction.

    (c) For negative controls, add 10 μl sterile distilled water to negative control tubes. The negative control(s) will provide a check for contamination occurring during the PCR set up.

9 Prepare amplification cocktail on ice:

    (a) Add 10% PCR mastermix (includes primers) from single or daily use aliquots to cocktail tube first.

    (b) Add calculated amount of sterile distilled water.

10 Add calculated amount of MgCl$_2$ *last*, close tube cap, and then VORTEX WELL.

11 Place all 0.5 ml thin-wall amplification tubes, or 96-well base with 0.2 ml tubes, into ice. Note: chilling tubes during set up will help avoid formation of primer–dimer.

12 Add amplification cocktail to tubes ON ICE, using a repeater pipettor (e.g. Easy Step with Combitip, Eppendorf repeater pipettor) or Pipetman.

13 Add sample/control DNA to appropriate tube or well, as described above under amplification cocktail calculations.

14 Add two drops of mineral oil to each thin-wall 0.5 ml PCR tube before capping, being careful not to touch the tip of the dropper to any surface. (Oil is not necessary for the 96-well 0.2 ml tubes.)

15 Cap all tubes. Use the special roller tool to firmly seat cap strips on the 96-well tubes.

B. In PCR laboratory

1 Place samples into thermal cycler(s), and start the amplification program(s). When the program is completed, remove the samples from the thermal cycler as soon as practical and store them at 4°C, to await further studies.

Protocol 1 continued

2 Before proceeding with typing protocol(s), verify negative and positive controls and the degree of amplification by running an agarose gel (3% Nusieve/1%GTG agar in TBE). From the agarose gel assay, check to be sure all negative controls are negative. If an amplification negative control is found to be positive, repeat the amplification.

3 Next, check to be sure all positive controls amplified correctly, with the appropriate base pair size, using the molecular marker lane. If positive controls do not amplify correctly, check to make sure the correct positive controls were chosen for amplification (this is especially important in group-specific amplifications).

4 Determine if there are sample amplification drop-outs, and if amplification is efficient. The criterion we use for accepting an amplification is that the band must be at least half as intense as the weakest band in the marker lane; this should give sufficient amplified material for typing. If the sample does not amplify or is not sufficient for typing, repeat the amplification.

Protocol 2

Immobilized probe strip hybridization

Equipment and reagents

- Shaking water-baths (e.g. Hot Shaker from Bellco)

- Automated hybridization/wash detection instruments (e.g. TECAN SLT Profiblot or DYNAL Autoreli 48)

- Typing trays (small and large) with lids (e.g. Perkin Elmer Oligonucleotide Typing Trays)

- Plastic, heat-sealable bags (e.g. Seal-A-Meal™)

- Heat sealer for plastic bags

- Glass dishes, various sizes (e.g. crystallizing dishes work well)

- Micropipettors and tips

- Vacuum aspirator set-up

- Polaroid camera and film or digitizing camera (e.g. Alpha Innotec System)

- Locus/test specific score sheets and overlays

- Locus/test specific genotyping software (e.g. DYNAL, Reli SSO A/B/C/DRB/DQB software)

- $20 \times$ SSPE (saline, sodium phosphate, EDTA buffer for hybridization and wash solutions): 0.2 M $NaH_2PO_4.H_2O$ pH 7.4, 3 M NaCl, and 0.02 M EDTA

- 20% SDS (sodium dodecyl sulfate, for hybridization (0.5%), wash solutions (0.1%), with SSPE)

- 0.1 M citrate buffer pH 5.0: 0.032 M citric acid-H_2O, 0.068 M Na_3citrate-$2H_2O$

- DYNAL Reli SSO kit SSPE concentrate

- DYNAL Reli SSO kit SDS concentrate

- DYNAL Reli SSO kit buffer C: 0.1 M citrate buffer pH 5.0

- DYNAL Reli SSO kit immobilized probe strips (for HLA-A, HLA-B, HLA-C, DRB1, 3, 4, 5, or DQB1 loci)

- DYNAL Reli SSO kit denaturant: 1.6% NaOH, thymol blue

- DYNAL Reli SSO kit streptavidin–HRP conjugate (SA-HRP)

- DYNAL Reli SSO kit substrate A: 0.1 M citrate buffer with 0.01% hydrogen peroxide (H_2O_2)
- DYNAL Reli SSO kit substrate B: 0.1% 3,3′,5,5′-tetramethylbenzidine (TMB) and 40% dimethylformamide (DMF)
- TMB: 2 mg/ml 3,3′,5,5′-tetramethylbenzidine in 100% ethanol
- 3% hydrogen peroxide
- Sterile distilled and deionized water (ddH_2O)
- 4 × SSPE + 0.5% SDS hybridization solution
- 1 × SSPE + 0.1% SDS wash solution

Method

1 Turn on the shaking water-bath(s). Set the temperature to 50 °C, and allow the temperature to equilibrate.

2 Pre-warm to 50 °C:
  (a) Hybridization solution: 4 × SSPE + 0.5% SDS.
  (b) Wash buffer: 1 × SSPE + 0.1% SDS sufficient to wash each probe strip with 10 ml.
  (c) Note: if the hybridization will be done in sealed plastic bags, pre-warm 1 × SSPE + 0.1% SDS wash buffer.

3 Have ready at room temperature:
  (a) 1 × SSPE + 0.1% SDS.
  (b) Citrate buffer.
  (c) Sterile ddH_2O.
  (d) Note: if the hybridization will be done in plastic bags, prepare four crystallizing dishes containing: 1 × SSPE + 0.1% SDS (wash buffer); 50 ml 1 × SSPE + 0.1% SDS (for conjugation step); 100 ml citrate buffer; sterile ddH_2O.

4 Denature the amplified DNA to be typed:
  (a) Pipette 50 μl of DYNAL Reli SSO kit denaturation solution (per sample or control) into the wells of a flexible assay plate using a repeat pipettor.
  (b) Add 50 μl of sample or control DNA to the denaturant. If taking samples from 96-well thermocycler plate, a multichannel pipettor may be used for this step.
  (c) Allow to denature at least 5 min at room temperature.

5 Wet the probe strips in sterile ddH_2O and add to hybridization container(s) with clean forceps. Hybridization may be done in sealed plastic bags or typing trays.

6 Set up the hybridization reaction:
  (a) Add 3 ml of pre-warmed hybridization solution (see step 2a) to each probe strip.
  (b) Add 70–100 μl denatured PCR product to the appropriate probe strip well in tray or to appropriate section/strip in plastic bags. Be careful to add the DNA directly to hybridization solution and not directly onto strip.

7 Begin the hybridization:
  (a) Cover the typing tray with lid. If using plastic bags, remove as many bubbles as possible by gently pressing upward on the bag to express bubbles. Seal the plastic bag across the top (2 ×) with a heat sealer.

Protocol 2 continued

    (b) Place the plastic bag(s) or tray in 50°C water-bath and weight it (them) down. Gently shake ~ 60 r.p.m. for at least 30 min.

8 Wash the probe strips when the hybridization is finished. The temperature and the timing of the stringent wash are critical. The wash buffer is $1 \times$ SSPE + 0.1% SDS.

    (a) Trays:

- Aspirate tray contents.
- Rinse strips with 10 ml wash buffer.
- Rock tray for several seconds at room temperature in wash buffer.
- Aspirate wash solution.
- Stringent wash: wash strips with shaking (60 r.p.m.) in 10 ml wash solution for 12 min at 50°C.
- Aspirate wash solution.

    (b) Plastic bags:

- Cut the bag open above the strips.
- Using filter forceps, remove the strips and place in a pre-warmed crystallizing bowl containing the wash solution for stringent wash.
- Stringent wash: wash the strips with shaking (60 r.p.m.) in wash solution for 12 min at 50°C.

9 Remove the strips and place into a crystallizing bowl containing 50 ml wash buffer ($1 \times$ SSPE + 0.1% SDS) at room temperature.

NOTE: ALL FURTHER STEPS ARE PERFORMED AT ROOM TEMPERATURE.

10 Set up the incubation reaction with the DYNAL Reli SSO streptavidin–HRP conjugate:

    (a) Trays:

- Add 5 ml of wash buffer ($1 \times$ SSPE + 0.1% SDS) and 5 μl of DYNAL Reli SSO streptavidin–HRP conjugate to each strip.
- Shake for 20 min at ~ 60 r.p.m.
- Aspirate the conjugate solution.
- Add 5 ml of wash buffer ($1 \times$ SSPE + 0.1% SDS) to the strips.
- Shake for 10 min at ~ 60 r.p.m.
- Aspirate the wash solution.

    (b) Plastic bags:

- Add 50 μl DYNAL/Reli streptavidin–HRP to the crystallizing bowl containing the strips and 50 ml of $1 \times$ SSPE + 0.1% SDS (see step 10a).
- Shake for 20 min at ~ 60 r.p.m.
- Remove the strips and place in a crystallizing bowl containing $1 \times$ SSPE + 0.1% SDS.
- Shake 10 min at ~ 60 r.p.m.

11 Prepare the colour developing solution (not more than 30 min before use). To 100 ml citrate buffer, add 5 ml of TMB. Add 100 μl of 3% peroxide to mix after adding the strips. Mix by swirling. Note: this is enough solution for 20 strips. If trays are used for typing, increase amounts proportionately for more strips.

12 Develop strips:

(a) Trays:

- Add 5 ml colour developing solution to each strip.
- Shake for 10 min at ∼ 60 r.p.m., or until blue colour develops on strips.
- Aspirate the tray contents.
- Wash the strips with shaking in 5 ml sterile ddH$_2$O for 5–10 min. Repeat.

(b) Plastic bags:

- Add the strips to a crystallizing bowl containing the colour developing solution.
- Shake for 10 min at ∼ 60 r.p.m., or until blue colour develops on strips.
- In a fresh crystallizing bowl, wash the strips with shaking in 5 ml sterile ddH$_2$O for 5–10 min.

13 Photograph the wet strips.

14 Determine and record the positive probes using the transparency for the specific locus assayed. Analyse the probe reactions for each sample or control using the DYNAL Reli SSO kit genotyping program specific for the locus analysed.

15 The DYNAL Reli SSO kit typing trays may be reused following this cleaning procedure (do not use detergents to clean trays):

(a) Add ∼ 10 ml of 95% EtOH or 70% isopropanol to each well. (Neither alcohol should have come in contact with a metal container.)

(b) Cover typing tray with lid and carefully agitate for 15–30 sec to dissolve any residual TMB chromogen. Let trays, with alcohol still in the wells, sit overnight for best results.

(c) Remove the lid and pour off alcohol. Visually inspect for presence of TMB chromogen (faint blue colour). If necessary, repeat steps 15a and 15b, until all blue is gone.

(d) Rinse each well in the tray and the tray lid thoroughly with dI or MilliQ water.

(e) Allow trays and lids to air dry. The trays are now ready for reuse.

Protocol 3

Dot blot membrane preparation

Equipment and reagents

- Vacuum source
- 96-well dot blotter (The Convertible Filtration Manifold System, Gibco BRL)
- Membrane (Biodyne-B from Pall)
- Reagent tubes (2 ml) in 96 sample/box array (e.g. USA Scientific)
- Reagent reservoirs
- Multichannel pipettor (12-channel) and tips
- Pipetmen and tips
- Repeat pipettor
- 3MM filter paper
- UV crosslinker (e.g. Stratalinker from Stratagene)

- Vacuum bubble tubing
- 3-way connectors
- Wash tubs
- Scrub brush
- Denaturant: 0.4 M NaOH, 25 mM EDTA pH 8.0
- Distilled water
- PCR product
- 0.1 M citrate buffer pH 5.0: 0.032 M citric acid-H_2O, 0.068 M Na_3citrate-$2H_2O$
- Bleach

Method

1 Connect the Gibco membrane base plate(s) to a vacuum source and add dot blot gaskets with raised ring side facing upward. Press gaskets firmly into place.

2 Calculate the number of membranes and total amount of denaturant cocktail to prepare for each sample: a portion of (or all) the PCR product will be denatured for membrane preparation. The number of membranes made is governed by the quantity of PCR product, and the number of probes to be used. If PCR product is robust and there are not more than ten probes, make as many membranes as there are probes to reduce the necessity of stripping the membranes before re-probing:

    (a) Count the number of membranes needed for expected probe analysis and add one 'extra' for pipetting error.

    (b) Determine if the PCR product is sufficient to accommodate the necessary membranes. If not, reduce the number of membranes to be made accordingly. If the PCR product is robust and there are not very many probes (i.e. six) to analyse, reduce the amount of PCR product added accordingly.

    (c) Calculate the amount of denaturant to add to each sample PCR product. For example, for six membranes: 50 μl $\times$ 7 membranes = 350 μl cocktail to prepare; 350 μl cocktail – X μl PCR product denatured = μl denaturant needed.

    (d) 50 μl denaturant–PCR product cocktail/dot is applied to each membrane.

3 Using a 96-well assay sheet, record the location and ID of each sample.

4 Set up 2 ml reagent tubes in the same pattern as the sample grid (see step 3).

5 Add the appropriate amount of denaturant (step 2b) to each tube using a repeating pipettor.

Protocol 3 continued

6 Add the appropriate amount (in μl) of PCR product (step 2b) to denaturant and mix by up/down sampling several times with pipette tip.

7 Allow at least 5 min for denaturation. During this time, label the membranes and apply membranes to the membrane base plate. Do not let the denaturation/sample mix stand for more than 30 min at RT. Refrigerate if longer times are needed before making membranes.

   (a) Trim membrane(s) as needed to fit onto base plate gasket.

   (b) Label each membrane using a Sharpie© extra fine point permanent marker.

   (c) Moisten with distilled water and set membrane onto gasket.

   (d) Add top plate and turn on vacuum. (Note: vacuum *must* remain on at all times.) Make sure vacuum seal is *tight*. CHECK the vacuum before starting sample application.

8 Add denatured samples to the apparatus wells using a 12-channel multipipetter set to deliver 50 μl/tip. Ensure sample/denaturant has been picked up in all appropriate channels before dispensing.

9 Apply sample to the membrane by turning the SAMPLE VACUUM dial to the ON position. An orange dot should be visible on the membrane after the sample has been applied.

10 Upon completion of the sample application, break the vacuum seal(s) and remove membrane(s). Place on a piece of clean 3MM filter paper.

11 Crosslink denatured sample(s) to membrane(s) with UV light:

   (a) Place filter paper containing the membrane(s) into the Stratagene Stratalinker.

   (b) Turn on power. Set energy to 500 μjoules × 100; press start. (The cycle lasts ~ 30 sec.)

   (c) When cycle is over, press reset. Turn off power and remove filter containing membranes.

   (d) Rinse membranes in distilled water or citrate buffer, and allow to dry. Use immediately or store together at 4°C in a plastic bag.

12 Wash membrane apparatus:

   (a) Soak all gaskets in HOT water and detergent for about 0.5 h. Do not use bleach on gaskets.

   (b) Soak all hard plastic parts in HOT water, detergent, and bleach, added to a final concentration of ~ 5%, for about 0.5 h.

   (c) After soaking time is complete, scrub all parts carefully with a stiff brush. Caution: any residual PCR product could contaminate future membrane preparation.

   (d) When washing is complete, rinse apparati and all parts three times with tapwater, followed by two rinses with distilled water.

   (e) Thoroughly air dry all parts before putting away the apparatus.

Protocol 4

Data interpretation

A. Immobilized probe assays

1 The DYNAL Reli SSO HLA strips have been striped with a number of probes (locus-specific) and include at least one control (one per exon amplified). The HLA type is assigned by reading the pattern of blue lines on the strip to determine which alleles are present in the DNA samples. This is done by using the locus-specific overlay and score sheet, which is subsequently read using either the DYNAL Reli SSO genotyping programs specific for each locus, or by manually genotyping using the HLA probe pattern charts.

2 The 'C' or internal control probe detects all of the HLA alleles at that locus and serves two functions:

(a) To indicate adequate amplification and hybridization of the sample. The 'C' line intensity is designed to be less than all other lines on the strip. Therefore, if the 'C' line is absent on the strip, an accurate determination of HLA locus-specific type cannot be made, since there is the possibility that other probe signals may not be detected. The presence of the 'C' line provides assurance that the appropriate probe lines are clearly visible. Any failure of the control will invalidate this portion of the testing. The failed portion must be repeated prior to release of results.

(b) To serve as an intensity threshold for true signal. The presence of visible lines with a signal intensity less than the 'C' line may indicate either procedural errors or DNA contamination.

3 If the data are interpreted by the software provided, the strip is displayed on the computer screen and the user simply types in the positive probes. The computer program then determines the HLA type.

B. Dot blot assays

1 Probe patterns from positive and negative controls are compared to known control patterns and aid in the determination of HLA type. Check to be sure all probes are working correctly (i.e. with the appropriate specificity) before continuing with typing samples. Use the appropriate controls for each probe and chart this for the locus under study. Any failure of controls will invalidate this portion of the testing. The failed portion must be repeated prior to release of results.

2 Record positive probe results for each sample (for very strong reactions, give a +, for weaker dots, record a ±, and for very weak dots). If there is no signal, do not give a mark for that probe and sample. Continue recording for all samples and probes on the chart. Using the sample results chart and DNA sequence alignments, determine the sample HLA locus genotype. It is also possible to develop probe pattern analysis and genotyping computer programs specific for each locus or allelic group for dot blot typing. Using this method, the data is interpreted by the software, a strip simulating probe hits is displayed on the computer screen and the user simply types in the positive probes. The computer then determines the HLA (locus-specific) type.

Protocol 4 continued

C. Failure of controls or tests

1   After the hybridization, wash, and detection procedures, the membranes are analysed and genotypes are interpreted from the probe hybridization patterns. Before genotyping samples, check to make sure that the positive controls are positive for the immobilized probe strips or dot blot membranes. In the event of unacceptable or ambiguous controls or testing results, repeat the assay. Group-specific amplifications to separate alleles and/or sequence analysis may be necessary if the probe pattern is ambiguous or difficult to interpret.

D. Resolving ambiguities in DNA-based HLA typing

1   As new alleles are continuously discovered in the HLA system, ambiguities can arise in HLA typing either by detection of new alleles through novel probe hybridization patterns, or by the generation of certain probe hybridization patterns that are consistent with more than one genotype. The following steps should be taken to resolve such ambiguities.

2   Novel probe hybridization patterns. Novel probe patterns can be generated by the loss of an expected probe reactivity, or the unexpected binding of a probe. The detection and reporting of novel HLA alleles is important to the HLA community and should be confirmed by sequencing.

3   Ambiguities that arise in HLA typing by detection of novel or ambiguous probe hybridization can be resolved by group-specific amplification to allow separate amplification of the two alleles in a heterozygote, and/or by sequence analysis of the alleles.

5.2.2 SSP/ASA/ARMS

Another PCR-based approach, based on the specificity of primer extension rather than that of probe hybridization, has also been applied to HLA typing. This method is known variously as allele-specific amplification (ASA) (44), sequence-specific priming (SSP) (45), and the amplification refractory mutation system (ARMS) (46, 47). Here, a specific primer pair is designed for each polymorphic sequence motif or pair of motifs and the presence of the targeted polymorphic sequence in a sample is detected as a positive PCR, typically identified as a band on a gel. In SSP typing, if the PCR is negative and no product is detected, the sample is assumed to lack one or both of the specific motifs. Since inhibition of the PCR or absence of template also yields a negative result, each reaction should include a positive control, that is, PCR primers for an unrelated monomorphic target sequence that produces a fragment that can be resolved from the HLA PCR product. SSP/ARMS typing has also been applied to class I typing (48–50) and robotics have, in some cases, simplified this procedure (51). Recently developed detection methods that are not based on visualizing a band in a gel and, can, therefore, eliminate the gel electrophoresis step, are just starting to be applied (see below). Although informative and relatively fast for small numbers of samples, the SSP approach requires many separate PCRs to achieve intermediate or high level typing and, in its current format, is not well suited to rapid through-put of large sample numbers. As noted above, allele-specific amplification can be used in conjunction with SSO probe typing for high resolution typing by allowing the separate amplification of the two alleles in a heterozygote.

5.2.3 PCR-RFLP, SSCP, SHA, DSCA

Other PCR-based methods involve the use of multiple restriction endonucleases and gel electrophoresis (PCR-RFLP) to characterize the polymorphisms in the PCR product; these approaches have been developed for class I and class II typing (53–56). Conformation-based gel mobility analyses, such as PCR-SSCP (single-strand conformation polymorphism) have also been applied (57, 58; see Chapters 4 and 6). Another conformation and mobility-based approach to HLA typing, PCR-DHA (directed heteroduplex analysis), has also been developed for class II typing (59) but these approaches, unlike SSO or SSP methods, are not widely used in clinical settings. A recent modification of the directed heteroduplex approach, termed double-stranded conformation analysis (DSCA), utilizes a fluor-escent single-stranded probe specific for a particular class I allele (i.e. A*0101) to hybridize to the class I PCR products (e.g. the two HLA-A alleles) amplified from the sample, thereby generating labelled heteroduplex molecules. The mobility of these molecules can be systematically compared to a standard set of markers for each allele (60).

5.2.4 Reverse hybridization with immobilized SSO probe arrays

A reverse hybridization approach to SSO probe analysis of HLA polymorphism has greatly facilitated PCR-based typing with multiple probes (61). The conventional dot blot involved an immobilized PCR product that is hybridized to each of many labelled SSO probes. The 'reverse blot' (or immobilized probe) method is based on the hybridization of PCR product, labelled with biotinylated primers during the amplification, to an array of immobilized probes on a membrane. Although initially the probes were immobilized by UV crosslinking polythy-midine 'tails' that had been added to the 3′ end of the probe with terminal transferase, a variety of immobilization methods can now be used (62). The pre-sence of the PCR product bound to a specific probe is detected using streptavidin–HRP and a chromogenic substrate. This procedure requires only a single PCR and a single hybridization reaction to obtain information from the entire SSO probe panel; all of the probe reactivity information is contained on a single membrane, making it amenable to automated data capture and interpretation. The critical challenge in this approach is to design a large number of SSO probes that will hybridize specifically under a single set of conditions. In addition, because the PCR product is denatured and hybridized in solution to the immobilized complementary probe, secondary structure in the labelled target single strand that would prevent binding to the probe must be minimized.

This approach has been applied to a variety of genetic typing systems, including direct mutation detection for beta-thalassemia and cystic fibrosis (61, 24) and was the basis for the first commercial PCR test, the Amplitype HLA-DQ-alpha Forensic test, introduced in 1990 and used, since that time, in hundreds of forensics cases. In order to accommodate more probes on the membrane, the probes are now immobilized as lines rather than as dots (62). A commercially available HLA-DRB test, the DYNAL/Reli HLA-DRB test, uses 36 probes and provides intermediate level typing for alleles at the DRB1, DRB3, DRB4, and DRB5 loci. Immobilized probe tests using the same PCR thermal profile and hybridization conditions have been developed for DQB1 and the HLA class I loci (9, 63, 64). Commercially available immobilized probe tests for an intermediate level of resolution are also available for DQB1 (DYNAL/Reli uses 25 DQB1 probes), HLA-A (DYNAL/Reli uses 37 HLA-A probes), and HLA-B (DYNAL/Reli uses 56 HLA-B probes). Our current higher resolution B locus typing system uses 89 probes for exons 2 and 3, which are co-amplified with two primer pairs. Our current higher resolution HLA-A typing system uses 57 immobilized probes. Two instruments to automate the hybridization, wash, and colour development of these immobilized probe strips are commercially available (SLT Profiblot and the DYNAL Autoreli48) as is software to read and interpret the probe reactivity patterns. The immobilized probe approach is well suited to the rapid typing of a few samples as well as to high-throughput typing of large sample numbers. Reverse hybridization approaches have also utilized the microtitre format (65) and other microtitre formats using biotinylated PCR product capture with streptavidin and hybridization with enzyme labelled SSO probes have been reported (66).

As noted above, high resolution typing often requires the separate amplification of the two alleles in a heterozygote. For this purpose, primers designed to polymorphic regions with many variants (i.e. codons 9–12 of DRB1, a region with 8 different sequence motifs) are valuable to carry out allele-specific amplification.

A table illustrating the probe reactivity patterns for individual alleles of the HLA-DQB1 locus is shown in *Figure 1*.

5.2.5 Sequence-based typing (SBT)

The application of semi-automated chain termination sequencing using either fluorescent primers or fluorescent dideoxy terminators, with the development of appropriate sequence analysis software, has become a powerful approach to allele-level HLA typing (67, 68). Several commercial approaches to automating the gel electrophoresis step are now available and recently, the introduction of modified thermostable DNA polymerases capable of efficiently incorporating fluorescent dideoxy NMPs has made sequencing a more robust typing method. The recent introduction of capillary-based systems (e.g. the ABI 310) has increased the throughput and decreased the cost of HLA sequence-based typing. High resolution typing by sequencing, which requires the separate amplification and analysis of the two alleles, is sometimes carried out for the final matching of bone marrow donor and recipient. However, in its current format, SBT is still a somewhat expensive procedure and not ideally suited to large scale typing or routine clinical typing.

6 HLA typing requirements

In general, the requirements for HLA typing and the desired performance characteristics of PCR-based typing methods will depend on the application. Bone marrow donor registry screening and recruitment requires a method that provides intermediate level resolution typing and that is low cost and high-throughput. The nature of the typing data and the level of resolution should be such to facilitate the storage and search of the donor typings in the registry for possible matches with the patient/recipient. The final HLA typing for matching bone marrow donors and recipients should be high resolution because, preliminary data suggest that the clinical outcomes (both survival and graft vs. host disease) can be influenced by allelic differences (i.e. DRB1*1101 vs. *1104) in subtypes within a given serotype (69). In this setting, cost and throughput are less critical issues. Solid organ transplantation, on the other hand, demands a fairly rapid typing method; here, speed, rather than cost and throughput is the critical issue and an intermediate level typing is probably sufficient. Research applications of HLA typing, such as disease associations or population genetics studies, should be carried out at a high level of resolution, when possible, because often a particular allele or haplotype, defined at the DNA sequence level, is much more strongly associated with a disease than is the serotype. Similarly, anthropological genetic analyses of populations are most informative when performed at the allele or haplotype level.

7 The problem of new alleles and of ambiguity

As more and more PCR-based HLA typing is being carried out in more and more populations, new (previously unreported) alleles at both class I and class II loci are being detected, leading to a slow but steady increase in the number of alleles at both class I and class II loci. The vast majority of these involve new combinations of previously known sequence motifs and thus, they can be identified without adding additional probes. Nonetheless, they can create problems for typing strategies. The identification of new alleles requires frequent updating of the files in the genotyping software that relate sequence motifs to alleles. The addition of these new alleles can lead to increased ambiguities in the genotype interpretation of the primary typing data, such as the SSO probe reactivity or SSP patterns. An additional consequence of these newly discovered alleles is to modify the interpretation of typing results obtained prior to their discovery. For example, a pattern of reactive SSO probes that was consistent with a given genotype, at one time, might, following the identification of the new allele, be consistent with additional genotypes. This ambiguity can, in principle, be avoided by complete sequencing of the two separated alleles in a heterozygous sample but this is not, at the moment, a practical solution for many clinical diagnostic settings or for large population genetics studies.

Most HLA typing systems, with the exception of sequencing separated alleles, can occasionally generate an ambiguous result; here, ambiguity is defined as HLA typing data (e.g. a probe reactivity pattern) consistent with more than one pair of alleles. The need to resolve these ambiguities is a function of the typing application. In some cases, if a given probe reactivity pattern (or other typing data) is consistent with either genotype X or Y, consideration of the genotype frequencies in the relevant populations and the likelihood that the sample is X or is Y may be appropriate in interpreting the typing data. For bone marrow transplantation, on the other hand, any ambiguity in the patient typing results should be resolved by additional typing. A proposal for storing intermediate level typing data in bone marrow donor registries by entering the probe reactivity patterns rather than the interpreted genotypes is one approach to dealing with ambiguity (70). This proposal solves some of the problems associated with storing typing data but the issue of interpreting these patterns as genotypes remains. As noted above, allele level resolution often requires the separate amplification of the two alleles in a heterozygote. This is most commonly carried out by performing a preliminary typing (e.g. DRB1*04/DRB1*08) and then using group-specific primers for the DRB1*04 group and the DRB1*08 group, based on the sequence variation in codons 9–12 of DRB1 to amplify the alleles separately.

PCR-based systems of HLA typing have evolved dramatically since the initial reports in the mid 1980s. New typing methods as well as new applications will provide valuable clinical and research data regarding these highly polymorphic loci.

Acknowledgements

We are grateful to our colleagues, Ann Begovich, Dory Bugawan, Ray Apple, Priscilla Moonsamy, Jim Novotny, Alan Blair, Sean Boyle, Cal Mano, and Joyce Ching for their contributions to the development of PCR-based HLA typing systems. I also thank Sean Boyle for his contribution of Figure 1 and for reviewing this manuscript, and Margaret Vinson for her assistance in constructing standard operating procedures.

References

1. Bodmer, J. G., Marsh, S. G. E., Albert, E. D., Bodmer, W. F., Vontrop, R. E., Charron, D., *et al.* (1997). *Tissue Antigens*, **49**, 297.
2. Bugawan, T. L., Saiki, R. K., Levenson, C. H., Watson, R. M., and Erlich, H. A. (1988). *Bio/Technology*, **6**, 943.
3. Saiki, R. K., Scharf, S., and Faloona, F. (1985). *Science*, **230**, 1350.
4. Saiki, R. K., Gelfand, D. A., Stoffel, S., Scharf, S. J., Higuchi, R., Horn, G., Mullis, K., *et al.* (1988). *Science*, **239**, 487.

5. Saiki, R. K., Chang, C., Levenson, C. H., Warren, T. C., Boehm, C. D., Kazazian, H. Jr., *et al.* (1988). *N. Engl. J. Med.*, **319**, 537.

6. Mullis, K. B. and Faloona, F. (1987). In *Methods in Enzymology*, Vol. 155, p. 335.

7. Li, H., Gyllensten, U. B., Cui, X., Saiki, R. K., Erlich, H. A., and Arnheim, N. (1988). *Nature*, **335**, 414.

8. Apple, R. J., Erlich, H. A., Klitz, W., Manos, M. M., Becker, T. M., and Wheeler, C. M. (1994). *Nature Genet.*, **6**, 157.

9. Bugawan, T. L., Apple, R., and Erlich, H. A. (1994). *Tissue Antigens*, **44**, 137.

10. Bugawan, T. L., Chang, J. D., Klitz, W., and Erlich, H. A. (1994). *Am. J. Hum. Genet.*, **54**, 331.

11. Blake, E., Mihalovich, J., Higuchi, R., Walsh, P. S., and Erlich, H. A. (1992). *J. Forensic Sci.*, **37**, 700.

12. Yu, J., Lazzeroni, L., Qin, J., Huang, M. M., Navidi, W., Erlich, H., *et al.* (1996). *Am. J. Hum. Genet.*, **59**, 1186.

13. Erlich, H. A., Zeidler, A., Chang, J., Shaw, S., Raffel, L. J., Klitz, W., *et al.* (1993). *Nature Genet.*, **3**, 358.

14. Caillat-Zucman, S., Garchon, H. J., Timsit, J., Assan, R., Boitard, C., Dkilali-Saiah, I., *et al.* (1992). *J. Clin. Invest.*, **90**, 2242.

15. Cucca, F., Muntoni, F., and Lampis, R. (1993). *Hum. Immunol.*, **37**, 85.

16. Scharf, S. J., Horn, G. T., and Erlich, H. A. (1986). *Science*, **223**, 1076.

17. Saiki, R. K., Bugawan, T. L., Horn, G. T., Mullis, K. B., and Erlich, H. A. (1986). *Nature*, **324**, 163.

18. Bjorkman, P. J., Saper, M. A., Samraoui, B., Bennett, W. S., Strominger, J. L., and Wiley, D. C. (1987). *Nature*, **329**, 506.

19. Bjorkman, P. J., Saper, M. A., Samraoui, B., Bennett, W. S., Strominger, J. L., and Wiley, D. C. (1987). *Nature*, **329**, 512.

20. Brown, J. H., Jardetzky, T. S., and Gorga, J. C. (1993). *Nature*, **364**, 33.

21. Hughes, A. L. and Nei, M. (1988). *Nature*, **335**, 167.

22. Hughes, A. L. and Nei, M. (1989). *Proc. Natl. Acad. Sci. USA*, **86**, 958.

23. Takahata, N. and Nei, M. (1990). *Genetics*, **124**, 967.

24. Erlich, H. A. and Gyllensten, U. (1991). *Immunol. Today*, **11**, 411.

25. Klein, J. and Figueroa, F. (1986). *Crit. Rev. Immunol.*, **6**, 295.

26. Bergstrom, T. F., Agnetha, J., Erlich, H. A., and Gyllensten, U. (1998). *Nature Genet.*, **18**, 237.

27. Bodmer, J. G., Marsh, S. G. E., Albert, E. D., Bodmer, W. F., Bontrop, R. E., Charron, D., *et al.* (1999). *Tissue Antigens*, **53**, 407.

28. Parham, P. (1997). *Tissue Antigens*, **50**, 318.

29. Schreuder, G. M. T., Hurley, C. K., Marsh, S. G. E., Lau, M., Maiers, M., Kollman, C., *et al.* (1999). *Tissue Antigens*, **54**, 409.

30. Terasaki, P. I., Mandell, M., Van de Water, J., and Edginton, T. E. (1964). *Ann. N. Y. Acad. Sci.*, **120**, 322.

31. Bach, F. H. and Noynow, N. K. (1966). *Science*, **153**, 545.

32. Wake, C. T., Long, E. O., and Mach, B. (1982). *Nature*, **300**, 372.

33. Erlich, H. A., Stetler, D., Sheng-Dong, R., Ness, D. G., and Grumet, C. (1983). *Science*, **222**, 72.

34. Angelini, G., Preval, C. D., Gorski, J., and Mach, B. (1986). *Proc. Natl. Acad. Sci. USA*, **83**, 4489.

35. Nevinny-Stickel, C., Bettinotti, M., and Andreas, A. (1991). *Hum. Immunol.*, **31**, 7.

36. Shaffer, A. L., Falk-Wade, J. A., and Tortorelli, V. (1992). *Tissue Antigens*, **39**, 84.

37. Scharf, S. J., Griffith, R. L., and Erlich, H. A. (1991). *Hum. Immunol.*, **30**, 190.

38. Bugawan, T. L. and Erlich, H. A. (1991). *Immunogenetics*, **33**, 163.

39. Bugawan, T. L., Begovich, A. B., and Erlich, H. A. (1990). *Immunogenetics*, **32**, 231.
40. Erlich, H. A., Bugawan, T., Begovich, A., Scharf, S., Griffith, R., Higuchi, R., *et al.* (1991). *Eur. J. Immunogenet.*, **18**, 33.
41. Erlich, H. A., Gelfand, D., and Sninsky, J. J. (1991). *Science*, **252**, 1643.
42. Oh, S. H., Fleischhauer, K., and Yang, S. Y. (1993). *Tissue Antigens*, **41**, 135.
43. Yoshida, M., Kimura, A., Numano, F., and Sasazuki, T. (1992). *Tissue Antigens*, **41**, 135.
44. Wu, D. Y., Ugozzoli, L., Pal, B. K., and Wallace, R. B. (1989). *Proc. Natl. Acad. Sci. USA*, **86**, 2757.
45. Olerup, O. and Zetterquist, H. (1992). *Tissue Antigens*, **39**, 225.
46. Newton, C. R., Graham, A., and Heptinstall, L. E. (1989). *Nucleic Acids Res.*, **17**, 2503.
47. Browning, M. J., Krausa, P., Rowan, A., Bicknell, D. C., Bodmer, J. G., and Bodmer, W. F. (1993). *Proc. Natl. Acad. Sci. USA*, **90**, 2842.
48. Krausa, P. and Browning, M. J. (1996). *Tissue Antigens*, **47**, 237.
49. Bunce, M. and Welsh, K. I. (1994). *Tissue Antigens*, **43**, 7.
50. Bunce, M., Fanning, G. C., and Welsh, K. I. (1995). *Tissue Antigens*, **45**, 81.
51. Bunce, M., O'Neill, C. M., and Barnardo, M. C. N. M. (1995). *Tissue Antigens*, **46**, 355.
52. Urya, N., Maeda, M., Ota, M., Tsuji, K., and Inolo, H. (1990). *Tissue Antigens*, **35**, 20.
53. Yunis, I., Salazar, M., and Unis, E. J. (1991). *Tissue Antigens*, **38**, 78.
54. Olerup, O. (1990). *Tissue Antigens*, **36**, 83.
55. Ota, M., Seki, T., and Nomura, N. (1991). *Tissue Antigens*, **38**, 60.
56. Maeda, M., Murayama, N., and Ishi, H. (1989). *Tissue Antigens*, **34**, 290.
57. Hoshino, S., Kimura, A., Fukuda, A., Dohi, K., and Sasazuki, T. (1992). *Hum. Immunol.*, **33**, 98.
58. Carrington, M., Miller, T., and White, M. (1992). *Hum. Immunol.*, **33**, 208.
59. Zimmerman, P. A., Carrington, M. N., and Nutman, T. B. (1993). *Nucleic Acids Res.*, **21**, 4541.
60. Arguello, J. R., Little, A., Pay, A. L., Gallardo, D., Rojas, I., Marsh, S. G. E., *et al.* (1998). *Nature Genet.*, **18**, 192.
61. Saiki, R. K., Walsh, P. S., Levenson, C. H., and Erlich, H. A. (1989). *Proc. Natl. Acad. Sci. USA*, **86**, 6230.
62. Begovich, A. and Erlich, H. A. (1995). *J. Am. Med. Assoc.*, **273**, 586.
63. Blair, A., Bugawan, T. L., and Erlich, H. A. (1997). *Hum. Immunol.*, **55**, 144.
64. Trachtenberg, E. A., Bugawan, T. L., Apple, R., Castro, R., and Erlich, H. A. (1994). *Hum. Immunol.*, **40**, 43.
65. Cros, P., Allibert, P., Mandrand, B., Tiercey, J. M., and Mach, B. (1992). *Lancet*, **340**, 870.
66. Lazaro, A. M., Fernandez-Vina, M. A., Liu, Z., and Stastny, P. (1993). *Hum. Immunol.*, **36**, 243.
67. McGinnis, M. D., Conrad, M. P., Bouwens, A. G. M., Tilanus, M. G. J., and Kronick, M. N. (1995). *Tissue Antigens*, **46**, 173.
68. Voorter, C. E. M., Rozemuller, E. H., de Bruyn-Geraets, D., van der Zwan, A. W., Tilanus, M. G. J., and van der Berg-Loonen, E. M. (1997). *Tissue Antigens*, **49**, 471.
69. Petersdorf, E. W., Kollman, C., Hurley, C., Dupont, B., Begovich, A., Hansen, J., *et al.* (1997). *Hum. Immunol.*, **55**, 30.
70. Hurley, C. K., Schreuder, M. T., Marsh, S. G. E., Lau, M., Middleton, D., and Noreen, H. (1997). *Tissue Antigens*, **50**, 401.

Chapter 8

Evolutionary analysis of molecular sequence data

Austin L. Hughes
Department of Biological Sciences, University of South Carolina, Columbia, SC 29208, USA.

Jack da Silva
Department of Biology, East Carolina University, Greenville, NC 27858, USA.

Federica Verra
Istituto di Parassitologia, Università di Roma 'La Sapienza', Piazzale Aldo Moro 5, 00185 Rome, Italy.

1 Introduction

In the 140 years since Darwin's *Origin of Species* was published, evolutionary ideas have formed an important part of the theoretical framework of biological research, but their practical consequences have been few for most of that period. The situation has changed since the advent of techniques for rapidly sequencing nucleic acids. Because evolution is nothing other than change in nucleotide sequences, the availability of sequence data enables us to study evolution far more directly than was previously possible. Molecular evolutionary analysis has now become an important part of the conceptual arsenal used by biologists in a wide variety of disciplines, including epidemiology.

Molecular evolutionary analysis is proving useful to epidemiologists in two major areas:

(a) Reconstructing the evolutionary relationships of pathogenic organisms.

(b) Understanding population processes within populations of such organisms, including their co-evolution with their hosts.

Most infectious agents responsible for human disease ('parasites' in the sense in which that term is used by evolutionary biologists; i.e. including not only parasitic protozoa and metazoan animals, but also parasitic fungi, bacteria, and viruses) are organisms with simple morphologies that provide relatively little information useful in reconstructing evolutionary relationships. Thus, if we are to understand the evolutionary relationships of these organisms, analyses based on molecular data are a necessity. Such understanding may be particularly important in cases where a strongly pathogenic strain of an otherwise relatively benign parasite suddenly emerges, causing an epidemic in the host population. Knowledge of such a strain's evolutionary origin is often a first step in devising strategies for its control.

It has long been speculated that parasites exert natural selection on their hosts, favouring adaptations that eliminate infection or minimize its effects (1). At the same time, the host's immune defences can be expected to exert natural selection on the parasite, favouring adaptations that evade immune recognition. Thus, a co-evolutionary race between host and parasite is predicted. Molecular data have made it possible to study host–parasite co-evolution directly.

The purpose of the present chapter is to review the conceptual background for some of the most commonly used methods of molecular sequence analysis and to illustrate their application to data of epidemiological relevance. We emphasize basic concepts rather than computational details. Those interested in a mathematical treatment of the issues covered here are referred to the texts of Nei and Kumar (2) and Li (3). Introductory treatments of this rapidly expanding area can be found in Graur and Li (4) and Hillis *et al.* (5). In addition, several computer packages designed for evolutionary analysis of sequence data are now available (6–8). The MEGA program (6) is particularly useful in that it computes numbers of nucleotide substitutions per site according to a variety of models as well as reconstructing phylogenies.

2 Comparing sequences

2.1 Rationale for statistical models

Often, molecular biologists compare sequences by computing the per cent similarity between them. This is sometimes called 'per cent homology,' but this usage is discouraged by biological editors. Two genes are homologous if they are descended from a common ancestral gene; thus, two genes either are homologous or they are not, and the idea of 'per cent homology' is meaningless. A frequent practice is to compute per cent similarity at the amino acid and nucleotide levels, as illustrated in *Table 1* for the nuclecapsid protein genes of three hantavirus isolates. As is usual for protein-coding genes, the per cent similarities at the amino acid level are greater than those at the nucleotide level (*Table 1*). This reflects the fact that not all mutations in coding regions change the amino acid sequence. Because of the redundancy of the genetic code, certain mutations in coding regions are 'synonymous' or 'silent' (those that do not change the amino acid encoded by a codon), while others are non-synonymous (those that do change the amino acid).

It is an important prediction of Motoo Kimura's Neutral Theory of Molecular Evolution that most non-synonymous mutations, because they are deleterious to protein structure, are quickly eliminated by natural selection (9). This kind of natural selection is called 'purifying selection'. By contrast, synonymous muta-

Table 1 Per cent similarity at DNA and amino acid level in pairwise comparisons among nucleocapsid genes of selected hantavirus isolates

Comparison	DNA	Amino acid
Sin Nombre vs. Convict Creek	90.6%	98.8%
Sin Nombre vs. New York	83.2%	93.7%
Convict Creek vs. New York	82.4%	92.5%

tions are selectively neutral in most cases (or nearly so). Thus, any synonymous mutation that occurs has some chance of becoming fixed over evolutionary time as a result of random genetic drift and some (much greater) chance of disappearing by drift. Thus, synonymous changes will accumulate more rapidly over evolutionary time than non-synonymous changes. The fact that homologous protein-coding genes are more similar at the amino acid level than at the DNA level is mainly due to the accumulation of synonymous changes and thus constitutes strong evidence in support of the Neutral Theory.

When we compare homologous sequences, we expect that on the average, more closely related sequences will be more similar than more distantly related sequences. For example, since the Sin Nombre and Convict Creek hantaviruses are considerably more similar to each other, at both nucleotide and amino acid levels, than either is to the New York hantavirus (*Table 1*), it seems reasonable to infer that the Sin Nombre and Convict Creek hantavirus are more closely related to each other than either is to New York hantavirus. In making such an inference, we are assuming that the sequence differences between any two of these viral nucleocapsid genes reflect mutations that became fixed over the time since their last common ancestor.

However, it is legitimate to ask whether the differences we observe between two present-day sequences represent all of the evolutionary changes that have occurred since their last common ancestor. For example, if we observe that two present-day sequences differ at a particular position, we cannot be certain that only a single change has occurred at that position over the time since the two sequences' last common ancestor. Perhaps multiple mutations have occurred at that site, many of which have become fixed in the populations, only to be replaced by yet other fixed mutations. But, of course, at the present time, we cannot observe any more than a single difference at any given site.

Molecular evolutionists have used statistical models to correct for unobserved changes in the past. Basically the idea is to start with the observed proportion of difference and then correct that value upward to account for unobserved past events. The choice of a statistical model involves a trade-off between realism of the assumptions and error of estimation. A very simple model will often make assumptions that are somewhat unrealistic. However, a simple model may be preferable even when its assumptions are violated, because the error of estimation tends to be relatively small when the model is simple. A more complicated model may have more realistic assumptions but it may require the estimation of multiple parameters. If so, the error of estimation may be large.

2.2 **Comparing amino acid sequences**

In the comparison of amino acid sequences, the simplest type of correction that is commonly employed is the Poisson correction for 'multiple hits' (that is, multiple amino acid replacements at a given site) (2, 6). This is based on the assumption of a Poisson model, which implies that the probability of an amino replacement is the same for all sites and that each site evolves independently of each other site. The most obvious factor leading to a violation of the assumptions of the Poisson model is rate variation among sites. In most amino acid sequences, certain sites that are important to protein function show little evolutionary change, while less functionally important sites are much freer to vary. The most commonly used model that takes into account rate variation in sites is based on the gamma distribution (10). This model includes a parameter (a) that is inversely related to the extent of rate variation among sites; the smaller a is, the greater the extent of rate variation.

2.3 **Comparing DNA sequences**

In the case of DNA sequences, the simplest statistical model is that of Jukes and Cantor (11). This model assumes that all four nucleotides are used with equal frequency and that each of the possible substitutions of one nucleotide for another occurs with equal frequency. Using Jukes and Cantor's model, we can correct the proportion of nucleotide differences not only for multiple hits but for convergent or parallel substitutions and forward and backward changes, by the following simple formula:

$$d = -\frac{3}{4}\ln\left(1 - \frac{4}{3}p\right) \qquad [1]$$

where d stands for the estimate of the number of nucleotide substitutions per site and p is the observed proportion of nucleotide difference between the two sequences.

The most commonly occurring violations of the assumptions of Jukes and Cantor's model are nucleotide content bias (unequal use of the four nucleotides); transitional bias (a tendency for transitional mutations to occur more frequently than transversional mutations); and rate variation among sites. Models have been developed to accommodate these more complex situations, some of them very complicated and including numerous parameters (2, 6). However, the most widely used of these models is the simplest, Kimura's two-parameter model (12), which estimates rates of transitional and transversional substitution separately. As with amino acid sequences, the simplest models are preferable unless the violations of their assumptions are very great. For example, when d is relatively low (less than about 0.3), Kumar *et al.* (6) recommend using the Jukes–Cantor correction rather than Kimura's two-parameter model even if the rate of transitions exceeds the rate of transversions as long as the transition/transversion ratio is less than 2:1. Under these conditions both corrections yield similar results, but the Jukes–Cantor model is preferable because its variance is lower. Note that, under the Jukes–Cantor model, the expected ratio of transitions to transversions is 1:2. Thus, when sequences are closely related, even a rather strong deviation from the assumptions of the Jukes–Cantor model has no practical effect.

One aspect of Equation 1 merits attention. When p = 0.75, Equation 1 becomes undefined. This makes intuitive sense because, under the assumption of equal use of all four nucleotides, two sequences that differ at three-quarters of their sites are no more similar to each other than are two random sequences. Thus, any two such sequences cannot be meaningfully compared; there is no evolutionary information in such a comparison. In such a case, the sequences are said to be *saturated* with changes. Note that Equation 1 becomes extremely unreliable even before complete saturation is reached; for example, when p is greater than about 0.55, then d is greater than 1. In other words, by Equation 1, we estimate that, on the average, more than one nucleotide substitution has occurred at each site. After so much change, little if any evolutionary information remains available from the sequence comparison.

Furthermore, if all four nucleotides are not used equally, saturation will occur even earlier. The malaria parasite *Plasmodium falciparum* provides an example of a species whose genome has a highly skewed nucleotide content. For genes of *P. falciparum* tabulated in the CUTG database (13), third positions of codons (the most free to vary because most mutations at third positions do not change the amino acid) are 41.6% A, 42.0% T, 8.2% C, and 8.2% G. Given this nucleotide composition, two sequences are no more similar than random sequences if they differ at 64% of sites.

2.4 Synonymous and non-synonymous substitution

As in the example shown in *Table 1*, most comparisons of protein-coding genes reveal greater similarity at the amino acid level than at the nucleotide level. As mentioned previously, this occurs because most non-synonymous mutations are deleterious to protein structure and thus are eliminated by purifying selection. However, there is a much more powerful and direct way of studying this phenomenon than merely computing similarity of nucleotide and amino acid sequences. This involves estimating the number of synonymous substitutions per synonymous site and the number of non-synonymous substitutions per non-synonymous site.

One of the basic equations of the Neutral Theory (9) states that the rate of fixation of selectively neutral alleles over evolutionary time equals the neutral mutation rate. This relationship can be expressed as follows:

$$k_0 = u_T f_0 \qquad [2]$$

where k_0 is the rate of substitution (fixation) of neutral mutants, u_T is the total mutation rate, and f_0 is the fraction of mutations which are neutral. This equation predicts differences among different sites in a genome with respect to their rate of evolution. For example, at a site which is essential for coding an amino acid necessary for the function of some important protein, f_0 will be close to zero. Thus, such a site will be unlikely to change over evolutionary time. On the other hand, at either a site in a non-coding region or a site in a coding region where a mutation will not affect the amino acid encoded, f_0 will be close to 1. When f_0 is equal to 1, the rate of substitution at a site will equal the mutation rate.

In coding regions, we expect to see a major difference in evolutionary rate between sites at which mutations change the amino acid and sites where they do not.

We can test this prediction by comparing the frequency of synonymous nucleotide substitution (i.e. substitution that does not change the amino acid) with that of non-synonymous nucleotide substitution (i.e. substitution that does change the amino acid). However, we cannot simply count synonymous and non-synonymous differences between homologous coding sequences because the opportunity for synonymous or non-synonymous mutation varies from one sequence to another and is dependent on the encoded protein's amino acid composition.

The difference among codons is best illustrated by examples. In the universal genetic code, ATG is the only methionine codon. Thus, any mutation at any of the three positions of an ATG codon will be non-synonymous, and we can count each of these positions as a non-synonymous site. In the case of the glycine codon GGC, any mutation at either of the first two positions will change the amino acid, while mutation to any of the three other nucleotides at the third position will not change the amino acid. Thus, the first two positions are counted as non-synonymous sites, and the third position as a synonymous site. The case of certain other codons is a little more complicated. Consider the lysine codon AAA. Any mutation at either of the first two positions will change the amino acid; thus, these can be counted as non-synonymous sites. However, at the third position, a mutation from A to G will not change the amino acid (since AAG also encodes lysine), but a mutation from A to T or C will change the amino acid.

In estimating the numbers of synonymous and non-synonymous substitutions per site, there are various ways of accounting for codons like those for lysine. (Codon sets like that of lysine are called 'twofold degenerate' because there are two possible synonymous mutations at the third position, in contrast to 'fourfold degenerate' codon sets like that for glycine.) The basic idea behind them is to count positions like the third position of a twofold degenerate codon as some fraction of a synonymous site and some fraction of a non-synonymous site, based on the relative likelihood of synonymous and non-synonymous mutation. The simplest method, that of Nei and Gojobori (14), counts the third position of a twofold degenerate codon as 1/3 of a synonymous site and 2/3 of a non-synonymous site, since one of the three possible mutations there is synonymous and the other two are non-synonymous.

More complicated methods, such as that of Li (15) and Zhang *et al.* (16) incorporate differences in the frequency of transitional and transversional mutations. The problem with using such methods in practice is that we do not generally know the transition/transversion ratio at the level of mutation. Simply estimating this ratio by counting transitional and transversional differences between sequences is problematic. For example, consider third positions in two-fold degenerate codons. The pattern of transitions and transversions observed at these sites will reflect both the mutational pattern and the effect of purifying selection. Because transversions at twofold degenerate sites change the amino acid, while transitions do not, transversions will often be eliminated by purifying selection. Thus, it seems most reliable to estimate the transition/transversion ratio from fourfold degenerate sites or from non-coding regions and to then apply that value to twofold degenerate sites. There is a second problem with methods like that of Zhang *et al.* (16). This method treats the transition/transversion ratio as a known quantity, not a parameter to be estimated. Thus, the standard error of estimation may be underestimated. For these reasons, Nei and Gojobori's (14) original method seems preferable to alternatives available at present except in cases where we have good quantitative knowledge of a strong genome-wide bias toward transitions.

Table 2 shows uncorrected proportions of synonymous (p_S) and non-synony-momous (p_N) differences among the hantavirus sequences from *Table 1*, plus estimated numbers of synonymous (d_S) and non-synonymous (d_N) substitutions per site, corrected by Equation 1. Clearly, the d_S values are much greater than the d_N values in all three comparisons. We can test the equality of d_S and d_N values statistically by a simple z-test:

$$z = (d_S - d_N) / \sqrt{(SE (d_S)^2 + SE (d_N)^2)} \qquad [3]$$

where SE (d_S) and SE (d_N) are the standard errors of estimation of d_S and d_N, respectively.

For a two-tailed test, this value can be compared with the value of the standard-normal distribution corresponding to $\alpha/2$. In *Table 2*, the d_S values are all significantly different from the corresponding d_N values ($P < 0.0001$).

In the case of most genes, d_S exceeds d_N. As pointed out by Kimura (17), this is predicted by Equation 2. In most organisms, all or nearly all possible synonymous mutations are expected to be selectively neutral. Thus, f_0 at synonymous sites should be close to 1, and the rate of substitution should be equal to the rate of mutation, or nearly so. At non-synonymous sites, clearly f_0 will vary from site to site, depending on how important the encoded amino acid is to the protein's function. But in any case, the average f_0 at non-synonymous sites is expected to

Table 2 Numbers of differences per synonymous site (p_S) and per non-synonymous site (p_N) and corrected estimates of the numbers of synonymous (d_S) and non-synonymous (d_N) substitutions per site, with their standard errors, in pairwise comparisons among hantavirus nucleocapsid genes

Comparison	p_S	p_N	d_S	d_N
Sin Nombre vs. Convict Creek	0.3955	0.0050	0.5619 ± 0.0604	0.0051 ± 0.0023
Sin Nombre vs. New York	0.5993	0.0409	1.2037 ± 0.1425	0.0420 ± 0.0066
Convict Creek vs. New York	0.6174	0.0454	1.2995 ± 0.1605	0.0469 ± 0.0070

be much lower than that at synonymous sites. The observation that $d_S > d_N$ in most genes is thus evidence in support of Equation 2 and of the Neutral Theory (2, 3, 9, 17). Comparison of d_S and d_N, as in Table 2, thus illustrates the same principle as per cent similarity at the nucleotide and amino acid levels in Table 1. However, it does so with much greater clarity and precision, since the computation of similarity at all nucleotide sites mixes together sites evolving at very different rates.

Another aspect of the values in *Table 2* is worth mentioning. The d_S estimates between the New York hantavirus and both the Sin Nombre and Convict Creek viruses are very high, over 1.2 substitutions per site. Thus, in these comparisons, synonymous sites are near saturation, and little evolutionary information can be provided by such sites. Yet in the same comparisons, the d_N values are much lower, and non-synonymous sites are far from saturation.

2.5 Mean nucleotide diversity

Frequently, it is of interest to compute mean d, d_S, or d_N ('mean nucleotide diversity') for all pairwise comparisons among a set of sequences. Because all pairwise comparisons are used and also because the sequences compared share an evolutionary relationship, these comparisons are not statistically independent. Thus, it is not appropriate to estimate the standard error of mean nucleotide diversity by the usual formula one uses for a sample from a normal distribution. Instead, methods have been developed to estimate the standard error of mean nucleotide diversity which take into account the covariance among these distances when computed for a set of sequences. The most commonly used method is that of Nei and Jin (18), implemented in the MEGA program for mean d_S and d_N (6). An alternative method developed by Ota and Nei (19) yields essentially identical results.

3 Reconstructing phylogenies

3.1 Overview of the problem

The evolutionary relationships among genes or among organisms can be represented by means of a diagram known as a phylogenetic tree. Frequently, the term 'operational taxonomic unit' (OTU) is used as a general designation for the entities whose relationships are described by a phylogenetic tree, indicating that these may be species, populations within species, or individual gene sequences. There are two types of phylogenetic trees: rooted and unrooted. In a rooted tree, there is one particular node called the root from which a unique path leads to any other node. The direction of each such path corresponds to evolutionary time, so the root is the common ancestor of each OTU in the tree.

Usually, we need some prior knowledge, independent of the tree itself, to determine the root of a tree. For example, *Figure 1* shows a phylogeny of alleles at the circumsporozoite protein (CSP) locus of the human malaria parasite *Plasmodium falciparum*. Other phylogenetic analyses have shown that the chimpan-

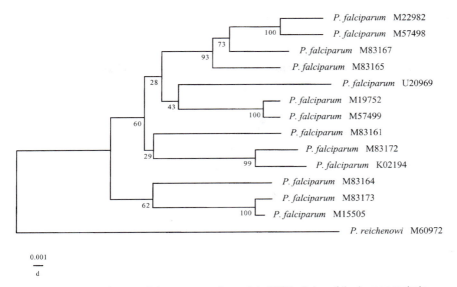

Figure 1 Phylogenetic tree of circumsporozoite protein (CSP) alleles of the human malaria parasite *Plasmodium falciparum*; the tree is rooted with a sequence from the chimpanzee parasite *P. reichenowi*. The tree was constructed by the NJ method on the basis of the number of nucleotide substitutions per site (d), estimated by the Jukes–Cantor method. Reliability of clustering patterns in the tree was tested by bootstrapping (1000 pseudo-samples). Numbers on the branches represent the percentage of pseudo-samples supporting that branch.

zee parasite *Plasmodium reichenowi* diverged from *P. falciparum* when the human and chimpanzee ancestors diverged 5–7 million years ago (20, 21) (see also Section 4.1). There is extensive polymorphism at the CSP locus in *P. falciparum*; the common ancestor of known CSP alleles has been dated at about 2.1 million years ago (22). As a consequence, the common ancestor of the *P. falciparum* CSP genes occurred well after the divergence of *P. falciparum* and *P. reichenowi*. Thus, the *P. reichenowi* CSP gene is what is called an 'outgroup' to the *P. falciparum* sequences, because it is known to have diverged from their common ancestor before they diverged from one another. An outgroup can be used to root a tree, as the *P. reichenowi* sequence is used to root the tree of *P. falciparum* CSP (*Figure 1*).

Even when a phylogenetic tree is unrooted because an outgroup is lacking, it is possible that one portion of the tree can be used to root an other portion of the tree. For example, *Figure 2* shows a phylogenetic tree of the anion exchanger (AE) and sodium bicarbonate exchanger (NBC) protein family of animals. In this phylogeny, the AE and NBC proteins form separate clusters. Thus, the NBC cluster can be used as an outgroup to root the AE cluster and vice versa (*Figure 2*).

One important distinction to make in considering phylogenetic analyses is the distinction between a gene tree and a species tree. A gene tree shows the relationships among genes. These may be alleles at a polymorphic locus within a population, as with the *P. falciparum* CSP alleles in *Figure 1*, or they may be members of a multigene family as in *Figure 2*. By contrast, a species tree shows the relationships among groups of organisms, such as species or populations.

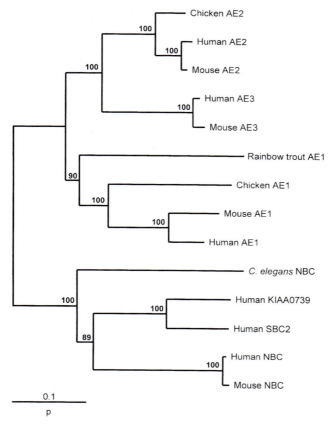

Figure 2 Phylogeny of selected vertebrate anion exchanger (AE) proteins, rooted with sodium bicarbonate exchanger (NBC) of vertebrates and the nematode worm *Caenorhabditis elegans*. The tree was constructed by the NJ method on the basis of the proportion of amino acid difference (p). Reliability of clustering patterns in the tree was tested by bootstrapping (1000 pseudo-samples). Numbers on the branches represent the percentage of pseudo-samples supporting that branch.

Typically, gene trees are used to infer species trees, but it is important to keep in mind that a gene tree is not necessarily equivalent to a species tree.

There are three main factors that cause gene trees not to be equivalent to species trees:

1 Use of paralogous loci. Gene loci which are homologous (descended from a common ancestral locus) can be classified as either orthologous (descended from a common ancestral locus without gene duplication) or paralogous (descended from a common ancestral locus by way of one or more gene duplication events). For example, in *Figure 2*, the AE1 genes of human, mouse, and chicken are all orthologous to one another; but AE1 genes are paralogous to AE2 and AE3. If we mistakenly believe that certain genes are orthologous when they are actually paralogous, we can infer an incorrect species tree

218

from a gene tree. (Note that these terms only apply to genetic loci, not to alleles at a given locus. Thus, although no gene duplication has intervened between the last common ancestor of two alleles at the same locus, they are not properly called 'orthologous' to each other, since they are alleles not loci.)

2 Polymorphism in the ancestral population. If there is polymorphism at a locus in an ancestral population, different alleles may be present in descendant species. If so, the phylogeny of these alleles will not in general correspond to the phylogeny of the species. Because most polymorphism is selectively neutral and thus is maintained for a relatively short time (9), this factor will usually only be a problem with phylogenies of closely related species. However, when balancing selection maintains polymorphisms, they can last for a much longer time (see Section 4), and in such cases the gene tree and the species tree can be markedly different.

3 Stochastic error. Because the accumulation of nucleotide substitutions is a random process, by chance a tree based on just one gene may not correspond to the species tree.

The process of phylogenetic tree reconstruction can best be viewed as consisting of two related processes of statistical estimation (23). The true tree, which represents the true evolutionary relationships among the OTUs, is in general not known to us; thus, we must use some statistical method to 'reconstruct' or 'estimate' it. Then, given an estimated tree, we can also use a statistical method to estimate the branch lengths within the tree, where the branch lengths correspond to numbers of substitutional events (i.e. nucleotide or amino acid substitutions) between the nodes of the tree. Finding the true tree is a difficult problem because, when the number of OTUs is moderately large, the number of possible trees is extremely large. For example, for 10 OTUs, there are over 2 million possible unrooted trees and over 34 million possible rooted trees.

3.2 Methods of phylogenetic reconstruction

The choice of method for phylogenetic reconstruction has been a contentious issue in certain circles, often needlessly so. A number of different methods have been created, starting from different philosophical and statistical bases, and each has strengths and weaknesses. Each can yield reliable results when applied to situations where its basic assumptions are applicable. There are three main approaches to choosing the 'best' tree:

1 The minimum evolution (ME) criterion. The ME criterion is applied to a data set consisting of a pairwise distance matrix among OTUs. In the case of molecular sequences, these distances include any of the amino acid or nucleotide distances discussed in Section 2. The ME tree is the tree with the smallest total sum of the branch lengths. In practice, finding the ME tree is quite time-consuming if the number of possible trees is large. However, the popular neighbour-joining (NJ) algorithm (24) provides a very quick way of finding a tree that is always quite close to the ME tree by means of a stepwise procedure. The phylogenetic trees in *Figures 1* and *2* are NJ trees. That in *Figure 1* is based on the Jukes–Cantor corrected estimate of the number of nucleotide substitutions per site, while that in *Figure 2* is based on the uncorrected proportion of amino acid differences.

2 The maximum parsimony (MP) criterion. The MP tree is the tree that assumes the smallest number of mutational steps. Again, if the number of OTUs is large, the process of finding the MP tree can be quite difficult, and heuristic search algorithms have been developed that find a tree close to the MP tree but perhaps not identical to it. Another complication is that, when the number of OTUs is large, there may be many equally parsimonious trees. However, these equally parsimonious trees often differ from one another only in a few details.

3 The maximum likelihood (ML) criterion. Assuming a given substitution model, it is possible to construct a statistical expression for the likelihood of the observed sequences given a particular phylogenetic tree. The ML method chooses the topology that gives the highest likelihood value.

Each of these methods has strengths and weaknesses. For example, the MP method is the only one that can easily incorporate insertion–deletion ('indel') events; thus it can make use of information ignored by the other methods. However, the MP method uses only information at so-called 'informative sites'; i.e. sites at which certain trees provide a more parsimonious explanation than other trees (see Chapter 2 for an example of a MP tree of sequences of Erwinia species). All evolutionary information at other sites which do not meet this definition is ignored by the MP method. Perhaps for this reason, the MP method has a tendency to provide poorer resolution of phylogenetic relationships than other methods. The MP method also does not incorporate any correction for 'multiple hits'. This can be a problem when sequences are distantly related.

The theoretical basis of the ML method is poorly understood. The likelihood function that is computed is conditional on both the substitution model and the topology. Thus, it is unclear whether comparison of likelihood functions for different topologies is really justified. The ML method is also computationally very time-consuming, a factor which has limited its use.

When an unbiased estimator is used for amino acid or nucleotide distance, it has been shown that the expected sum of branch lengths is smallest for the true topology (25). This finding provides a theoretical foundation for the ME method. It is still unknown, however, how choice of an inappropriate distance can affect the likelihood of this method's recovering the true tree.

In spite of such limitations and unanswered questions, all three of these methods produce very similar results when they are applied judiciously. In terms of practical application of phylogeny reconstruction, it seems that the most commonly encountered problems arise from two sources:

(a) Lack of rate constancy in different branches of the tree.

(b) Saturation of synonymous sites.

The NJ algorithm is known to be relatively robust when rate constancy differs among branches of a tree (24). By contrast, other widely used algorithms for reconstructing a phylogeny from a distance matrix do not have this property. Among these, the UPGMA method, which explicitly assumes a constant rate of evolution ('molecular clock') and constructs a rooted tree based on this assumption, is extremely likely to give erroneous results when there is rate variation among sites (24). Unfortunately, the UPGMA algorithm is included in a number of popular sequence analysis computer packages. The MP method also seems to be somewhat sensitive to lack of rate constancy; thus results of MP analysis should be treated with caution when rate variation among branches is present.

3.3 Testing phylogenies

When we have reconstructed the phylogenetic relationships among a number of sequences, it is desirable to have some way of assessing how reliable our reconstruction is. Since we do not know the true tree in most cases, the best we can do is to ascertain how strongly our data themselves support the tree we have reconstructed. One approach to doing this involves 'bootstrapping', a term used by statisticians to refer to a variety of techniques for creating 'pseudo-samples' by sampling at random from a data set (26). In a molecular sequence data set involving n sites, bootstrapping involves sampling n sites with replacement to create a pseudo-sample. For example, the AE phylogeny shown in *Figure 2* was based on 724 aligned amino acid residues. For this data set, each bootstrap pseudo-sample would consist of 724 sites sampled with replacement from these sites.

The pseudo-sample is then used as the basis of tree construction; and this process is repeated a large number of times, preferably at least 1000 (27). For any given branch, the percentage of bootstrap pseudo-samples supporting that branch (called the 'bootstrap confidence percentage' or 'bootstrap percentage') gives an indication of the strength of support in the data for that branch. The bootstrap method can be taken as a test of the hypothesis that the branch length equals zero. We reject the null hypothesis at the 5% significance level, when the bootstrap percentage is greater than 95%. Computer simulations have suggested that bootstrapping provides a conservative test of this hypothesis (28).

The phylogeny of CSP sequences in *Figure 1* illustrates the results of bootstrapping. In this phylogeny, bootstrap support for the deep branches in the cluster of *P. falciparum* CSP alleles is generally quite low. High bootstrap percentages are only seen on the terminal branches; for example, the clustering of M22982 and M57498 receives 100% bootstrap support (*Figure 1*).

Bootstrapping can theoretically be applied to any method of phylogenetic reconstruction. It is often applied to NJ trees, and sometimes to MP trees. In the case of ME trees, if the branch lengths are estimated by the ordinary least squares method, an alternative method can be used to test the hypothesis that a branch length is equal to zero (29). This method provides an estimate of the standard error of the branch length. Assuming approximate normality, the ratio of the branch length to its standard error can be compared to the standard normal distribution; thus, the null hypothesis will be rejected at the 5% level when this ratio is greater than 1.96, the value of the Z-statistic for a two-tailed test at the 5% level. The standard error test is in general more powerful (less conservative) than the bootstrap test.

4 Applications

4.1 Phylogenetic analysis

Phylogenetic analysis has by now become a widely used tool in the study of organisms causing human disease. By reconstructing the relationships of pathogenic organisms, researchers have been able to answer many different questions about the origin and transmission of infections. These questions have involved a variety of time frames. For example, in the case of human immunodeficiency viruses (HIV), phylogenetic analyses have been used to address questions ranging from the forensic (e.g. the origin of specific infections) to the origin of HIV-1 as a human pathogen. Thus, the time frames have ranged from a few months to several decades. In the case of other human pathogens, including the malaria parasites, phylogenetic analyses have been used to address questions involving time frames of millions of years.

Probably the most famous example of the use of phylogenetic analysis in a forensic case was that of the Florida dentist suspected of infecting certain of his patients with HIV. In the initial report on this case, Ou *et al.* (30) sequenced a small portion of the *env* gene of the virus from the dentist, from seven infected patients, and from a number of HIV-positive individuals from the same area ('local controls') (30). In the initial paper, the authors presented an MP tree including only two sequences from each patient and two from the dentist; these sequences were said to represent the most divergent pair from each host (30). Their tree showed that sequences from five of the patients clustered with those of the dentist, while those of two other patients did not. The five patients whose sequences clustered with those of the dentist had no known risk factors for HIV, while the other two patients did have known risk factors (30). Thus, the authors concluded that their results pointed to the dentist as the likely source of the infection in the five patients lacking other risk factors.

This conclusion generated a great deal of controversy, legal as well as scientific (31–33). *Figure 3* shows the NJ tree based on all sequences generated by Ou *et al.*'s (30) study. As in the original tree, the sequences from five of the patients (A, B, C, E, and G) clustered with sequences from the dentist, while the other two (D and F) fall outside this cluster (*Figure 3*). The five patients clustering with the dentist are those with no other known risk factors. The clustering of these sequences with the dentist receives fairly strong bootstrap support (90%). When the standard error test of branch lengths was applied, this branch was significant at the 1% level.

This example illustrates the greater power of the standard error test compared to bootstrapping, but both analyses support the conclusion that the

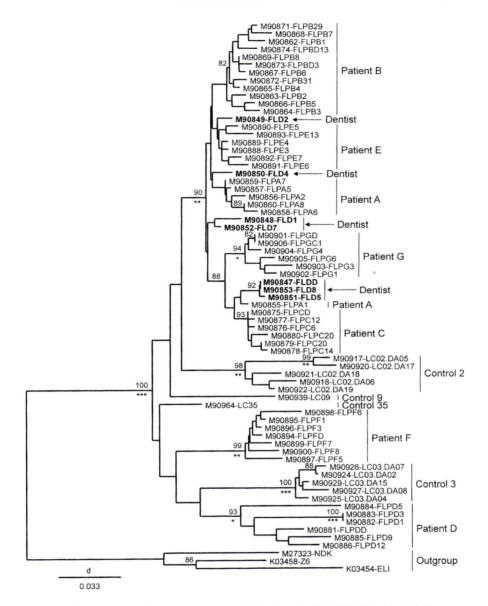

Figure 3 Phylogeny of partial *env* sequences of HIV-1 from the Florida dentist, his patients, and local controls. The tree is rooted with selected HIV-1 subtype D sequences. The tree was constructed by the NJ method on the basis of the number of nucleotide substitutions per site (d), estimated by the Jukes–Cantor method. Reliability of clustering patterns in the tree was tested by bootstrapping (1000 pseudo-samples) and by the standard error test of branch lengths. Numbers on the branches represent the percentage of pseudo-samples supporting that branch. Only bootstrap percentages > 80% are indicated. Significance levels of the standard error test are indicated as follows: * P < 0.05; ** P < 0.01; *** P < 0.001.

dentist was the source of these five patients' infection. The NJ tree thus shows much clearer resolution of this problem than did Ou *et al.*'s (30) original MP tree. Contrary to the conclusion of Brown (33), the MP analysis was not 'about as good as it gets'. Indeed, one cannot help wondering whether there would have been less controversy in this case if an analysis like that of *Figure 3* had been applied in the original paper. Note also that the sequences from the dentist are scattered among those of patients A, B, C, E, and F (*Figure 3*), just as would be expected if the dentist's viral population were the founding population from which these patients' viral populations were independently derived.

An example of a phylogenetic question of epidemiological relevance involving a much greater extent of time is that of the origin of the most virulent of human malaria parasites, *Plasmodium falciparum*. On the basis of a phylogenetic tree in which *P. falciparum* clustered with a *Plasmodium* species parasitic on birds, it was previously believed that *P. falciparum* was recently transferred to humans from a bird host (34). This was an appealing hypothesis to parasitologists because of their belief that parasites inevitably evolve in the direction of commensalism and that therefore virulent parasites are always recently acquired. However, though widely held, this view is not necessarily true in every case (35); for example, natural selection will favour virulence as long as it is correlated with transmission rate (36).

In the case of *P. falciparum,* phylogenetic analyses of both small subunit ribosomal RNA (SSU rRNA) (20) and circumsporozoite protein (21) revealed a close relationship with the chimpanzee parasite *P. reichenowi*. These results supported the hypothesis that *P. falciparum* has been in the hominid lineage at least since the last common ancestor of human and chimpanzee (5–7 million years ago). However, it was not clear from these analyses whether the common ancestor of *P. falciparum* and *P. reichenowi* might have transferred to a primate host from a bird host.

Figure 4 shows an NJ tree based on conserved domains of asexual-stage SSU rRNA sequences of *Plasmodium* species. Non-conserved domains were excluded because these domains are saturated with changes in the more distant comparisons. The tree is rooted with sequences from related genera of Apicomplexa (*Figure 4*). In this tree, grouping of *P. falciparum* with *P. reichenowi* is strongly supported (100% bootstrap support). Bird malarias group outside all mammalian malarias, and reptile malarias outside mammal and bird malarias (*Figure 4*). However, the bootstrap support for the position of the bird (50%) and reptile (77%) malarias was not strong (*Figure 4*). Nonetheless, the tree provides no support for transfer of the ancestor of *P. falciparum* and *P. reichenowi* from a bird host.

4.2 Testing for positive selection

By now there is substantial evidence that most polymorphism in natural populations of organisms is selectively neutral and that most events of fixation of polymorphic variants at the DNA level occur as a result of genetic drift, not natural selection (2, 3, 9). Nonetheless, we expect that natural selection favouring certain

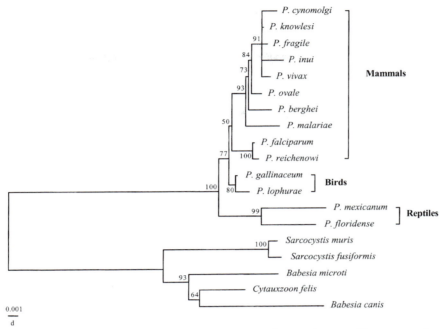

Figure 4 Phylogeny of asexual-stage SSU rRNA of *Plasmodium* species parasitic on mammals, birds, and reptiles. The tree is rooted with sequences from other genera of Apicomplexa. The tree was constructed by the NJ method on the basis of the number of nucleotide substitutions per site (d) in conserved gene regions, estimated by the Jukes–Cantor method. Reliability of clustering patterns in the tree was tested by bootstrapping (1000 pseudo-samples). Numbers on the branches represent the percentage of pseudo-samples supporting that branch.

variants must sometimes occur. We observe that organisms possess characteristics adapting them to their environment, and since Darwin it has been believed that natural selection is the most likely explanation for the origin of such traits (37). In molecular evolutionary studies, it is customary to use the term 'positive Darwinian selection' to refer to cases in which natural selection acts on molecular variation. This term is used to contrast with purifying selection or 'negative selection', which merely removes deleterious mutations from a population. Positive selection includes both balancing selection, which maintains a polymorphism, and directional selection, which favours fixation of a beneficial allele.

As mentioned previously, the fact that d_S exceeds d_N in most protein-coding genes is evidence for the omnipresence of purifying selection. On the other hand, when natural selection favours change at the amino acid level, we can see a reversal of this pattern. Comparing d_S and d_N thus is a powerful method of testing for positive selection at the molecular level (37, 38). This method has been applied to a wide variety of cases in the past decade. Probably not surprisingly, many of the cases for which there is the strongest evidence of positive selection involve molecules of the vertebrate immune system that are involved in recognition of and/or defence against pathogens and molecules of pathogens that are recognized by the host immune system (37).

The genes of the vertebrate major histocompatibility complex (MHC) were among the first cases to which this approach was applied (37–43). The MHC gene family includes a number of highly polymorphic loci whose products present peptides to T cells (see Chapter 7). On the basis of early evidence that different MHC gene products present different antigens (i.e. peptides), Doherty and Zinkernagel (44) proposed that MHC polymorphism is maintained by the type of balancing selection called 'overdominant selection' or 'heterozygote advantage' relating to the ability of heterozygotes to present a wider array of peptides than homozygotes and thus to be resistant to a broader array of pathogens. Comparison of rates of synonymous and non-synonymous nucleotide substitution provided strong support for this hypothesis. In the codons encoding the peptide binding region of the MHC molecules, d_N greatly exceeds d_S, whereas in other gene regions $d_S > d_N$ as in most genes (37–43). This indicates that MHC polymorphism is maintained by a form of balancing selection that favours diversity in peptide binding, as predicted by Doherty and Zinkernagel.

The comparison of synonymous and non-synonymous rates of nucleotide substitution has also become a powerful tool in studying the evolution of parasitic organisms. If natural selection favours the host's ability to recognize a diverse array of foreign antigens, it is to be expected that it will favour mutations in genes encoding parasite antigens that evade immune recognition. For example, a pattern of $d_N > d_S$ has been reported for a number of surface proteins of *Plasmodium falciparum* (21, 45, 46). Particularly interesting are the cases where natural selection has been shown to favour diversity in the regions of *Plasmodium* antigens known to be bound by host MHC molecules (21, 45). Such a pattern supports the hypothesis that host MHC and T cell recognition are the factors driving selection for diversity in the parasite.

Balancing selection is expected to maintain polymorphism for a much longer time than neutral polymorphisms are typically maintained (47). In the case of the MHC, phylogenetic analyses of sequences from humans and other primate species have been used to show that some allelic lineages have been maintained since the common ancestor of human and chimpanzee (42). There is also evidence that certain polymorphisms of *Plasmodium falciparum* have been maintained for millions of years (21, 22, 46). Even in the absence of other evidence, phylogenetic evidence of long-term (for example, over two million years) maintenance of a polymorphism in any cellular organism is evidence of balancing selection.

Sometimes, examining patterns of nucleotide substitution can provide evidence regarding which portions of an antigenic protein are subject to selection by the host's immune system. This, in turn, has implications both for understanding the population dynamics of the pathogen and, possibly, for therapeutic strategies. We will discuss an example involving human immunodeficiency virus-1 (HIV-1). The structure of the envelope glycoprotein gp120 has recently been elucidated (48). Some features of the structure are illustrated in *Figure 5*. Using data sampled over time from an individual patient with a strong antibody response (49), we computed mean d_S and d_N within each time sample for four distinct regions of gp120:

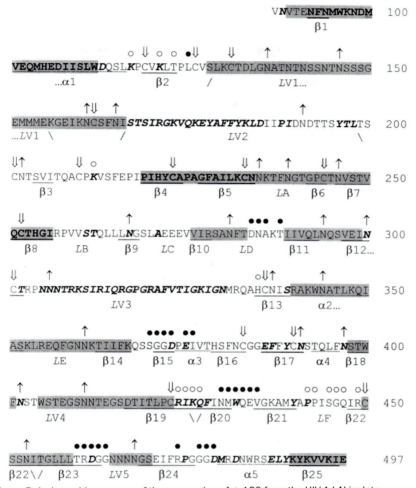

Figure 5 Amino acid sequence of the core region of gp120 from the HIV-1 LAI isolate. Secondary structural elements are indicated as follows: beta-strands (straight) and alpha-helices (wavy) are underlined, and loops are labelled L. Glycosylation sites (↑) and disulfide bond sites (⇓) are also indicated, as are putative CD4 binding sites (●) and CCR5 binding sites (○). Segments forming the non-neutralizing face of the folded protein are in bold font and are shaded; segments forming the silent face are in regular font and are shaded; the remaining segments within the core form the neutralizing face. Neutralizing Mab epitope sites are in bold italics.

(a) Antibody epitopes in the highly polymorphic V3 loop.

(b) Other epitopes for neutralizing antibodies outside the V3 loop.

(c) The remainder of the neutralizing face, the region of the molecule to which neutralizing antibodies attach.

(d) The silent face, a region of the molecule rich in *N*-glycosylation sites which does not bind antibodies.

The results are shown in *Figure 6*. In the V3 loop, for the first three years of infection, mean d_S was greater than mean d_N (*Figure 6A*). However, after about three years, d_N exceeded d_S; and in the samples taken at 48 and 53 months post-infection, there was a highly significant difference between d_N and d_S (*Figure 6A*). None of the other regions of gp120 showed strong differences between d_S and d_N, though mean d_S exceeded mean d_N in a majority of samples (*Figure 6B–D*). Because the evidence for positive selection is confined to the V3 epitopes, these results implicate host antibodies as the source of selection favouring diversity in gp120 of HIV-1, particularly antibodies recognizing epitopes in the V3 loop.

4.3 Nucleotide diversity and population structure

One of the most important concepts in population genetics is that of effective population size (2). The effective size of a given population is the size of an ideal-ized population that would behave, with respect to genetic drift, in the same manner as that population. The effective population size is generally lower—and sometimes much lower—than the census population size; that is, the number we would get if we counted all living individuals in the population. A number of factors can contribute to reducing the effective population size including the following:

(a) Unequal contribution by members of the two sexes to reproduction.

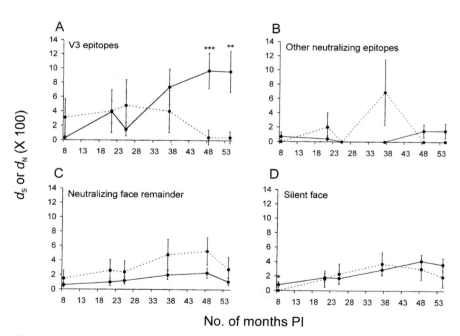

Figure 6 Mean d_S (dashed line) and mean d_N (solid line) (with standard error bars) in different regions of gp120 in samples taken over the course of infection of an AIDS patient with a strong antibody response. Significant differences between d_S and d_N are indicated as follows: ** P < 0.01; *** P < 0.001.

(b) Overlapping generations (because some individuals in the population may be pre-reproductive and some post-reproductive).

(c) Long-term variation in population size over time.

One common example of the latter would be a so-called 'population bottleneck', which occurs when the population reduces to a very small number and then recovers.

Effective population size is important because it is the major factor affecting the amount of polymorphism that can be maintained. This includes both selectively neutral polymorphism and balanced polymorphisms. In general, we have no direct way of measuring effective population size. If a given species is highly abundant at the present time, it may still have undergone a severe bottleneck in the past. However, sequence comparisons enable us to obtain evidence regarding such past events.

For example, Rich and colleagues (50) recently proposed that the human malaria parasite *Plasmodium falciparum* went through a very recent and very extreme population bottleneck. In fact, they proposed that all *P. falciparum* in the world today are descended from a single haploid genotype which existed between 27500 and 57500 years ago. If true, this would have important epidemiological consequences. It would mean that world-wide this species should have an extremely low level of polymorphism—good news for the designers of antimalarial vaccines, which would not have to cope with the complexities of polymorphic antigens in the parasite population.

Unfortunately, Rich *et al.*'s (50) hypothesis is demonstrably false. Sequence comparisons provide powerful evidence for testing the hypothesis of a recent bottleneck, and in this case the evidence indicates overwhelmingly that no such bottleneck occurred in *P. falciparum*. As mentioned previously, there is evidence that polymorphism at certain loci encoding *P. falciparum* surface antigens has been maintained for millions of years, contradicting the idea of a single recent ancestral haploid genome (21, 22, 45, 46).

Furthermore, there is evidence that even neutral polymorphism is quite high in this species, suggesting a large effective population size.

Table 3 shows mean d_S values in the mitochondrial cytochrome *b* (*cyt b*) gene for pairwise comparisons among *P. falciparum* isolates; for comparisons between *P. falciparum* and the chimpanzee parasite *P. reichenowi*; for pairwise comparison

Table 3 Mean numbers of synonymous substitutions per site ($d_S \pm$ SE) among mitochondrial *cyt b* alleles of *Plasmodium falciparum*; between *P. falciparum* and *P. reichenowi*; and between human and chimpanzee (*Pan troglodytes*)[a]

	vs. *P. falciparum*	vs. *P. reichenowi*
P. falciparum	0.00336 ± 0.00258	0.10954 ± 0.02249
	vs. Human	**vs. Chimpanzee**
Human	0.01124 ± 0.00339	0.47611 ± 0.05112

[a] Numbers of sequences compared are as follows: *P. falciparum* 5, *P. reichenowi* 1, human 21, chimpanzee 20.

of human *cyt b* alleles; and for comparisons between human and chimpanzee. Since these data involve only synonymous changes, they are expected to be selectively neutral and to reflect the mutation rate. Mean d_S between human and chimpanzee *cyt b* genes is about 4.3 times as great as mean d_S between *P. falciparum* and *P. reichenowi cyt b* genes (*Table 3*). Assuming the *P. falciparum* and *P. reichenowi* diverged at the same time as human and chimpanzee (about 5–7 million years ago), this suggests that the *cyt b* gene in primates has a mutation rate about 4.3 times as high as that of the homologous gene in *Plasmodium*.

Mammalian mitochondrial genomes are known to have a high mutation rate, about ten times that of nuclear genes (3). Assuming a divergence time of six million years for human and chimpanzee, the data in *Table 3* give a rate of 7.9×10^{-8} substitutions/site/year, which is quite close to published estimates for the mutation rate of mammalian mitochondrial genes (3, 51). Assuming the same divergence time for *P. falciparum* and *P. reichenowi*, we get a rate of 1.8×10^{-8} substitutions/site/year.

Mean d_S among human *cyt b* genes is about 3.3 times as high as that among *P. falciparum cyt b* genes. Given that the extent of neutral polymorphism is a function of effective population size, we might be led to conclude that the effective population size of humans is considerably larger than that of *P. falciparum*. However, we must also take into account the fact that the extent of neutral polymorphism is a function of the mutation rate. Since the mutation rate of this gene is about 4.3 times as high in primates as in *Plasmodium*, we would expect mean d_S in *P. falciparum* to be less than a quarter of that in humans even if the effective population sizes of the two species are identical. In fact, mean d_S in *P. falciparum* is nearly a third that in humans, suggesting that the effective population size of *P. falciparum* is as large as that of humans or even larger.

Using our estimation of the substitution rate in primate *cyt b*, we conclude that the most divergent pair of human *cyt b* genes in our sample ($d_S = 0.0249$) diverged 315 000 years ago, well within the range estimated by others for the time of the human mitochondrial ancestor (51). Similarly, we estimate that the most divergent pair of *P. falciparum cyt b* genes ($d_S = 0.0084$) diverged 470 000 years ago. If the ancestor of all *P. falciparum* really occurred only 57 500 years ago, we would require a substitution rate of 1.5×10^{-7} substitutions/site/year to accumulate this degree of divergence. Then we would have to explain why the substitution rate in *P. falciparum* should be an order of magnitude greater than that between *P. falciparum* and *P. reichenowi*.

This example illustrates how even a small amount of nucleotide sequence data can provide insight into major questions in population biology which are of interest to epidemiologists. Clearly, a more extensive data set from *P. falciparum* would shed still further light on the extent of polymorphism and thus the effective population size of this species. In general, the more extensively we sample a population by sequencing and the longer the stretch of sequence we examine, the greater will be our power to resolve evolutionary questions. It is true in general with sequence data—whether our interests are in reconstructing phylogeny, in testing for positive Darwinian selection, or simply examining the extent of neutral polymorphism present in a population—the more data we have the more accurate our conclusions will be.

References

1. Haldane, J. B. S. (1949). *Ricerca scientifica*, (Suppl) **19**, 2.
2. Nei, M. and Kumar, S. (2000). *Molecular evolution and phylogenetics*. Oxford University Press, New York.
3. Li, W.-H. (1997). *Molecular evolution*. Sinauer, Sunderland MA.
4. Graur, D. and Li, W.-H. (2000). *Fundamentals of molecular evolution*, 2nd edn. Sinauer, Sunderland MA.
5. Hillis, D. M., Moritz, C., and Mable, B. K. (1996). *Molecular systematics*, 2nd edn. Sinauer, Sunderland MA.
6. Kumar, S., Tamura, K., and Nei, M. (1993). *MEGA: Molecular evolutionary genetic analysis*. Version 1.0. Pennsylvania State University, University Park.
7. Maddison, W. and Maddison, D. (1992). *MacClade 3*. Sinauer, Sunderland MA.
8. Swofford, D. L. (1999). *PAUP* 4.0*. Sinauer, Sunderland MA.
9. Kimura, M. (1983). *The neutral theory of molecular evolut*ion. Cambridge University Press, New York.
10. Ota, T. and Nei, M. (1994). *J. Mol. Evol.*, **38**, 642.
11. Jukes, T. H. and Cantor, C. R. (1969). In *Mammalian protein metabolism* (ed. H. N. Munro), p. 21. Academic Press, New York.
12. Kimura, M. (1980). *J. Mol. Evol.*, **16**, 111.
13. Nakamura, Y., Gojobori, T., and Ikemura, T. (1998). *Nucleic Acids Res.*, **26**, 334.
14. Nei, M. and Gojobori, T. (1986). *Mol. Biol. Evol.*, **3**, 418.
15. Li, W.-H. (1993). *J. Mol. Evol.*, **36**, 96.
16. Zhang, J., Rosenberg, H. F., and Nei, M. (1998). *Proc. Natl. Acad. Sci. USA*, **95**, 3708.
17. Kimura, M. (1977). *Nature*, **267**, 275.
18. Nei, M. and Jin, L. (1989). *Mol. Biol. Evol.*, **6**, 290.
19. Ota, T. and Nei, M. (1994). *Mol. Biol. Evol.*, **11**, 613.
20. Escalente, A. A. and Ayala, F. (1994). *Proc. Natl. Acad. Sci. USA*, **91**, 11373.
21. Hughes, M. K. and Hughes, A. L. (1995). *Mol. Biochem. Parasitol.*, **71**, 99.
22. Hughes, A. L. and Verra, F. (1998). *Genetics*, **150**, 511.
23. Nei, M. (1996). *Annu. Rev. Genet.*, **30**, 371.
24. Saitou, N. and Nei, M. (1986). *Mol. Biol. Evol.*, **4**, 406.
25. Rzhetsky, A. and Nei, M. (1993). *Mol. Biol. Evol.*, **10**, 1073.
26. Felsenstein, J. (1985). *Evolution*, **39**, 783.
27. Hedges, S. B. (1992). *Mol. Biol. Evol.*, **9**, 336.
28. Sitnikova, T. (1996). *Mol. Biol. Evol.*, **13**, 605.
29. Rzhetsy, A. and Nei, M (1992). *Mol. Biol. Evol.*, **9**, 945.
30. Ou, C.-Y., Ciesielski, C. A., Myers, G., Bandea, C. I., Luo, C.-C., Korber, B. T. M., *et al.* Laboratory Investigation Group, and Epidemiologic Investigation Group. (1992). *Science*, **256**, 1165.
31. DeBry, R. W., Abele, L. G., Weiss, S. H., Hill, M. D., Bouzas, M., Lorenzo, E., *et al.* (1993). *Nature*, **361**, 691.
32. Hillis, D. M. and Huelsenbeck, J. P. (1994). *Nature*, **369**, 24.
33. Brown, D. (1996). *Ann. Intern. Med.*, **124**, 255.
34. Waters, A. P., Higgins, D. G., and McCutchan, T. F. (1991). *Proc. Natl. Acad. Sci. USA*, **88**, 3140.

35. May, R. M. (1985). In *Ecology and genetics of host-parasite interactions* (ed. D. Rollinson and R. M. Anderson), p. 243. Academic Press, London.

36. MacKinnon, M. J. and Read, A. F. (1999). *Evolution*, **53**, 689.

37. Hughes, A. L. (1999). *Adaptive evolution of genes and genomes*. Oxford University Press, New York.

38. Hughes, A. L. and Nei, M. (1988). *Nature*, **335**, 167.

39. Hughes, A. L. and Nei, M. (1989). *Proc. Natl. Acad. Sci. USA*, **86**, 958.

40. Hughes, A. L., Hughes, M. K., Howell, C. Y., and Nei, M. (1994). *Phil. Trans. R. Soc. Lond. B Biol. Sci.*, **345**, 359.

41. Hughes, A. L. and Hughes, M. K. (1995). *Immunogenetics*, **42**, 233.

42. Hughes, A. L. and Yeager, M. (1998). *Annu. Rev. Genet.*, **32**, 415.

43. Yeager, M. and Hughes, A. L. (1999). *Immunol. Rev.*, **167**, 45.

44. Doherty, P. C. and Zinkernagel, R. (1975). *Nature*, **256**, 50.

45. Hughes, A. L. (1991). *Genetics*, **127**, 345.

46. Hughes, A. L. (1992). *Mol. Biol. Evol.*, **9**, 381.

47. Takahata, N. and Nei, M. (1990). *Genetics*, **124**, 967.

48. Wyatt, R., Kowng, P. D., Desjardins, E., Sweet, R. W., Robinson, J., Hendrickson, W. A., *et al.* (1998). *Nature*, **393**, 705.

49. Wolinksky, S. M., Korber, B. T., Neumann, A. U., Daniels, M., Kunstman, K. J., Whetsell, A. J., *et al.* (1996). *Science*, **272**, 537.

50. Rich, S. M., Licht, M. C., Hudson, R. R., and Ayala, F. J. (1998). *Proc. Natl. Acad. Sci. USA*, **95**, 4425.

51. Tamura, K. and Nei, M. (1993). *Mol. Biol. Evol.*, **10**, 512.

List of Suppliers

Amersham Pharmacia Biotech, Inc.,
800 Centennial Avenue, Piscataway,
NJ 08855-1327, USA. Tel: 732 457 8000
Fax: 732 457 8000
URL: http://www.apbiotech.com

Anderman and Co. Ltd., 145 London Road,
Kingston-upon-Thames, Surrey KT2 6NH, UK.
Tel: 0181 541 0035
Fax: 0181 541 0623

Applied Biosystems, Inc., Division
Headquarters, 850 Lincoln Centre Drive,
Foster City, CA 94404, USA.
Tel: 650 638 5800, 800 345 5224
Fax: 650 638 5884
URL: http://www.appliedbiosystems.com
Applied Biosystems, 7 Kingsland Grange,
Woolston, Warrington, Cheshire WA1 7SR,
UK.
Tel: 44 1925 825650
Fax: 44 1925 282502

Applied Scientific, 154 West Harris Avenue,
S. San Francisco, CA 94080, USA.
Tel: 650 244 9851
Fax: 650 244 9866
URL: http://www.appliedsci.com

Appligene-Oncor, Purchase, NY, USA.

Beckman Coulter (UK) Ltd., Oakley Court,
Kingsmead Business Park, London Road, High
Wycombe, Buckinghamshire HP11 1JU, UK.
Tel: 01494 441181
Fax: 01494 447558
URL: http://www.beckman.com

Beckman Coulter Inc., 4300 N Harbor
Boulevard, PO Box 3100, Fullerton,
CA 92834-3100, USA.
Tel: 001 714 871 4848
Fax: 001 714 773 8283
URL: http://www.beckman.com

Becton Dickinson and Co., 21 Between
Towns Road, Cowley, Oxford OX4 3LY, UK.
Tel: 01865 748844
Fax: 01865 781627
URL: http://www.bd.com
Becton Dickinson and Co., 1 Becton Drive,
Franklin Lakes, NJ 07417-1883, USA.
Tel: 001 201 847 6800
URL: http://www.bd.com

Bio 101 Inc., c/o Anachem Ltd., Anachem
House, 20 Charles Street, Luton, Bedfordshire
LU2 0EB, UK.
Tel: 01582 456666
Fax: 01582 391768
URL: http://www.anachem.co.uk
Bio 101 Inc., PO Box 2284, La Jolla,
CA 92038-2284, USA.
Tel: 001 760 598 7299
Fax: 001 760 598 0116
URL: http://www.bio101.com

Bio-Rad Laboratories Ltd., Bio-Rad House,
Maylands Avenue, Hemel Hempstead,
Hertfordshire HP2 7TD, UK.
Tel: 0181 328 2000
Fax: 0181 328 2550
URL: http://www.bio-rad.com

Bio-Rad Laboratories Ltd., Division Headquarters, 1000 Alfred Noble Drive, Hercules, CA 94547, USA.
Tel: 001 510 724 7000
Fax: 001 510 741 5817
URL: http://www.bio-rad.com

CP Instrument Co. Ltd., PO Box 22, Bishop Stortford, Hertfordshire CM23 3DX, UK.
Tel: 01279 757711
Fax: 01279 755785
URL: http://www.cpinstrument.co.uk

Dupont (UK) Ltd., Industrial Products Division, Wedgwood Way, Stevenage, Hertfordshire SG1 4QN, UK.
Tel: 01438 734000
Fax: 01438 734382
URL: http://www.dupont.com
Dupont Co. (Biotechnology Systems Division), PO Box 80024, Wilmington, DE 19880-002, USA.
Tel: 001 302 774 1000
Fax: 001 302 774 7321
URL: http://www.dupont.com

Eastman Chemical Co., 100 North Eastman Road, PO Box 511, Kingsport, TN 37662-5075, USA.
Tel: 001 423 229 2000
URL: http://www.eastman.com

Equilibrium, Three Harbours Drive, Ste. 111, Sausalito, CA 94965, USA.
Tel: 415 332 4343, 800 524 8651
Fax: 415 332 4433
URL: http://www.equilibrium.com

Fisher Scientific UK Ltd., Bishop Meadow Road, Loughborough, Leicestershire LE11 5RG, UK.
Tel: 01509 231166
Fax: 01509 231893

URL: http://www.fisher.co.uk
Fisher Scientific, Fisher Research, 2761 Walnut Avenue, Tustin, CA 92780, USA.
Tel: 001 714 669 4600
Fax: 001 714 669 1613
URL: http://www.fishersci.com

Fluka, PO Box 2060, Milwaukee, WI 53201, USA.
Tel: 001 414 273 5013
Fax: 001 414 2734979
URL: http://www.sigma-aldrich.com
Fluka Chemical Co. Ltd., PO Box 260, CH-9471, Buchs, Switzerland.
Tel: 0041 81 745 2828
Fax: 0041 81 756 5449
URL: http://www.sigma-aldrich.com

Gentra Systems, Minneapolis, MN, USA.

Hitachi Instruments, Inc., 3100 N First Street, San Jose, CA 95134, USA.
Tel: 408 432 0520, 800 548 9001
Fax: 408 432 0704
URL: http://www.hii.hitachi.com

Hoefer/Pharmacia Biotech, see Pharmacia Biotech
Tel: 800 526 3593
Fax: 800 FAX 3593
URL: http://www.hpb.com

Hybaid Ltd., Action Court, Ashford Road, Ashford, Middlesex TW15 1XB, UK.
Tel: 01784 425000
Fax: 01784 248085
URL: http://www.hybaid.com
Hybaid US, 8 East Forge Parkway, Franklin, MA 02038, USA.
Tel: 001 508 541 6918
Fax: 001 508 541 3041
URL: http://www.hybaid.com

HyClone Laboratories, 1725 South HyClone Road, Logan, UT 84321, USA.
Tel: 001 435 753 4584
Fax: 001 435 753 4589
URL: http://www.hyclone.com

Idaho Technology, Inc., 390 Wakara Way, Salt Lake City, UT 84108, USA, Tel: 801 736 6354, 800 735 6544 Fax: 801 588 0507 URL: http://www.idahotech.com

Invitrogen Corp., 1600 Faraday Avenue, Carlsbad, CA 92008, USA. Tel: 001 760 603 7200 Fax: 001 760 603 7201 URL: http://www.invitrogen.com Invitrogen BV, PO Box 2312, 9704 CH Groningen, The Netherlands. Tel: 00800 5345 5345 Fax: 00800 7890 7890 URL: http://www.invitrogen.com

Life Technologies Ltd., PO Box 35, Free Fountain Drive, Incsinnan Business Park, Paisley PA4 9RF, UK. Tel: 0800 269210 Fax: 0800 838380 URL: http://www.lifetech.com Life Technologies Inc., 9800 Medical Center Drive, Rockville, MD 20850, USA. Tel: 001 301 610 8000 URL: http://www.lifetech.com

Merck Sharp & Dohme, Research Laboratories, Neuroscience Research Centre, Terlings Park, Harlow, Essex CM20 2QR, UK. URL: http://www.msd-nrc.co.uk MSD Sharp and Dohme GmbH, Lindenplatz 1, D-85540, Haar, Germany. URL: http://www.msd-deutschland.com

Millipore (UK) Ltd., The Boulevard, Blackmoor Lane, Watford, Hertfordshire WD1 8YW, UK. Tel: 01923 816375 Fax: 01923 818297 URL: http://www.millipore.com/local/UK.htm Millipore Corp., 80 Ashby Road, Bedford, MA 01730, USA. Tel: 001 800 645 5476 Fax: 001 800 645 5439 URL: http://www.millipore.com

MJ Research, Inc., 590 Lincoln Street, Waltham, MA 02451, USA. Tel: 617 972 8000, 888 735 8437 Fax: 617 923 8080 URL: http://www.mjr.com

Molecular Devices, 1311 Orleans Avenue, Sunnyvale, CA 94089-1136, USA. Tel: 800 635 5577 Fax: 408 747 3602 URL: http://www.moleculardevices.com Molecular Devices, Ltd., 135 Wharfedale Road, Winnersh Triangle, Winnersh, Wokingham RG41 5RB, UK. Tel: +44 118 944 8000 Fax: +44 118 944 8001

Molecular Dynamics, 928 East Arques Avenue, Sunnyvale, CA 94086-4520, USA. Tel: 408 773 1222, 800 333 5703 Fax: 408 773 1493 URL: http://www.mdyn.com

Molecular Probes, Inc., 4849 Pitchford Avenue, Eugene, OR 97402-9165, USA. Tel: 541 465 8300 Fax: 541 344 6504 URL: http://www.probes.com

National Diagnostics, 305 Patton Drive, Atlanta, GA 30336, USA. Tel: 800 526 3867 Fax: 404 699 2077 URL: http://www.nationaldiagnostics.com National Diagnostics, Unit 4, Fleet Business Park, Itlings Lane, Hessle, Hull HU13 9LX, UK. Tel: 44 01482 646022/20 Fax: 44 01482 646013

New England Biolabs, 32 Tozer Road, Beverley, MA 01915-5510, USA. Tel: 001 978 927 5054

New England Nuclear, Life Science Products, Boston, MA 02118-2512, USA. New England Nuclear, B-1930 Zaventem, Belgium.

Nikon Inc., 1300 Walt Whitman Road,
Melville, NY 11747-3064, USA.
Tel: 001 516 547 4200
Fax: 001 516 547 0299
URL: http://www.nikonusa.com
Nikon Corp., Fuji Building, 2-3, 3-chome,
Marunouchi, Chiyoda-ku, Tokyo 100, Japan.
Tel: 00813 3214 5311
Fax: 00813 3201 5856
URL: http://www.nikon.co.jp/main/index_e.htm

Nycomed Amersham plc, Amersham Place,
Little Chalfont, Buckinghamshire HP7 9NA,
UK.
Tel: 01494 544000
Fax: 01494 542266
URL: http://www.amersham.co.uk
Nycomed Amersham, 101 Carnegie Center,
Princeton, NJ 08540, USA.
Tel: 001 609 514 6000
URL: http://www.amersham.co.uk

Operon Technologies, Inc., 1000 Atlantic Ave,
St. 108, Alameda, CA 94501, USA.
Tel: 510 865 8644, 800 688 2248
Fax: 510 865 5255
URL: http://www.operon.com

Orca Research, Bothell, WA, USA.

Pegasus Scientific, Inc., 15779 Columbia
Pike, 760 Burtonsville, Maryland 20866, USA.

Perkin Elmer Ltd., Post Office Lane,
Beaconsfield, Buckinghamshire HP9 1QA,
UK.
Tel: 01494 676161
URL: http://www.perkin-elmer.com

Pharmacia Biotech (Biochrom) Ltd., Unit 22,
Cambridge Science Park, Milton Road,
Cambridge CB4 0FJ, UK.
Tel: 01223 423723
Fax: 01223 420164
URL: http://www.biochrom.co.uk

Pharmacia and Upjohn Ltd., Davy Avenue,
Knowlhill, Milton Keynes, Buckinghamshire
MK5 8PH, UK.
Tel: 01908 661101
Fax: 01908 690091
URL: http://www.eu.pnu.com

Promega UK Ltd., Delta House, Chilworth
Research Centre, Southampton SO16 7NS,
UK.
Tel: 0800 378994
Fax: 0800 181037
URL: http://www.promega.com
Promega Corp., 2800 Woods Hollow Road,
Madison, WI 53711-5399, USA.
Tel: 001 608 274 4330
Fax: 001 608 277 2516
URL: http://www.promega.com

Qiagen UK Ltd., Boundary Court, Gatwick
Road, Crawley, West Sussex RH10 2AX, UK.
Tel: 01293 422911
Fax: 01293 422922
URL: http://www.qiagen.com
Qiagen Inc., 28159 Avenue Stanford,
Valencia, CA 91355, USA.
Tel: 001 800 426 8157
Fax: 001 800 718 2056
URL: http://www.qiagen.com

Research Genetics, 2130 Memorial Parkway,
Huntsville, AL 35801, USA.
Tel: 800 533 4363   Fax: 256 536 9016
URL: http://www.resgen.com

Robbins Scientific, 1250 Elko Drive,
Sunnyvale, CA 94089-2213, USA.
Tel: 408 734 8500
Fax: 408 734 0300, 800 752 8585
URL: http://www.robsci.com
Robbins Scientific, Molecular Biology
Laboratories Genetic Research
Instrumentation, Ltd., Gene House,
Queensborough Lane, Rayne, Braintree,
Essex CM7 8TF, UK.
Tel: 44 1376 332800   Fax: 44 1376 344724

Roche Diagnostics Ltd., Bell Lane, Lewes,
East Sussex BN7 1LG, UK.
Tel: 01273 484644
Fax: 01273 480266
URL: http://www.roche.com
Roche Diagnostics Corp., 9115 Hague Road,
PO Box 50457, Indianapolis, IN 46256, USA.
Tel: 001 317 845 2358
Fax: 001 317 576 2126
URL: http://www.roche.com
Roche Diagnostics GmbH, Sandhoferstrasse
116, 68305 Mannheim, Germany.
Tel: 0049 621 759 4747
Fax: 0049 621 759 4002
URL: http://www.roche.com

Roche Molecular Systems, Pleasanton, CA,
USA.

Sarstedt, Inc., PO Box 468, Newton,
NC 28658-0468, USA.
Sarstedt, Inc., 6373 Des Grades Prairies,
St-Leonard, Quebec H1P 1A5, Canada.

Schleicher and Schuell Inc., Keene, NH
03431A, USA.
Tel: 001 603 357 2398

Shandon Scientific Ltd., 93-96 Chadwick
Road, Astmoor, Runcorn, Cheshire WA7 1PR,
UK.
Tel: 01928 566611
URL: http://www.shandon.com

Sigma-Aldrich Co. Ltd., The Old Brickyard,
New Road, Gillingham, Dorset XP8 4XT, UK.
Tel: 01747 822211
Fax: 01747 823779
URL: http://www.sigma-aldrich.com
Sigma-Aldrich Co. Ltd., Fancy Road, Poole,
Dorset BH12 4QH, UK.
Tel: 01202 722114
Fax: 01202 715460
URL: http://www.sigma-aldrich.com

Sigma Chemical Co., PO Box 14508, St Louis,
MO 63178, USA.
Tel: 001 314 771 5765
Fax: 001 314 771 5757
URL: http://www.sigma-aldrich.com

Stratagene Inc., 11011 North Torrey Pines
Road, La Jolla, CA 92037, USA.
Tel: 001 858 535 5400
URL: http://www.stratagene.com
Stratagene Europe, Gebouw California,
Hogehilweg 15, 1101 CB Amsterdam
Zuidoost, The Netherlands.
Tel: 00800 9100 9100
URL: http://www.stratagene.com

Transgenomic, 2032 Concourse Drive,
San Jose, CA 95131, USA.
Tel: 408 432 3230
URL: http://www.transgenomic.com

United States Biochemical, PO Box 22400,
Cleveland, OH 44122, USA.
Tel: 001 216 464 9277

Varian, Inc., 3120 Hansen Way, Palo Alto,
CA 94304-1030, USA.
Tel: 650 213 8000
URL: http://www.varianinc.com

Wolfram Research, Corporate Headquarters,
100 Trade Center Drive, Champaign,
IL 61820-7237, USA.
Tel: 217 398 0700, 800 965 3726
Fax: 217 398 0747
URL: http://www.wolfram.com
Wolfram Research Europe, Ltd., 10 Blenheim
Office Park, Lower Road, Long Hanborough,
Oxfordshire OX8 8LN, UK.
Tel: 44 01993 883400
Fax: 44 01993 883800

Index

affected family-based controls (AFBAC) 127
AIDS *see* HIV
allele frequency determination
  kinetic PCR 132–4
  single nucleotide polymorphisms (SNPs) 129–34
allele image patterns (AIPs), microsatellite data analysis 127–9
allele-specific amplification (ASA) 201–2
allele-specific directional hypothesis (ASDH) 129
alleles
  discriminating by DHPLC 158
  discriminating by gel electrophoresis
    ethidium bromide staining 172
    non-denaturing GE 170
    preparing polyacrylamide gels 168
    sample preparation 170
    silver staining 171
  discriminating by primer length (ADPL) 154
  methods of detection compared 158
amino acids, evolutionary analysis of molecular sequence data 212
amplicons, gel electrophoresis 43
amplification fragment length polymorphism (AFLP), vs RAPD 33

amplification refractory mutation system (ARMS) 201–2
anion exchanger (AE) proteins, sodium bicarbonate exchanger (NBC) 218
association mapping 113–43
  (*see* DNA pooling)
Azospirillum, PAGE 51

bacterial chromosome
  DNA sequence analysis of *Erwinia ompA* gene 57–63
  PCR-based fingerprinting 33–44
    analysis and interpretation 44
    freeze-fracture, cell lysates from Gram+ bacteria 35
    gel electrophoresis of amplicons 43
    high quality DNA for RFLP analysis 36–7
    RAPD-PCR 41–3
    rapid cell lysates, Gram- bacteria 34–5
    repetitive fingerprinting 40–1
    ribotyping 32, 33, 38–40
    set-up strategy, amplification-based 38
  RFLP *see* restriction fragment length polymorphism
  see also pulsed field gel electrophoresis
bacterial typing 29–66

molecular markers for strain differentiation 31–2
PCR advantages 31
balancing selection 226
biotin probes 186
blood, HIV DNA qualitative assay 75
  dried blood spot extraction 78
  extraction of DNA from PBMCs 77
  preparation of cell pellets from whole blood 75
bootstrapping 221, 222–4

Caenorhabditis elegans, anion exchanger (AE) proteins 218
capillary array electrophoresis (CAE) 117
case-control studies 3, 10–13
  example: tuberculosis and *NRAMP1* 12–13
  pooled DNA amplification of microsatellite markers 126–7
causality, Bradford-Hill's criteria 18–20
cell pellet preparation 75
chemokine receptors in HIV disease progression, cohort study 8–9
chimpanzee
  ancestor divergence 217
  Plasmodium reichenowi 217
  synonymous substitutions 229–30

coated microwell plates 81-2
cohort studies 3, 4-10
  attributable risk 9-10
  cumulative incidence 5-7
  example: chemokine
    receptors in HIV disease
    progression 8-9
  incidence 7-8
  prospective vs retrospective 4
colorimetric microwell plates 82
confounding, linkage
  disequilibrium 18
consensus primers 69
Cox proportional hazards
  regression 18
cross-sectional studies 14-15

D6S291 175
denaturing DHPLC 97-8, 103-10
  allele detection 158
  interpretation of reslts 110
  mutation detection 104-8
denaturing gradient gel
  electrophoresis (DGGE)
  119, 170
denaturing polyacrylamide gel
  see polyacrylamide gel
digoxigenin probes 186
DNA analysis, evolutionary,
  molecular sequence data
  212-13
DNA digestion
  PFGE analysis 54
  RFLP analysis 47
DNA fingerprinting see
  PCR-based fingerprinting
DNA pooling, association
  mapping 113-43
  experimental design 134-40
  gel electrophoresis 119-21
    samples using automatic
    sequencer 120-1
  human genome 140-1
  microsatellite data analysis
    121-9
    allele image patterns (AIPs)
    127-9
    nuclear family-based
    samples 127
    stutter and differential
    amplification 122-5
  PCR amplification
    elimination of A-overhang
    119

fluorescence detection
  115-16
  microsatellite markers 118
  sample quantitation
  115-16
SNP allele frequency
  determination 129-34
  see also single nucleotide
    polymorphisms (SNPs)
DNA quantitation
  DNA assay 92-3
  samples for pooled
    amplification 116
DNA sequence analysis
  bacterial ompA gene
    interpretation 62-3
    preparation and storage
    of competent bacterial
    cells 60
    strategy for the molecular
    cloning of PCR products
    61
  Jukes and Cantor model
    212-13
dot blot typing
  data interpretation 200-1
  dot blot membrane
    preparation 198-9
  DQB1 and DPB1 group-
    specific primers 190
  DQB1 probe reactivity
    patterns 191
  DRB1 group-specific primers
    188-9
  locus-specific primers 188
dye intercalation 94-5

epidemiological studies
  associations 16
  candidate genes 24-5
  case-control studies 3, 10-13
  cohort studies 3, 4-10
  cross-sectional studies 14-15
  future prospects 25-6
  interpretation 15
  sources of error 17-24
  whole-genome association
    studies 25-6
error
  Bradford-Hill's criteria on
    causality 18-20
  confounding 17-18
  interactions 23-4
  multiple comparisons 21-2

random error 20
stochastic errors 219
systematic errors 20
Type-1 21-2
Type-2 21, 22-3
Erwinia spp.
  BOX PCR analysis 44-5
  ompA gene, bacterial DNA
    sequence analysis
    amplification of locus 58-9
    cloning and sequencing
    59-60
    phylogenetic tree 63
    ribotype banding 38-40, 42
evolutionary analysis of
  molecular sequence
  data 209-32
  applications 222-31
  comparing sequences 210-16
    amino acids 212
    DNA 212-13
    mean nucleotide diversity
    216
    statistical models 210-11
    synonymous and
    non-synonymous
    substitution 213-16
  minimum evolution (ME)
    criterion 219
  reconstructing phylogenies
    216-21
  testing phylogenies 221-2

fluorescence activated cell
  sorting (FACS) 146,
  148, 150
fluorescence detection, DNA
  pooling, association
  mapping 116

$[\gamma\text{-}^{32}P]$-dATP 162
$[\gamma\text{-}^{32}P]$-probes 186
gel electrophoresis
  amplicons 43
  automatic sequencer 120-1
  discriminating alleles 168-72
  see also denaturing
    polyacrylamide gel
gene trees, and species trees
  218-19
gene—environment
  interactions 23-4
genetic drift 224

genomic DNA, preparation
    from Gram negative
    bacteria 34–5
glycoprotein gp120 226, 227–8
Gram positive/negative bacteria,
    preparation of cell
    lysates 34–5

haemochromatosis, pooled
    DNA amplification of
    microsatellite markers
    126–7
hantavirus isolates, per cent
    similarity 210–11
haploid DNA, whole genome
    amplification 153–4
hazard
    Cox proportional hazards
        regression 18
    see also risk
heteroduplex analysis (HA)
    106–8
    see also single-stranded
        conformation
        polymorphism (SSCP)
HIV
    amplification target, DNA
        vs RNA 72–3
    assay sensitivity and
        specificity 70–1
    disease progression,
        chemokine receptors,
        study 8–9
    evaluation of assay
        performance 75
    HIV-1 and HIV-2,
        classification 67
    internal controls and
        quantitation standards
        (IC/QS) 73–4
    mismatches 68
    primer and probe design
        69–70
    qualitative vs quantitative
        assays 73
HIV DNA assay, qualitative
    75–83
    colorimetric microwell plate
        detection for qualitative
        DNA assay 82
    DNA amplification 80
    dried blood spot extraction 78
    extraction of DNA from
        PBMCs 77

preparation of cell pellets
    from whole blood for
    HIV DNA PCR 75
preparation of coated
    microwell plates 81
preparation of Ficoll-Hypaque
    separated cells for DNA
    PCR 76
sample collection 75
HIV DNA assay, quantitative
    91–3
    total DNA 92
HIV infection, forensic
    phylogenetic analysis
    222–4
HIV RNA assay, quantitative
    83–91
    amplification 87–8
    colorimetric detection of
        amplified products 88
    extraction of RNA from
        plasma: GuSCN 84–6
    extraction of RNA from
        plasma: ultrasensitive
        method 86
    processing plasma for HIV
        RNA PCR 84
    results
        calculation 89
        interpretation 90–1
HLA loci 182–3
HLA typing
    DNA-based techniques
        185–204
    dot blot membrane
        preparation 198–9
    high throughput PCR
        amplification 191–4
    immobilized probe strip
        hybridization 194–7
    PCR-RFLP, SSCP, SHA,
        DSCA 202
    reverse hybridization with
        immobilized SSO probe
        arrays 202–3
    sequence-based typing
        (SBT) 203–4
    sequence-specific
        oligonucleotides (SSO)
        186–91
    SSP/ASA/ARMS 201–2
    markers for genome
        association 137–8
    new alleles 204–5
    nomenclature of HLA 184
    PCR-based methods 181–207

requirements 204
sequence diversity 183–4
serological/cellular methods
    185
HPLC see denaturing HPLC
human diseases
    affected family-based controls
        (AFBAC) 127
    genetic factor detection
        114–15
    linkage disequilibrium 113
    nuclear family-based samples
        127
    see also DNA pooling
human genome, DNA pooling,
    association mapping
    140–1
hypotheses, generation vs
    confirmation 22

interactions,
    gene—environment 23–4
internal controls, and
    quantitation standards
    (IC/QS) 73–4
isolation of single sperm,
    fluorescence activated
    cell sorting 149, 150

Jukes—Cantor correction, DNA
    sequence analysis
    212–13

linkage analysis 25
    see also sperm, single-sperm
        typing
linkage disequilibrium 18,
    113–15
logistic regression 18

malaria
    bird and reptile 224
    Plasmodium spp., phylogenetic
        analysis 224–5
    and sickle-cell anaemia 25
    see also Plasmodium spp.
Mantel—Haenzsel odds ratio 18
maximum likelihood (ML)
    criterion 220
maximum parsimony (MP)
    criterion 220–1
    tree analysis 222–4

measures of association,
    summary 16
meta-analyses 22
MHC polymorphism 226
microsatellite markers
    analysis of data 121–9
        stutter and differential
            amplification 122–5
    names and websites 138
    pooled DNA amplification
        113–15, 118–20
        case-control study 126–7
microwell plates, colorimetric
    detection 81
minimum evolution (ME)
    criterion 219
mismatch tolerance, thermal
    cycling parameters 70
MOGCA 175
molecular sequence data
    209–32
    evolutionary analysis, neutral
        theory of Kimura
        210–11
    see also evolutionary analysis
multiple comparisons 21–2
multiple PCR-RFLP 202
multiplex PCR 156
    allele detection 158
    options 157
mutation detection
    SSCP and DHPLC 97–111
        applications and
            sensitivity 108

natural selection 225
neighbour-joining (NJ)
    algorithm 219–20, 222–4
neutral theory
    comparing sequences,
        synonymous and non-
        synonymous substitution
        213–16
    Kimura 210–11
NRAMP1, and tuberculosis
    12–13
nucleotides
    diversity and population
        structure 228–31
    mean nucleotide diversity 216

oligonucleotide primers,
    radiolabelling 100, 162

oligonucleotides, PCR-based
    fingerprinting of
    bacterial chromosome 39
ompA gene, bacterial DNA
    sequence analysis 57–63
    phylogenetic tree 63
operational taxonomic unit
    (OTU) 216–19

paralogous loci, gene trees and
    species trees 218–19
parasites, see also human
    diseases; Plasmodium spp.
PCR
    dye intercalation 94–5
    preventing false positives
        from carryover 71–2
    products, determination of
        melting temperature 106
    real time detection faults
        93–5
    for SSCP/HA 98–103
    TaqMan technology 93–4, 130
    see also bacterial typing
PCR amplification
    elimination of A-overhang
        119
    HLA typing 181–207
    kinetic, allele frequency
        determination 132
    microsatellite markers
        113–15, 118–20
PCR-RFLP 202
PEP see primer extension pre-
    amplification
PFGE see pulsed field gel
    electrophoresis
phylogenetic algorithms 32
phylogenetic analysis 222–4,
    242–3
    anion exchanger (AE)
        proteins, sodium
        bicarbonate exchanger
        (NBC) in C. elegans 218
    malarial parasite (Plasmodium
        spp.) 217
    maximum parsimony (MP)
        criterion 63, 220–1,
        222–4
Plasmodium spp.
    CSP locus 216–17
    maintenance of
        polymorphisms 226
    P. reichenowi 217

phylogenetic analysis 217,
    224–6
    bird and reptile 224–5
    skewed nucleotide content
        213
    SSU rRNA 225
    synonymous substitutions
        229–30
polyacrylamide gel 168–9
polyacrylamide gel
    electrophoresis (PAGE)
    allele detection 158
    denaturing GE 119, 170
    discriminating alleles by
        GE 168
    ethidium bromide staining of
        DNA 172
    non-denaturing GE 171
    restriction digests 48–50
    silver staining of DNA 171
    SSCP GE 170
    see also denaturing gradient
        gel electrophoresis
polymorphisms, gene trees and
    species trees 219
positive selection 224–8
primer extension pre-
    amplification (PEP) 146,
        153–4
    reaction products 154–66
        gamma-[S]32[s]PdATP 162
        first round, STRs only 159
        second round (nested)
        SNPs only 165
        STRs only 161
        single round, SNPs only
            164
primer and probe design
    consensus primers 69
    reaction conditions and
        cycling parameters 70
primer-dimers 71
primers, discrimination by
        primer length (ADPL)
        154
pulsed field gel electrophoresis
    (PFGE) analysis
    bacterial chromosome
        50–7
        agarose concentration 52
        analysis and interpretation
            56–7
        digestion of bacterial DNA
            for PFGE analysis 54
        electrophoretic conditions
            55–6

genomic DNA quality 53
preparation of DNA in
agarose plugs 53
restriction enzymes 54
purifying selection 210
quantitation standards (QS)
73-4
quantitative DNA assay
quantification of HIV DNA 93
samples for pooled
amplification,
fluorescence detection
116
total DNA determination 92

radiolabelling
allele detection 158
oligonucleotide primers,
gamma-[S]32[s]PdATP
100, 162
randomly amplified
polymorphic DNA,
PCR-based fingerprinting
of bacterial chromosome
41-3
rDNA, small subunit sequences
32
real time detection faults, PCR
93-5
recombination freqencies see
sperm, single-sperm
typing
restriction enzymes, PFGE,
bacterial chromosome 54
restriction fragment length
polymorphism (RFLP) of
bacterial chromosome
44-50
analysis and interpretation
50
digestion of DNA for RFLP
analysis 47-8
enzymes 47
PAGE 48-50
polyacrylamide gel
electrophoresis of
restriction digests 49
preparation of genomic
DNA 46
reverse hybridization with
immobilized SSO probe
arrays, HLA typing
202-3
ribotyping 32, 33

risk
attributable risk 9-10, 16
hazard ratio 16
incidence rate ratio 16
odds ratio 16
risk ratio 16
segregation analysis 25
selection
balancing selection 226
natural selection 225
positive selection 224-8
purifying selection 210
sequence-based typing (SBT),
HLA typing 203-4
sequence-specific
oligonucleotides (SSO)
HLA typing 186-91
immobilized probe arrays
202-3
sequence-specific priming (SSP)
201-2
short tandem repeats (STRs)
154-62
mutation rate 155
use in sperm typing 156
sickle-cell anaemia, and
malaria 25
significance 21
see also error
single nucleotide
polymorphisms (SNPs)
allele frequency
determination 129-34
kinetic PCR 132
pooled DNA samples 132
databases, names and
websites 138
maps 114-15
PCR amplification 162-6
second round (nested)
165
single round 164
single-stranded conformation
polymorphism (SSCP)
97-111, 154, 167-9
and heteroduplex analysis
(HA)
PCR set up and
optimization 99
preparing an SSCP/HA
gel 100
HLA typing 202
preparing a polyacrylamide
gel 168-9
small subunit ribosomal RNA
(SSU rRNA) 224-5

sodium bicarbonate exchanger
(NBC), anion exchanger
(AE) proteins 218
species trees, and gene trees
218-19
sperm, single-sperm typing
145-79
interpretation of data 172-7
false recombinants 176-7
recombination data 174-7
single-sperm haplotype
scoring 173-4
isolation of sperm 147-51
PCR amplification 154-66
statistical models, evolutionary
analysis of molecular
sequence data 210-11
statistics
confidence interval 20
see also error
stratification 18
Suppliers, list 233-8
synonymous and
non-synonymous
substitution, neutral
theory 213-16

TaqMan technology 93-4, 93-4,
130
thermal cycling parameters,
mismatch tolerance 70
transmission—disequilibrium
test (TDT) 127
tuberculosis and NRAMP1, case-
control study 12-13

UING, uracil-N-glycosylase

viral targets 67-96
sequence heterogeneity and
PCR 68
see also HIV
visualizing alleles 158

whole-genome amplification,
haploid DNA, primer
extension pre-
amplification (PEP)
153-4
whole-genome association
studies 25-6